Part 1

Neoplastic Disorders

1

Outcomes Following Gamma Knife for Metastases

Henry S. Park[1], James B. Yu[1], Jonathan P.S. Knisely[2] and Veronica L.S. Chiang[1]
[1]*Yale University School of Medicine*
[2]*Hofstra North Shore-LIJ School of Medicine*
USA

1. Introduction

Brain metastases occur in approximately 20-40% of all cancer patients, with an annual incidence of 170,000-200,000 cases, outnumbering primary brain tumors by a factor of ten to one (Gavrilovic, 2005; Posner, 1992). The management of brain metastases has evolved significantly in the past 10-20 years. These changes are attributable not only to improvements in the fields of neurosurgery and radiation oncology but also to refinements in diagnostic imaging and systemic therapy. Management of brain metastases requires a multidisciplinary approach. In this chapter, we will explore the evolving role of radiosurgery in the treatment of brain metastases and the controversies that have surrounded this promising therapeutic modality, especially in the context of evolving systemic management protocols.

2. Whole brain radiation therapy

While up to 20% of patients can present with brain metastases as their first sign of cancer, most typically occur later in the course of disease. The finding of a brain metastasis in a cancer patient has historically indicated a continued progression of systemic disease, portending a poor prognosis and shifting the primary goal of treatment to relief of symptomatology. Treatment of brain metastases was therefore, by definition, palliative. Prior to the availability of computerized axial tomographic scanning (CT scan) and magnetic resonance imaging (MRI), brain metastases were diagnosed when they caused symptomatology, including seizures, the effects of increased intracranial pressure, or focal neurological deficits from mass effect on critical structures. Without treatment, the survival rate after diagnosis averaged approximately 4-6 weeks (Al-Shamy & Sawaya, 2009) despite the use of glucocorticoids and ongoing systemic therapy.

This dismal view of brain metastases outcomes began to change with the introduction of whole brain radiation therapy (WBRT). One of the first reports of radiation therapy for brain metastases was by Lenz & Fried (1931) for the palliation of breast cancer patients with intracranial metastases. The initial reasoning behind WBRT was to treat clinically symptomatic metastatic disease, and the ability to control presumed, clinically silent, and radiographically occult metastatic lesions was a bonus. With the advent of megavoltage, skin-sparing radiotherapy equipment that could deliver treatment rapidly, efficiently, and with acceptable acute morbidity, WBRT became accepted as a standard management approach. More recent retrospective studies have documented WBRT to be effective at reducing brain metastasis growth (Cairncross, 1980; Coia, 1992), improving neurologic symptom relief (Lassman & DeAngelis, 2003), and prolonging median survival to 3-6 months (Berk, 1995; Mintz, 1996; Order, 1968; Patchell, 1990; Vecht, 1993).

Despite the rapid adoption of WBRT, it was soon recognized that there were limitations to its use. Patients undergoing WBRT experienced the acute effects of hair loss, scalp irritation, nausea, debilitating fatigue, anorexia and sometimes worsening neurological function due to increased cerebral edema for possibly up to a month after starting treatment. In addition, in patients living beyond the 3-6 month expected survival duration, two main problems arose. The first was that it was possible for brain metastases to regrow either at previously treated sites or in new locations in the brain (Patchell, 1998). While there are reports of salvage repeat WBRT (Son, 2011; Wong, 1996), the cognitive consequences of radiation-induced leukoencephalopathy were not insignificant. Second, cerebral leukoencephalopathy can also be seen after a single course of WBRT in patients surviving longer than 12 months. A report from the Memorial Sloan-Kettering Cancer Center reported an 11% rate of progressive dementia, ataxia, and urinary incontinence among WBRT patients who survived for at least one year (DeAngelis, 1989a, 1989b). The current relevance of this study has been questioned, however, since hypofractionated regimens of 3-6 Gy to a total dose of 25-39 Gy were used, while smaller fractions are used more commonly today. Multiple phase III RTOG clinical trials evaluating numerous potential WBRT schedules from 10-54 Gy in 1-34 fractions have shown that many fractionation schemes are equivalent in overall survival, neurologic improvement, and overall toxicity, though neurocognitive toxicities have often not been well evaluated (Borgelt, 1980; Borgelt, 1981; Komarnicky, 1991; Kurtz, 1981; Murray, 1997; Sause, 1990).

Several other factors besides WBRT treatment may also contribute to a decline in neurocognitive function in brain metastasis patients, including the tumor itself, neurosurgical procedures, chemotherapy, medical therapy like corticosteroids and anticonvulsants, systemic progression, and paraneoplastic effects. It has been difficult for investigators to resolve these contributing factors (Khuntia, 2006). Though the evidence is limited and sometimes conflicting, the risks of long-term cognitive deficits due to WBRT have raised the controversial possibility that it may be reasonable to delay upfront WBRT when focal therapy is applied for selected patients.

3. Neurosurgery and diagnostic imaging

Neurosurgical resection of apparently isolated brain metastases was one of the first areas in which brain metastasis management standards changed over the past several decades and was a direct result of improved lesion detection with cross-sectional imaging. Beginning in the 1970s, advances in imaging facilitated an increasingly clear visualization of the lesions themselves. Based on early CT scans, retrospective case series began to report a survival benefit following neurosurgical resection of single brain metastases in selected patients. The role of surgical resection remained controversial until the early 1990s, when two randomized controlled studies validated the advantage of the use of resection for single brain metastasis management. The first study enrolled 48 patients with KPS scores ≥70, including 25 for surgical resection followed by WBRT and 23 with biopsy followed by WBRT (Patchell, 1990). Compared to patients receiving WBRT alone, patients receiving surgical resection with WBRT had longer median overall survival (40 vs. 15 weeks, $p<0.01$), longer median duration of functional independence (38 vs. 8 weeks, $p<0.005$), lower rates of local intracranial recurrence (20% vs. 52%, $p<0.01$), and lower rates of mortality due to neurologic causes (26 vs. 62 weeks, $p<0.001$).

A second randomized trial by Vecht et al. (1993) of 63 patients (with resection+WBRT vs. WBRT alone) confirmed the findings of overall survival benefit for the surgical group (10 vs. 6 months, $p=0.04$), with a non-significant trend of functionally independent survival benefit for the surgical group (7.5 vs. 3.5 months, $p=0.06$). Interestingly, a novel twice-a-day fractionation scheme was used (2 Gy bid x 10 days to a total of 40 Gy), and none of the nine long-term survivors developed late neurological side effects, though detailed neuropsychological assessments were not performed. The subgroup receiving the largest benefit from surgical resection was comprised of patients without active extracranial disease (median overall survival 12 vs. 7 months, functionally independent survival 9 vs. 4 months).

These two studies demonstrated the benefit of focal therapy in appropriately chosen individuals, i.e. those with good performance status (KPS>70) and good extracranial disease control. A third trial by Mintz et al. (1996) failed to show a survival advantage, but the impact of the first two trials established the indispensible role of surgical resection in the management of single brain metastases. Surgical resection can achieve tissue diagnosis, relieve mass effect, improve intracranial hypertension, and rapidly decrease the need for corticosteroids, especially for tumors that are large, radioresistant, or located in the posterior fossa (Vogelbaum & Suh, 2006). However, multiple craniotomies have been rarely offered for multiple brain metastases, given the excessive risk of morbidity.

Gadolinium-enhanced magnetic resonance imaging (Gd-MRI) has further revolutionized the detection and management of brain metastases in several ways. First, many patients who appear to have a single visible intracranial lesion on computerized tomography (CT) have subsequently been found to have multiple lesions on Gd-MRI (Bronen & Sze, 1990; Davis, 1991). Further, increased gadolinium dose and increased MRI scan resolution results in the detection of further additional lesions in 30-40% of patients (Engh, 2007; Hanssens, 2011; Patel, 2011b). The finding of multiple lesions may alter plans for potential surgical management. Second, surveillance use of Gd-MRI allows for the detection of lesions long before the development of symptomatology. Treatment of these lesions is therefore prophylactic and therefore must carry a low-risk profile. Finally, Gd-MRI allows the neurosurgeon to visualize the presence or absence of gross residual tumor after resection. For patients in whom gross total resection is achieved for a truly single brain metastasis, it may be reasonable to avoid further therapy, including WBRT, unless tumor were to recur locally or at a distant intracranial site.

To address this last issue, the role of postoperative WBRT was evaluated by a randomized, controlled trial (Patchell, 1998). This study of 95 patients demonstrated that patients receiving postoperative WBRT had a reduction in local recurrence (10% vs. 46%, $p<0.001$), distant intracranial recurrence (14% vs. 37%), and neurologic cause of death (14% vs. 44% of patients who died, $p=0.003$). The trial did not show a significant difference in overall survival (48 vs. 43 weeks) or the length of time patients remained independent, though this may have been due to the early death by systemic progression in the majority of patients that prevented definitive determination of brain metastasis control. In addition, 61% of patients in the resection-only group crossed over to receive delayed WBRT, and so the impact of withholding WBRT altogether could not be adequately assessed.

With the frequent findings of multiple asymptomatic brain metastases and of lesions too small to warrant craniotomy in cancer patients when scanned with Gd-MRI, a tool superior to craniotomy that could treat small lesions (either single or multiple) was required. Despite the effectiveness of WBRT and the temporary nature of its acute side effects, the risk of subacute and delayed neurologic sequelae of WBRT remain concerning. Furthermore, timing of the use of WBRT has become an issue. One of the fundamental radiobiological principles states that the likelihood of tumor control decreases with increasing number of tumor cells, i.e. tumor size. This means that brain metastases would be best treated at their smallest size, earlier in the course of their disease. However, early treatment with WBRT puts patients at risk for cognitive decline long before onset of symptomatology from metastases as well as leaving them with no other good options for treatment when new small brain metastases develop later along their course. Therefore, the ideal treatment would occur when tumors are small and asymptomatic, but distinguishable from normal brain tissue, and would optimally spare normal brain from unnecessary irradiation.

4. The changing face of cancer care

Advances in the management of solid organ cancers have occurred alongside the advances in neurosurgery and radiation oncology.

The most common primary sources of brain metastases in descending frequency are: lung cancers, breast cancers, colon cancers, melanoma, and renal cell carcinomas. Over the past few decades, it has become increasingly recognized that outcome is affected not only by the cancer histopathology itself but also by subtypes within each histopathology and by therapies targeted specifically at each histopathology type. It has been shown repeatedly that the identification of HER2/Neu receptor positivity in a breast cancer patient is associated with a survival advantage and that targeted systemic agents such as trastuzumab can result in long-term control of breast cancer. Epidermal growth factor receptor (EGFR) inhibition in non-small cell lung cancer has also been shown repeatedly to improve survival in a subset of patients whose tumors have EGFR mutations. Small molecule tyrosine kinase inhibitors such as sorafenib and sunitinib have also been found to be very effective in some patients with renal cell cancer, while immunomodulation agents such as interleukin-2 and ipilimumab are prolonging survival in melanoma patients. Furthermore, the identification of patients whose tumors have specific genetic markers for responsiveness to targeted treatment has improved survival for a subset of patients with stage IV disease. Median survival durations of 1-3 years have been reported in the literature for these patients (Bafford, 2009; Eichler, 2010; Robert, 2011; Sperduto, 2011; Webber, 2011).

With the improved ability of medical oncologists to control systemic disease, the previously nihilistic approach to brain metastases has also changed. As an example of changing medical oncology practices, one publication compared 103 patients with brain metastases treated from 1983-1989 with a similar cohort treated from 2005-2009 in 3 institutions in Germany and Norway (Nieder, 2010). Compared with the historical group, contemporary patients were more likely to present with brain metastases simultaneous to their cancer diagnosis (30% vs. 18%) or have an increased time from cancer diagnosis to brain metastasis diagnosis (8 vs. 3 months). Additionally, contemporary patients typically had more frequent findings of multiple brain metastases (61% vs. 29%) and extracranial metastases (52% vs. 23%). This reflects an increased use of MRI resulting in an improved ability to detect metastases over the 20-year period. With regards to cancer therapy, the authors reported concomitantly increased use of focal treatments such as surgery or SRS for brain metastases and decreased use of WBRT. Compared to the 1980s, when it was common to cease administration of systemic treatments after the diagnosis of brain metastases (76%), 55% of contemporary patients received systemic therapy after brain metastasis diagnosis and 13% of contemporary patients (vs. 0% in the historical group) received third line chemotherapy. One-year survival was doubled in the contemporary group compared to the historical group (34% vs. 15%).

Because some stage IV cancer patients may enjoy a prolonged survival, it has now become essential to identify these patients and to offer treatments that carry minimal side effects with the most durable cancer control to provide optimal quality-of-life. It is also increasingly important to offer treatment options that do not interfere with systemic therapy in order to maintain the best systemic control possible, thereby decreasing the chance of developing metastases.

5. Patient selection and prognostic indices

There has been a growing recognition that pre-treatment patient variables may play a major role in determining patient prognosis. One of the most important variables is patient functionality and activity, otherwise known as performance status. Two classifications are widely used (Table 1): the Karnofsky performance status (KPS) and the Eastern Cooperative Oncology Group (ECOG) performance status (PS), the latter of which was adopted by the World Health Organization (WHO) (Karnofsky & Burchenal, 1949; Oken, 1982).

In an attempt to determine patient prognosis following WBRT, Gaspar et al. (1997) published a seminal prognostic index for patients with brain metastases, known as the Radiation Therapy Oncology Group (RTOG) Recursive Partitioning Analysis (RPA). Using data from 1,200 patients in three consecutive clinical trials (RTOG 7916, 8528, 8905), an interactive, nonparametric statistical method was used to classify patients in three groups depending on four criteria. Patients younger than 65 years with good performance status (KPS≥70), a well-controlled primary tumor, and no extracranial metastases were assigned to RPA Class I (median survival 7.1 months), those with KPS<70 were assigned to RPA Class III (median survival 2.3 months), and all others to Class II (median survival 4.3 months). Despite its widespread validation and adoption, one of the major criticisms of the RPA system was the inhomogeneity of Class II and III, which are based primarily on the KPS, which may not be an entirely objective measure of functionality. Thus, several other research groups have created indices to try to more accurately and reproducibly classify patients into prognostic categories (Table 2).

KPS	Description	ECOG / WHO PS	Description
100	Normal, no signs of disease	0	Fully active, able to carry on all pre-disease performance without restriction
90	Capable of normal activity, few symptoms or signs of disease		
80	Normal activity with some difficulty, some symptoms or signs	1	Restricted in physically strenuous activity but ambulatory and able to carry out work of a light or sedentary nature, e.g. light house work, office work
70	Caring for self, not capable of normal activity or work		
60	Requiring some help, can take care of most personal requirements	2	Ambulatory and capable of all self-care but unable to carry out any work activities, up and about more than 50% of waking hours
50	Requiring help often, requiring frequent medical care		
40	Disabled, requiring special care and help	3	Capable of only limited self-care, confined to bed or chair more than 50% of waking hours
30	Severely disabled, hospital admission indicated but no risk of death		
20	Very ill, urgently requiring admission and supportive measures or treatment	4	Completely disabled, cannot carry on any self-care, totally confined to bed or chair
10	Moribund, rapidly progressive fatal diseases processes		
0	Dead	5	Dead

Table 1. Descriptions of the Karnofsky performance status (KPS) and the Eastern Cooperative Oncology Group (ECOG)/World Health Organization (WHO) performance status (PS).

Most recently, the Graded Prognostic Assessment (GPA) was developed using data from 1,960 patients from RTOG trials 7916, 8528, 8905, 9104, and 9508 (Sperduto, 2008). It was the first index to remove primary tumor control and systemic disease stability as prognostic indicators, due to subjectivity in the assessment of these factors, which may vary widely based on type, technique, and timing of restaging studies. Additionally, the GPA added number of intracranial metastases as a prognostic factor, due to the findings of RTOG 9508 showing a survival advantage for patients with 1 vs. 2-3 metastases (Andrews, 2004). This study showed that across all histopathology types, patients with age<50 years, KPS 90-100, a single brain metastasis, and no evidence of extracranial metastases survived a median of 11.0-21.7 months, while patients with age>60 years, KPS<70, >3 brain metastases, and evidence of extracranial metastases had median survivals of 2.6-3.0 months.

Prognostic index	Prognostic factors	Score
RTOG Recursive Partitioning Analysis **[RPA]** (Gaspar, 1997)	4 (age, KPS, systemic disease status, extracranial metastases)	-Class I: Age<65, KPS≥70, no extracranial metastases, primary tumor controlled -Class III: KPS<70 -Class II: all others
Rotterdam Index (Lagerwaard, 1999)	3 (ECOG PS, systemic disease status, response to steroids)	-"good": ECOG 0/1, no/limited systemic tumor activity, good steroid response -"poor": ECOG 2/3, limited/ extensive systemic tumor activity, little steroid response -"moderate": all others
Score Index for Radiosurgery **[SIR]** (Weltman, 2000)	5 (age, KPS, systemic disease status, number of metastases, volume of largest lesion)	Summation of individual scores (0, 1, 2) to total score of 0-10
Basic Score for Brain Metastases **[BSBM]** (Lorenzoni, 2004)	3 (KPS, systemic disease status, extracranial metastases)	Summation of individual scores (0, 1) to total score of 0-3
Graded Prognostic Assessment **[GPA]** (Sperduto, 2008)	4 (age, KPS, extracranial metastases, number of metastases)	Summation of individual scores (0, 0.5, 1) to total score of 0-4
Diagnosis-Specific Prognostic Assessment **[DS-GPA]** (Sperduto, 2010)	-Lung: 4 (age, KPS, extracranial metastases, number of metastases) -Breast: 3 (age, KPS, cancer subtype) -Melanoma/Renal: 2 (KPS, number of metastases) -GI: 1 (KPS)	-Lung: Summation of individual scores (0, 0.5, 1) to total score of 0-4 -Melanoma/Renal: Summation of individual scores (0, 0.5, 1) to total score of 0-2 -Breast/GI: Summation of individual scores (0, 1) to total score of 0-4
RTOG = Radiation Therapy and Oncology Group; KPS = Karnofsky Performance Status; GI = gastrointestinal		

Table 2. Summary of major prognostic indices for brain metastases in the past 15 years.

Subsequently, a retrospective, multi-institutional database of 5,067 patients was then undertaken to identify histology-specific prognostic factors to create the Diagnosis-Specific Graded Prognostic Assessment (DS-GPA) (Sperduto, 2010). For non-small cell and small cell lung cancer, all four of the original GPA prognostic factors remained significant. For breast cancer, 3 factors determined prognosis: age, tumor subtype and KPS but not number of brain metastases. However, for melanoma and renal cell cancer, only KPS and number of metastases remained significant, while for gastrointestinal cancer, only KPS remained significant. For every histology, a DS-GPA score of 3.5-4.0 was associated with median survival durations of >12 months (13.2 months for melanoma to 18.7 months for breast cancer). This data emphasizes yet another layer of heterogeneity of patients with brain metastases, in that not all of the prognostic factors were significant for tumors of different histologies and different prognostic factors carried different weights in the prediction of outcome. More importantly, it showed that studies investigated results of treatment must take these varying prognostic indicators into account.

6. Stereotactic radiosurgery and the gamma knife

With the increasing duration of survival in cancer patients, the overall incidence of brain metastases will likely continue rising, making improved therapies for treating brain metastases even more valuable. As discussed previously, WBRT is associated with transient but often not insignificant acute side effects, and may be associated with significant delayed cognitive side effects. It is essentially used only once during the course of a patient's disease, and the appropriate time to intervene with this therapy is still debated in many clinical settings. If WBRT has been used previously, it cannot be repeated with any expectation of significant efficacy for most tumors at the time of intracranial disease recurrence, and most radiation oncologists are hesitant to deliver a second full dose of radiation because of fears of cumulative toxicity. Craniotomy carries significantly higher morbidity and mortality risks than any radiation-based procedure and is also limited by the inability to treat multiple lesions at the same time.

The marriage between the neurosurgical and radiation oncology specialties resulted in the development of stereotactic radiosurgery (SRS), which is a method to deliver a single, high-dose fraction of ionizing radiation treatment to a precisely defined focal target volume. Gamma Knife radiosurgery (GK-SRS), initially developed by Lars Leksell and Borje Larsson (Leksell, 1951), delivers treatment using multiple gamma radiation beams from Cobalt-60 sources that simultaneously converge on a single focus point known as an isocenter. Stereotaxis is achieved with a fixed alignment of the patient to a physical coordinate system, via stereotactic head frame for GK-SRS. GK-SRS is the gold standard system for delivery of stereotactic radiosurgery to the brain, and the latest version of the Gamma Knife, the Perfexion, was specifically designed to facilitate radiosurgical treatment of multiple metastases.

Advantages of GK-SRS include its non-invasiveness, except for the application of the head frame, and association with excellent tolerability. It can be used to treat lesions in any region of the brain and is better tolerated than surgery in eloquent cortical areas (Dea, 2010; Elliott, 2010). Small and multiple lesions can be treated in one setting, minimizing the need for interruption from systemic therapy, unlike WBRT or surgery. GK-SRS treatments are also highly conformal, sparing radiation effects to much of the normal brain.

Disadvantages of SRS treatment include its inability to treat lesions >3 cm in diameter, a relative delay in symptomatic relief from mass effect, and the possibility of inducing a delayed leukoencephalopathic process that is often difficult to distinguish from tumor recurrence (Rauch, 2011). In addition, neither SRS nor surgical resection address the risk of developing further metastases outside the focused field of therapy that WBRT can achieve, though SRS can be used repeatedly for salvage therapy. The delivery of GK-SRS treatment itself is also expensive and labor-intensive compared with standard WBRT.

For brain metastases, SRS was first evaluated for potential effectiveness as a salvage treatment for inoperable, recurrent, and/or persistent lesions. One of the earliest publications reported data from 12 patients with solitary, deep, and radioresistant brain metastases treated with LINAC in Heidelberg (Sturm, 1987). Patients received 20-30 Gy to the 80% isodose surface, and all patients had an arrest in tumor growth and a marked improvement in clinical condition beginning a few days after irradiation, with all but one of these patients being free from side effects at last follow-up. Another study from the Dana-Farber Cancer Institute analyzed data from 18 patients with 21 recurrent or persistent metastases treated with 9-25 Gy to the 70-90% isodose surface with LINAC (Loeffler, 1990). After a median follow-up of 9 months (range 1-39 months), all lesions were well-controlled, and rapid clinical and radiographic improvement was observed with no cases of radiation necrosis despite previous exposure to radiotherapy. One of the first reports of GK-SRS for brain metastases was a case study from the Karolinska Institute of a patient with a solitary recurrent renal cell carcinoma metastasis treated with 25 Gy to the 35% isodose surface without WBRT (Lindquist, 1989). Shrinkage of this growth was observed and no regrowth was evident when the patient expired from his systemic disease 11 months later.

Since these original studies, several authors have reported superior metastasis control rates using SRS or SRS+WBRT when compared with WBRT alone. One-month local control rates of 93-96% have been reported for SRS with or without WBRT compared with 88% for WBRT, while 1-year local control rates of 80-90% have been reported for WBRT+SRS vs. 65-75% for SRS alone vs. 0-30% for WBRT alone (Elaimy, 2011). Two multi-arm studies showed a significant survival advantage for SRS alone and SRS+WBRT over WBRT alone (Li, 2000; Wang, 2002). One large retrospective study of 1,702 patients comparing SRS+WBRT to WBRT alone also reported a significant survival benefit for patients receiving SRS for all three RPA classes (Sanghavi, 2001). Three other studies comparing SRS alone to WBRT alone found that SRS patients lived significantly longer (Kocher, 2004; Lee, 2008; Rades, 2007b), while one found no significant survival difference (Datta, 2004).

Factors that have been shown to affect lesional responses to SRS include lesion volume, 10-12 Gy treatment volumes, marginal treatment dose, histopathology, and time since SRS (Hasegawa, 2003; Hatiboglu, 2011; Shehata, 2004; Yang, 2011), although lesion volume has been the only factor consistent among the varying studies. Typically, lesions <2 cm diameter respond well to 20 Gy of SRS. However, doses have varied from 16 to 24 Gy depending on lesional size and location. One of the additional advantages of SRS over WBRT is the relative uniformity of response of different histopathological tumors to the same SRS treatment dose (Kim, 2011; Powell, 2008, Varlotto, 2003; Wegner, 2011).

Time since SRS has also been shown to play a role in lesion control rates, falling from 93-96% at 1 month to 80-90% at 1 year to 69% at 3 years and 5 years in a study by Varlotto et al. (2005). Local control rates are determined by serial imaging, and local control failure is typically defined as an increase in the size of lesion after SRS. One of the difficulties with interpreting local control has been the demonstration that up to one third of lesions can transiently increase in size following SRS but if followed, many will regress again without further treatment (Patel, 2011a). This study reported that while a significant number of lesions showed transient enlargement 9-18 months following SRS, 2-3 year follow-up showed a local control rate of 99%. This suggests that in previous studies, a significant number of patients may have been classified incorrectly as having local failure.

The first randomized clinical trial to examine the potential benefit of SRS boost for brain metastasis patients was conducted in Pittsburgh (Kondziola, 1999). A total of 27 patients (13 with SRS+WBRT vs. 14 with WBRT alone) with 2-4 brain metastases (all ≤2.5 cm in diameter) and KPS≥70 were enrolled in the study. GK-SRS was utilized for all patients receiving SRS. Compared to WBRT alone, patients receiving SRS+WBRT had significantly lower local failure rates (8% vs. 100%, $p=0.002$), longer median time to local failure (36 vs. 6 months, $p<0.001$), and longer median time to any brain failure (34 vs. 5 months, $p=0.002$). There was also a non-significant trend favoring the patients receiving SRS boost in terms of median overall survival (11 vs. 7.5 months, $p=0.02$). No neurologic or systemic morbidity related to SRS was noted.

A larger, multi-institutional trial (RTOG 9508) was then undertaken to define the role of SRS boost for a limited number of metastases (Andrews, 2004). A total of 333 patients with 1-3 brain metastases (≤4 cm in diameter for the largest lesion and ≤3 cm for the remainder) and KPS≥70 were randomized to SRS+WBRT (167 patients) and WBRT alone (164 patients). Overall, there was no significant difference in median overall survival between the two arms (6.5 months for SRS+WBRT vs. 5.7 months for WBRT alone, $p=0.14$) or overall intracranial disease control ($p=0.13$), although SRS was associated with superior local control ($p=0.013$), stability or improvement of KPS score at 6 months follow-up ($p=0.033$), and decrease in steroid requirement ($p=0.016$). Among patients with single brain metastases, however, those receiving SRS+WBRT had a higher median overall survival than those receiving WBRT alone (11.6 vs. 9.6 months, $p=0.045$).

One of the major criticisms of the RTOG 9508 trial includes the lack of follow-up neuroimaging review on 43% of the patients. Another was the large bilateral crossover rate, as 19% of patients in the SRS+WBRT arm (mostly in RPA Class II) did not receive their planned SRS, while 17% of patients in the WBRT arm received salvage SRS. Despite these limitations, the superiority of SRS in survival for selected patients with 1 brain metastasis and in local control and KPS maintenance for 1-3 metastases shown by the RTOG 9508 trial, combined with the benefit in local control for 2-4 metastases demonstrated by the Pittsburgh trial, have provided level I evidence for the use of SRS as standard-of-care treatment for patients with a limited number of metastases and KPS≥70.

7. Controversies related to stereotactic radiosurgery

7.1 SRS vs. surgical resection for single metastases

Given that both surgery and SRS can treat single metastases effectively, the question has arisen as to which focal therapy might result in a better outcome. In choosing a focal therapy to use with or without WBRT, SRS and surgical resection each have their own advantages. As described previously, surgical resection is effective in single, large, and surgically accessible lesions, can rapidly relieve mass effect, and obtain tissue diagnosis. However, SRS requires no general anesthesia, is minimally invasive and can be used for small lesions located in nearly any area of the brain, including deep or highly functional regions. Nevertheless, for patients with overlapping indications (i.e. single, accessible lesions without an emergent need for resection in patients who are reasonable surgical candidates), the question of which focal therapy would yield better outcomes continues to be debated.

Several retrospective studies have been performed to evaluate this question. When comparing SRS+WBRT vs. resection+WBRT, a significant survival advantage for SRS+WBRT patients was found in three studies (Garell, 1999; Rades, 2011; Schoggl, 2000), for resection+WBRT patients in one study (Bindal, 1996), and for neither group in one study (O'Neill, 2003). Median time to local recurrence was longer for SRS+WBRT in two studies (Rades, 2011; Schoggl, 2000) and for resection+WBRT in one study (Bindal, 1996). For SRS alone vs. resection+WBRT, no significant survival or local recurrence difference was found in two studies (Muacevic, 1999; Rades, 2007a), while resection+WBRT was favored in survival and local recurrence in one study (Shinoura, 2002).

Given the contradictory conclusions of these retrospective studies, one prospective, randomized clinical trial was performed comparing SRS alone vs. resection+WBRT (Muacevic, 2008). Sixty-four patients (31 SRS alone vs. 33 resection+WBRT) with a single surgically accessible brain metastasis ≤3 cm in diameter and KPS≥70 were enrolled in the study. Between the patients receiving SRS alone vs. resection+WBRT, there was no significant difference in median survival (10.3 vs. 9.5 months, $p=0.8$), neurologic death rates (11% vs. 27%, $p=0.3$), and 1-year local control (97% vs. 82%, $p=0.06$). An increased rate of distant intracranial recurrence was initially observed among SRS patients (26% vs. 3%, $p<0.05$), but this difference no longer persisted following salvage SRS treatment. SRS was also associated with fewer grade 1 or 2 early or late radiation complications ($p<0.01$). Although the study was likely underpowered or biased from poor accrual (25% of target), it appears that SRS, even without WBRT but with the availability of future SRS salvage treatments, is not inferior to surgery with WBRT for highly functional patients with a single operable brain metastasis, and may be preferred due to the shorter hospital stay, less frequent and shorter duration of steroid application, and lower frequency of complications. Patients with stage IV cancer are often reluctant to undergo major surgical procedures and it may not be realistic to design a study to answer this question.

7.2 Omission of WBRT from SRS treatment for limited metastases

Given the previously discussed side effects of WBRT, the possibility of prolonged survival in patients with a limited number of brain metastases, and the demonstrated ability of SRS to provide equivalent local control of brain metastases compared with WBRT, the question of deferring WBRT at initial time of brain metastasis treatment has been raised. Despite their inherent biases, retrospective studies have raised the possibility that the SRS-alone approach may be viable for a limited number of metastases. When first proposed, many studies demonstrated that freedom from intracranial disease progression at 1 year, predominantly at sites distant than those treated with SRS, was significantly worse for SRS alone than SRS+WBRT (Chidel, 2000; Hoffman, 2001; Noel, 2003; Pirzkall, 1998). A single-institution review of 105 patients with 1-4 brain metastases, however, showed that the addition of WBRT to SRS did not result in improvement in survival or local control if salvage therapy was available for recurrence after SRS alone (Sneed, 1999). This lack of a statistically significant difference in overall survival was confirmed by seven other retrospective cohort studies (Chidel, 2000; Hoffman, 2001; Jawahar, 2002; Noel, 2003; Pirzkall, 1998; Sneed, 2002; Varlotto, 2005) and one prospective cohort study (Li, 2000), while one study showed a survival benefit for SRS alone (Combs, 2004) and another showed a survival benefit for SRS+WBRT (Wang, 2002). Among these 10 retrospective cohort studies, only one reported a statistically significant worsening in local tumor control for patients treated with SRS alone compared to SRS+WBRT (Varlotto, 2005). Despite the excellent outcomes demonstrated by these retrospective studies, their potential for selection bias increased the need for randomized trials to compare SRS alone to SRS+WBRT.

The first randomized trial comparing SRS alone vs. SRS+WBRT was a multi-institutional phase III study (JROSG 99-1) from Japan (Aoyama, 2006). A total of 132 patients (67 SRS alone vs. 65 SRS+WBRT) with KPS scores ≥70 and 1-4 newly diagnosed brain metastases <3 cm in maximum diameter were accrued. Median follow-up was 7.8 months for all patients and 49.2 months for survivors. Overall survival for all patients was not significantly affected by the addition of WBRT (median survival 8 months for SRS alone vs. 7.5 months for SRS+WBRT, p=0.42). Intracranial failure rates, however, were considerably higher in those patients who did not receive WBRT compared with those who did (1-year distant intracranial recurrence 63.7% vs. 41.5%, p=0.003; 1-year overall intracranial recurrence 76.4% vs. 46.8%, p<0.001) as was the use of salvage treatment (43.3% vs. 15.4%, p<0.001). Death attributable to neurologic cause and 1-year systemic functional preservation as defined by a decrease in KPS score to ≤70 were not significantly different between the two arms.

To determine if the increased rate of distant intracranial failure or WBRT affected cognitive function, a secondary analysis was performed for 82 patients for whom baseline Mini-Mental Status Examination (MMSE) scores were >27 and who also had follow-up MMSE testing (Aoyama, 2007). The 1-year, 2-year, and 3-year actuarial MMSE preservation rates were 59.3%, 51.9%, and 51.9% for SRS alone, and 76.1%, 68.5%, and 14.7% for SRS+WBRT, respectively (p=0.73) suggesting that the addition of WBRT resulted in better control of central nervous system (CNS) disease and therefore improved cognitive function. The mean time to 3-point MMSE deterioration was also shorter for SRS alone compared to SRS+WBRT (7.6 vs. 16.5 months, p=0.005). MMSE recovery, however, was observed after successful salvage treatment in patients who had SRS alone and whose MMSE had deteriorated with the development of new brain metastases. Similar improvements were not seen for MMSE deterioration in patients who had received SRS+WBRT and who required protracted steroid therapy for CNS symptoms. These results suggest that progression of CNS disease as seen at time of intracranial distant failure can result in a reversible cognitive decline if successfully treated, compared with an irreversible decline following WBRT.

A second phase III trial at the M.D. Anderson Cancer Center was conducted to further evaluate the neurocognitive effects of SRS vs. SRS+WBRT (Chang, 2009). A total of 58 patients (30 SRS alone vs. 28 SRS+WBRT) with 1-3 newly diagnosed brain metastases and KPS scores ≥70 were accrued, before the trial was stopped early because planned interim analysis indicated that patients randomized to SRS+WBRT were significantly more likely to have learning and memory function deficits at 4 months post-treatment. Baseline characteristics between the two groups were similar, as were the median prescription target volume ratio and median prescription isodose. Median follow-up was 9.5 months for all patients. Patients receiving WBRT were significantly more likely to show a decline in cognitive function as measured by learning and memory function at 4-month follow-up compared to those treated using SRS alone, particularly in Hopkins Learning Test-Revised (HVLT-R) total recall (mean posterior probability of decline 24% for SRS alone vs. 52% for SRS+WBRT) and delayed recall and recognition. The decline in total recall was also found to persist at 6 months. As a secondary finding, median survival was also found to be significantly higher for patients with SRS alone compared to SRS+WBRT (15.2 vs. 5.7 months, p=0.003), despite their having significantly lower 1-year local tumor control (67% vs. 100%, p=0.012), distant tumor control (45% vs. 73%, p=0.02), and freedom from CNS recurrence (27% vs. 73%, p=0.0003). Salvage therapy was necessary in 87% of patients receiving SRS alone (33% surgical resection, 20% SRS, 33% WBRT), compared to only 7% of those receiving SRS+WBRT. There was no difference between the two groups in neurological cause of death or rate of treatment toxicities. The difference in survival reported in this study is contrary to most other previous studies and was possibly explained by post-hoc analysis showing that patients who received SRS alone underwent systemic therapy over one month earlier and received a median of two cycles more systemic therapy than patients who received additional WBRT. This finding will need further study for validation.

A third randomized clinical trial, EORTC 22952-26001, was performed in Europe to evaluate functional independence and quality-of-life, which are not adequately captured by neurocognitive function alone (Kocher, 2011). A total of 353 patients with 1-3 brain metastases ≤3.5 cm (≤2.5 cm each for multiple metastases), stable extracranial disease, and WHO PS scores of 0-2 were recruited into the study. They were then randomized into two treatment arms: one without WBRT (100 patients SRS alone vs. 79 resection alone) and one with WBRT (99 SRS+WBRT vs. 81 resection+WBRT). There were no significant differences in baseline characteristics between patients not receiving WBRT vs. those receiving WBRT. Median follow-up for surviving patients was 40 months for those not receiving WBRT and 49 months for those receiving WBRT. The median time to decline in functional independence to a WHO PS>2 was not significantly different between patients without WBRT vs. patients with WBRT (10.0 months vs. 9.5 months, p=0.71), nor was overall survival significantly different between the two groups (10.7 months vs. 10.9 months, p=0.89). While median progression-free survival was slightly shorter for the no WBRT group compared to those undergoing WBRT (3.4 months vs. 4.6 months, p=0.02), overall intracranial progression at 2 years was significantly higher for the non-WBRT arm (78% vs. 48%, p<0.001), as was having intracranial failure as a component of cause of death (44% vs. 28%, p<0.002). No differences in toxicity rates were seen.

Several limitations of these trials have been noted by the authors and other observers. Though two of the three major randomized trials showed no difference in overall survival, they may have been underpowered to do so (Patchell, 2006). The increased survival for patients treated with SRS only compared to SRS+WBRT despite increased rates of intracranial recurrence with the omission of WBRT shown in the M.D. Anderson trial (Chang, 2009) may have been due to a much higher utilization of salvage therapies overall (87%), and particularly surgical salvage (33% of patients treated with SRS alone and 0% of patients who also underwent WBRT) as well as a possible difference in chemotherapeutic treatment.

The neurocognitive outcomes in the M.D. Anderson trial have also been called into question for two reasons. First, patients with terminal cancer are known to experience profound neurocognitive dysfunction (Lawlor, 2000; Pereira, 1997); thus, since overall survival was decreased in the arm receiving WBRT, the decreased neurocognitive function could itself be partially explained by the decreased overall survival and not by the additional WBRT the patients received. What may ultimately impact patient survival and function is the decrease in delay of effective systemic therapy that SRS-only treatment affords - a factor that has not been studied to date. Second, the choice of a single time point for assessment of neurocognitive function at 4 months post-treatment as the primary outcome in the Chang et al. study is controversial. Previous studies have shown that neurocognitive function often reaches its nadir at 2-4 months post-treatment but subsequently rebounds in patients who survive beyond 4 months, and recurrence of intracranial disease tends to affect neurocognitive function more profoundly (Armstrong, 2000; Li, 2007). It is possible to postulate that while WBRT may cause a worsened subacute neurocognitive decline, its ability to control disease recurrence in long-term survivors may ultimately be superior if there is neurocognitive recovery.

Lastly, all three studies are limited by their choice of neurocognitive and functional assessment tools. While the MMSE and HTLV-R tests may be excellent screening tests for neurocognitive dysfunction, the MMSE has been criticized for having low sensitivity and specificity, while the HTLV-R can produce abnormal results in patients with focal neurological deficits that may not accurately reflect neurocognitive dysfunction (Meyers, 2003). Along the same lines, the WHO performance status has also not been validated as a measure of functional independence in patients with brain metastases and has been noted to be subject to inter-observer and intra-observer bias and variability, particularly in a non-blinded setting (Mehta, 2011). In addition, none of these tests have been specifically validated for patients with brain metastases.

In summary, for patients presenting with 1-4 newly diagnosed brain metastases, all three clinical trials discussed above appear to indicate a lack of detriment in neurocognition or quality-of-life with the omission of WBRT despite significantly worsened intracranial tumor control that would require additional salvage therapy (additional SRS, WBRT, or resection) in almost all patients. While the addition of WBRT clearly and reproducibly results in improved local and distant brain disease control, there is insufficient data to conclude definitively if this improved control translates into long-term improved neurocognitive function, functional independence, and quality of life. Thus, the use of SRS alone for the initial treatment of patients with 1-4 newly diagnosed brain metastases in a patient with KPS>70 may be a reasonable strategy in conjunction with frequent serial surveillance and the availability of salvage treatments, though further validation is needed to answer these questions more definitively.

7.3 SRS with or without WBRT for extensive metastases

In patients presenting with ≥5 brain metastases, the evidence for using SRS while deferring WBRT is scarce and primarily limited to retrospective data that mostly use GK-SRS. Two publications reported that patients with 1-10 and 2-20 brain metastases, respectively, treated with GK-SRS only without WBRT had longer overall survival than those treated with WBRT only (Serizawa, 2000; Park, 2009), with the first study also showing improved neurological and qualitative survival (interval from date of initial diagnosis to date of impaired quality-of-life) in those treated with GK-SRS only. Moreover, in patients with ≥10 brain metastases, two other studies reported that the use of GK-SRS alone allowed the achievement of "acceptable" tumor control with low morbidity, and high patient-reported satisfaction with regards to brain metastasis-related symptom management and quality-of-life (Kim, 2008; Suzuki 2000). Another study noted that GK-SRS treatment of 10-43 lesions in 80 patients with ≥10 brain metastases resulted in acceptable WBRT doses on the order of 2.16-8.51 Gy (Yamamoto, 2002).

Recently, retrospective studies have begun to report that the number of brain metastases does not necessarily predict survival. One study retrospectively compared 130 patients with 1-3 vs. ≥4 brain metastases in patients receiving GK-SRS, and found that only RPA class and neither multiplicity of brain metastases nor receipt of WBRT affected survival (Nam, 2005), while another showed that for 205 patients with ≥4 brain metastases receiving a single SRS procedure, it was the total treatment volume and not the number of metastases that was associated with survival (Bhatnagar, 2006). The largest series to date showed that in their 1,885 patients undergoing 2,448 total GK-SRS treatment, no significant differences were found in median survival among patients with 2, 3-4, 5-8, or ≥9 brain metastases (Karlsson, 2009). Similarly, two other studies showed no significant difference in survival or intracranial recurrence among 778 patients who received GK-SRS without prophylactic WBRT with 1, 2, 3-4, 5-6, or 7-10 brain metastases (Serizawa, 2010) or among 323 patients with 1-5, 6-10, 11-15, and 16-20 brain metastases (Chang, 2010), though in the second study, patients with ≥16 metastases appeared to have an increased risk of distant intracranial recurrence.

For ≥5 brain metastases, no publications were found that specifically address direct comparisons of SRS only vs. SRS+WBRT. It appears that in patients with up to 10-20 metastases, the number of metastases may not be a factor that independently predicts survival. A recent survey of radiosurgeons at two major international meetings revealed that 55-83% of respondents considered it "reasonable" to extend the use of SRS as an initial treatment for ≥5 brain metastases, though there was no clear consensus regarding a reasonable maximum number of brain metastases to treat with SRS alone (Knisely, 2010). However, prospective analyses specifically studying SRS vs. SRS+WBRT for ≥5 brain metastases are still needed to validate this approach.

7.4 SRS as post-resection tumor bed consolidation

Another area of controversy surrounds the use of SRS as a consolidative tool to the tumor bed after microneurosurgical resection of a brain metastasis as an alternative to WBRT. As discussed previously, Patchell et al. (1990) demonstrated the value of resection of a single brain metastasis in improving survival, local control, and functional independence compared with WBRT alone. In a subsequent study, WBRT following resection resulted in superior intracranial metastasis control relative to resection alone (Patchell, 1998), and resection+WBRT has since been the standard approach for patients with single metastases. Despite WBRT, tumor bed recurrences can still occur, and Patchell's studies observed a 10-20% local and distant failure rate with a median follow-up of less than one year. Roberge et al. (2009) reported that an SRS boost with a 10 Gy marginal dose to the area recurring after resection+WBRT could be delivered safely with a 94% local control rate at 2 years.

Due to the potential delayed neurocognitive side effects of WBRT, investigators suggested the use of SRS in lieu of WBRT for consolidation of surgical resection cavities reserving WBRT for salvage therapy. Mathieu et al. (2008) reported on the use of SRS alone following surgical resection of single metastases. In 80% of the cases, a gross total resection was achieved and GK-SRS was administered a median of 4 weeks after surgery. Median margin dose administered was 16 Gy and this resulted in a local control rate of 73% at 13 months follow-up. At the time of SRS, 33% of patients had additional non-resected lesions treated using GK-SRS at the time of surgical bed GK-SRS. Ultimately, only 16% of patients needed salvage WBRT. Similarly, Jagannathan et al. (2009) reported post-resection GK-SRS to 47 patients, all of whom had gross total resection. Mean marginal doses of 19 Gy were administered for a mean of 14 days after surgery, and local control rate was 94% at 14 months. The most recent series by Jensen et al. (2011) in 106 patients reported an 80% 1-year local control rate when marginal doses of 17 Gy were administered for a mean of 24 days after surgery.

Both Jensen et al. and Jagannathan et al. reported that increased size of resection cavity resulted in decreased local control. Several factors varied within these studies, however. First was marginal dose; unlike most other radiosurgical targets, the post-operative resection bed has its highest tumor burden peripherally where radiosurgical dose is lowest. Thus, it would seem reasonable that the higher the marginal dose, the more effective the local control, as suggested by the previously described three studies and one additional study (Iwai, 2008), which reported superior local control when doses ≥18 Gy were used. Second was time from surgery to SRS; it has been documented that rim enhancement of non-neoplastic resection cavities can show enhancement for 30 days after surgery (Sato, 1997). While this rim enhancement is typically thin and linear in the first 5 days post-operatively, it may become thick and nodular until at least 30 days post-operatively. It may therefore be difficult to determine which parts of the resection cavity are merely post-operative change and which are areas needing treatment for tumor. This may explain why larger lesions are more difficult to control and why two non-GK-SRS studies by Soltys et al. (2008) and Do et al. (2009) in fact recommend adding a 1-3 mm margin around the enhancing lesion to decrease conformality and improve local control. Third was extent of surgical resection; the highest local control rate was seen in the study by Jagannathan et al., in which all the lesions had gross total resection, compared with the other two studies which included subtotal resection cases also. Thus, it is important to determine if differing treatment protocols are required to maximize outcome based on extent of resection. No publications have addressed this question to date.

Only one retrospective study directly comparing resection+SRS with resection+WBRT has been published (Hwang, 2010). For the 43 patients (25 GK-SRS vs. 18 WBRT) treated at Tufts following tumor resection, there were non-significant trends towards superior survival for patients receiving GK-SRS (15 vs. 7 months, p=0.008) and local control (100% vs. 83%). Though the groups were well-balanced in histology, mean number of metastases, and resection extent, the study was severely limited by the lack of other important clinical variables, including performance status, measures of neurological function, cause of death, and control of systemic disease.

Despite these somewhat promising results regarding local tumor control following SRS post-resection boost without initial WBRT, distant intracranial failures appear to occur frequently, requiring high rates of salvage SRS or WBRT. Additional evidence from both retrospective and prospective studies demonstrating noninferiority in survival and preferably overall intracranial control is needed before the substitution of SRS for WBRT as initial post-resection consolidation becomes standard treatment.

8. Conclusions

Several conclusions can be drawn from this chapter. First, WBRT remains the cornerstone of treatment for most patients with brain metastases, since it is highly effective in the palliative setting, and since many patients with brain metastases present in poor functional condition and would not likely benefit from aggressive focal therapy. Second, the addition of focal therapy with either surgical resection or SRS confers benefit in local control, neurologic symptoms, functional independence, and survival for selected patients with good functional status, good systemic control, and a single brain metastasis (and possibly for those with a limited number of multiple metastases). Third, several other questions remain controversial, including the role of SRS in substituting for surgical resection for operable single metastases, serving as definitive treatment without upfront WBRT for a limited number of multiple metastases, complementing or substituting for WBRT for an extensive number of multiple metastases, and substituting for WBRT in the post-resection setting. The key to some of these questions would be clarifying whether or not WBRT truly plays an independent role in contributing to permanent neurocognitive deficits, and if so, whether or not survival and local control outcomes would allow its deferral in various settings. There continues to be a need for well-designed prospective and retrospective studies to evaluate these controversial topics further.

The outcome of treatment of brain metastases using SRS cannot be studied in isolation and must be interpreted in the context of changing systemic cancer care and evolving prognostic indicators. Clinical trials of combined modality approaches with SRS and agents capable of penetrating the blood-brain barrier will likely be mounted in the future. These studies may include chemotherapy, radiation sensitizers, monoclonal antibodies, and other tumor-specific targeted agents, as researchers and clinicians obtain a deeper understanding of the molecular drivers of different subtypes of cancers that metastasize to the brain. As these therapies continue to develop and improve, the potential for more durable systemic control and overall survival may warrant an increase in the utilization of SRS, making a more thorough understanding of its potential indications even more critical.

9. References

Al-Shamy, G. & Sawaya, R. (2009). Management of brain metastases: the indispensible role of surgery. *J Neurooncol*, Vol. 92, No. 3, pp. 275-282, ISSN 0167-594X

Andrews, D.; Scott, C.; Sperduto, P.; et al. (2004). Whole brain radiation therapy with or without stereotactic radiosurgery boost for patients with one to three brain metastases: phase III results of the RTOG 9508 randomised trial. *Lancet*, Vol. 363, No. 9422, pp. 1665-1672, ISSN 0140-6736

Aoyama, H.; Shirato, H.; Tago, M.; et al. (2006). Stereotactic radiosurgery plus whole-brain radiation therapy vs stereotactic radiosurgery alone for treatment of brain metastases: a randomized controlled trial. *JAMA*, Vol. 295, No. 21, pp. 2483-2491, ISSN 0098-7484

Aoyama, H.; Tago, M.; Kato, N.; et al. (2007). Neurocognitive function of patients with brain metastasis who received either whole brain radiotherapy plus stereotactic radiosurgery or radiosurgery alone. *Int J Radiat Oncol Biol Phys*, Vol. 68, No. 5, pp. 1388-1395, ISSN 0360-3016

Armstrong, C.; Corn, B.; Ruffer, J.; et al. (2000). Radiotherapeutic effects on brain function: double dissociation of memory systems. *Neuropsychiatry Neuropsychol Behav Neurol*, Vol. 13, No. 2, pp. 101-111, ISSN 0894-878X

Bafford, A.; Burstein, H.; Barkley, C.; et al. (2009). Breast surgery in stage IV breast cancer: impact of staging and patient selection on overall survival. *Breast Cancer Res Treat*, Vol. 115, No. 1, pp. 7-12, ISSN 0167-6806

Berk, L. (1995). An overview of radiotherapy trials for the treatment of brain metastases. *Oncology (Williston Park)*, Vol. 9, No. 11, pp. 1205-1212, ISSN 0890-9091

Bhatnagar, A.; Flickinger, J.; Kondziolka, D.; et al. (2006). Stereotactic radiosurgery for four or more intracranial metastases. *Int J Radiat Oncol Biol Phys*, Vol. 64, No. 3, pp. 898-903, ISSN 0360-3016

Bindal, A.; Bindal, R.; Hess, K.; et al. (1996). Surgery versus radiosurgery in the treatment of brain metastasis. *J Neurosurg*, Vol. 84, No. 5, pp. 748-754, ISSN 0022-3085

Borgelt, B.; Gelber, R.; Kramer, S.; et al. (1980). The palliation of brain metastases: final results of the first two studies by the Radiation Therapy Oncology Group. *Int J Radiat Oncol Biol Phys*, Vol. 6, No. 1, pp. 1-9, ISSN 0360-3016

Borgelt, B.; Gelber, R.; Larson, M.; et al. (1981). Ultra-rapid high dose irradiation schedules for the palliation of brain metastases: final results of the first two studies by the Radiation Therapy Oncology Group. *Int J Radiat Oncol Biol Phys*, Vol. 7, No. 12, pp. 1633-1638, ISSN 0360-3016

Bronen, R. & Sze, G. (1990). Magnetic resonance imaging agents: theory and application to the central nervous system. *J Neurosurg*, Vol. 73, No. 6, pp. 820-839, ISSN ISSN 0022-3085

Cairncross, J.; Kim, J. & Posner, J. (1980). Radiation therapy for brain metastases. *Ann Neurol*, Vol. 7, No. 6, pp. 529-541, ISSN 0364-5134

Chang, E.; Wefel, J.; Maor, M.; et al. (2007). A pilot study of neurocognitive function in patients with one to three new brain metastases initially treated with stereotactic radiosurgery alone. *Neurosurgery*, Vol. 60, No. 2, pp. 277-283, ISSN 0148-396X

Chang, E.; Wefel, J.; Hess, K.; et al. (2009). Neurocognition in patients with brain metastases treated with radiosurgery or radiosurgery plus whole-brain irradiation: a randomised controlled trial. *Lancet Oncol*, Vol. 10, No. 11, pp. 1037-1044, ISSN 1470-2045

Chang, W.; Kim, H.; Chang, J.; et al. (2010). Analysis of radiosurgical results in patients with brain metastases according to the number of brain lesions: is stereotactic radiosurgery effective for multiple brain metastases? *J Neurosurg*, Vol. 113 (Supplement), pp. 73-78, ISSN 0022-3085

Chidel, M.; Suh, J.; Reddy, C.; et al. (2000). Application of recursive partitioning analysis and evaluation of the use of whole brain radiation among patients treated with stereotactic radiosurgery for newly diagnosed brain metastases. *Int J Radiat Oncol Biol Phys*, Vol. 47, No. 4, pp. 993-999, ISSN 0360-3016

Coia, L. (1992). The role of radiation therapy in the treatment of brain metastases. *Int J Radiat Oncol Biol Phys*, Vol. 23, No. 1, pp. 229-238, ISSN 0360-3016

Combs, S.; Schulz-Ertner, D.; Thilmann, C.; et al. (2004). Treatment of cerebral metastases from breast cancer with stereotactic radiosurgery. *Strahlenther Onkol*, Vol. 180,No. 9, pp. 590-596, ISSN 0179-7158

Datta, R.; Jawahar, A.; Ampil, F.; et al. (2004). Survival in relation to radiotherapeutic modality for brain metastasis: whole brain irradiation vs. Gamma Knife radiosurgery. *Am J Clin Oncol*, Vol. 27, No. 4, pp. 420-424, ISSN 0277-3732

Davis, P.; Hudgins, P.; Peterman, S.; et al. (1991). Diagnosis of cerebral metastases: double-dose delayed CT vs. contrast-enhanced MR imaging. *AJNR Am J Neuroradiol*, Vol. 12, No. 2, pp. 293-300, ISSN 0195-6108

Dea, N.; Borduas, M.; Kenny, B.; et al. (2010). Safety and efficacy of Gamma Knife surgery for brain metastases in eloquent locations. *J Neurosurg*, Vol. 113 (Supplement), pp. 79-83, ISSN 0022-3085

DeAngelis, L.; Delattre J. & Posner, J. (1989). Radiation-induced dementia in patients cured of brain metastases. *Neurology*, Vol. 39, No. 6, pp. 789-796, ISSN 0028-3878

DeAngelis, L.; Mandell, L.; Thaler, H.; et al. (1989). The role of postoperative radiotherapy after resection of single brain metastases. *Neurosurgery*, Vol. 24, No. 6, pp. 798-805, ISSN 0148-396X

Do, L.; Pezner, R.; Radany, E.; et al. (2009). Resection followed by stereotactic radiosurgery to resection cavity for intracranial metastases. *Int J Radiat Oncol Biol Phys*, Vol. 73, No. 2, pp. 486-491, ISSN 0360-3016

Eichler, A.; Kahle, K.; Wang, D.; et al. (2010). EGFR mutation status and survival after diagnosis of brain metastasis in non-small cell lung cancer. *Neuro Oncol*, Vol. 12, No. 11, pp. 1193-1199, ISSN 1522-8517.

Elaimy, A.; Mackay, A.; Lamoreaux, W.; et al. (2011). Clinical outcomes of stereotactic radiosurgery in the treatment of patients with metastatic brain tumors. *World Neurosurg*, Vol. 75, No. 5-6, pp. 673-683, ISSN 1878-8750

Elliott, R.; Rush, S.; Morsi, A.; et al. (2010). Neurological complications and symptom resolution following Gamma Knife surgery for brain metastases 2 cm or smaller in relation to eloquent cortices. *J Neurosurg*, Vol. 113 (Supplement), pp. 53-64, ISSN 0022-3085

Engh, J.; Flickinger, J.; Niranjan, A.; et al. (2007). Optimizing intracranial metastasis detection for stereotactic radiosurgery. *Stereotact and Funct Neurosurg*, Vol. 85, No. 4, pp. 162-168, ISSN 1011-6125

Flickinger, J.; Kondziolka, D.; Lunsford, L.; et al. (1994). A multi-institutional experience with stereotactic radiosurgery for solitary brain metastasis. *Int J Radiat Oncol Biol Phys*, Vol. 28, No. 4, pp. 797-802, ISSN 0360-3016

Garell, P.; Hitchon, P.; Wen, B.; et al. (1999). Stereotactic radiosurgery versus microsurgical resection for the initial treatment of metastatic cancer to the brain. *J Radiosurg*, Vol. 2, No. 1, pp. 1-5, ISSN 1096-4053

Gaspar, L.; Scott, C.; Rotman, M.; et al. (1997). Recursive partitioning analysis (RPA) of prognostic factors in three Radiation Therapy Oncology Group (RTOG) brain metastases trials. *Int J Radiat Oncol Biol Phys*, Vol. 37, No. 4, pp. 745-751, ISSN 0360-3016

Gaspar, L.; Scott, C.; Murray, K.; et al. (2000). Validation of the RTOG recursive partitioning analysis (RPA) classification for brain metastases. *Int J Radiat Oncol Biol Phys*, Vol. 47, No. 4, pp. 1001-1006, ISSN 0360-3016

Gavrilovic, I. & Posner, J. (2005). Brain metastases: epidemiology and pathophysiology. *J Neurooncol*, Vol. 75, No. 1, pp. 5-14, ISSN 0167-594X

Hanssens, P.; Karlsson, B.; Yeo, T.; et al. (2011). Detection of brain micrometastases by high-resolution stereotactic magnetic resonance imaging and its impact on the timing of and risk for distant recurrences. *J Neurosurg*, Vol. 111, Epub ahead of print, ISSN 0022-3085

Hasegawa, T.; Kondziolka, D.; Flickinger, J.; et al. (2003). Brain metastases treated with radiosurgery alone: an alternative to whole brain radiotherapy? *Neurosurgery*, Vol. 52, No. 6, pp. 1318-1326, ISSN 0148-396X

Hatiboglu, M.; Chang E.; Suki, D.; et al. (2011). Outcomes and prognostic factors for patients with brainstem metastases undergoing stereotactic radiosurgery. *Neurosurgery*, Epub ahead of print (April 2011), ISSN 0148-396X

Hoffman, R.; Sneed, P.; McDermott, M.; et al. (2001). Radiosurgery for brain metastases from primary lung carcinoma. *Cancer J*, Vol. 7, No. 2, pp. 121-131, ISSN 1528-9117

Hwang, S.; Abozed, M.; Hale, A.; et al. (2010). Adjuvant Gamma Knife radiosurgery following surgical resection of brain metastases: a 9-year retrospective cohort study. *J Neurooncol*, Vol. 98, No. 1, pp. 77-82, ISSN 0167-594X

Iwai, Y.; Yamanaka, K. & Yasui, T. (2008). Boost radiosurgery for treatment of brain metastases after surgical resections. *Surg Neurol*, Vol. 69, No. 2, pp. 181-186, ISSN 0090-3019

Jagannathan, J.; Yen, C.; Ray, D.; et al. (2009). Gamma Knife radiosurgery to the surgical cavity following resection of brain metastases. *J Neurosurg*, Vol. 111, No. 3, pp. 431-438, ISSN 0022-3085

Jawahar, A.; Willis, B.; Smith, D.; et al. (2002). Gamma Knife radiosurgery for brain metastases: do patients benefit from adjuvant external-beam radiotherapy? An 18-month comparative analysis. *Stereotact and Funct Neurosurg*, Vol. 79, No. 3-4, pp. 262-271, ISSN 1011-6125

Jensen, C.; Chan, M.; McCoy, T.; et al. (2011). Cavity-directed radiosurgery as adjuvant therapy after resection of a brain metastasis. *J Neurosurg*, Vol. 114, No. 6, pp. 1585-1591, ISSN 0022-3085

Kalani, M.; Filippidis, A.; Kalani, M.; et al. (2010). Gamma Knife surgery combined with resection for treatment of a single brain metastasis: preliminary results. *J Neurosurg*, Vol. 113 (Supplement), pp. 90-96, ISSN 0022-3085

Karlovits, B.; Quigley M.; Karlovits, S.; et al. (2009). Stereotactic radiosurgery boost to the resection bed for oligometastatic brain disease: challenging the tradition of adjuvant whole-brain radiotherapy. *Neurosurg Focus*, Vol. 27, No. 6, pp. E7, ISSN 1092-0684

Karlsson, B.; Hanssens, P.; Wolff, R.; et al. (2009). Thirty years' experience with Gamma Knife surgery for metastases to the brain. *J Neurosurg*, Vol. 111, No. 3, pp. 449-457, ISSN 0022-3085

Karnofsky, D. & Burchenal, J. (1949). The clinical evaluation of chemotherapeutic agents in cancer, In: *Evaluation of Chemotherapeutic Agents*, MacCleod (ed), p. 196, Columbia University Press, ISBN B002JNAA42, p., New York, NY

Khuntia, D.; Brown, P.; Jing, L.; et al. (2006). Whole-brain radiation in the management of brain metastases. *J Clin Oncol*, Vol. 24, No. 8, pp. 1295-1304, ISSN 0732-183X

Kim, C.; Im, Y.; Nam, D.; et al. (2008). Gamma Knife radiosurgery for ten or more brain metastases. *J Korean Neurosurg Soc*, Vol. 44, No. 6, pp. 358-363, 1225-8245

Kim, P.; Ellis, T.; Stieber, V.; et al. (2006). Gamma Knife surgery targeting the resection cavity of brain metastasis that has progressed after whole-brain radiotherapy. *J Neurosurg*, Vol. 105 (Supplement), pp. 75-78, ISSN 0022-3085

Kim, W.; Kim, D.; Han, J.; et al. (2011). Early significant tumor volume reduction after radiosurgery in brain metastases from renal cell carcinoma results in long-term survival. *Int J Radiat Oncol Biol Phys*, Epub ahead of print (June 2011), ISSN 0360-3016

Knisely, J.; Yamamoto, M.; Gross, C.; et al. (2010). Radiosurgery alone for 5 or more brain metastases: expert opinion survey. *J Neurosurg*, Vol. 113 (Supplement), pp. 84-89, ISSN 0022-3085

Kocher, M.; Maarouf, M.; Bendel, M.; et al. (2004). Linac radiosurgeyr versus whole brain radiotherapy for brain metastases: a survival comparison based on the RTOG recursive partitioning analysis. *Strahlenther Onkol*, Vol. 180, No. 5, pp. 263-267, ISSN 0179-7158

Kocher, M.; Soffietti, R.; Abacioglu, U.; et al. (2010). Adjuvant whole-brain radiotherapy versus observation after radiosurgery or surgical resection of one to three cerebral metastases: results of the EORTC 22952-26001 study. *J Clin Oncol*, Vol. 29, No. 2, pp. 134-141, ISSN 0732-183X

Komarnicky, L.; Phillips, T.; Martz, K.; et al. (1991). A randomized phase III protocol for the evaluation of misonidazole combined with radiation in the treatment of patients with brain metastases (RTOG 79-16). *Int J Radiat Oncol Biol Phys*, Vol. 20, No. 1, pp. 53-58, ISSN 0360-3016

Kondziolka, D.; Patel, A.; Lunsford, L.; et al. (1999). Stereotactic radiosurgery plus whole brain radiotherapy versus radiotherapy alone for patients with multiple brain metastases. *Int J Radiat Oncol Biol Phys*, Vol. 45, No. 2, pp. 427-434, ISSN 0360-3016

Kurtz, J.; Gelber, R.; Brady, L.; et al. (1981). The palliation of brain metastases in a favourable patient population: a randomized clinical trial by the Radiation Therapy Oncology Group. *Int J Radiat Oncol Biol Phys*, Vol. 7, No. 7, pp. 891-895, ISSN 0360-3016

Lagerwaard, F.; Levendag, P.; Nowak, P.; et al. (1999). Identification of prognostic factors in patients with brain metastases: a review of 1292 patients. *Int J Radiat Oncol Biol Phys*, Vol. 43, No. 4, pp. 795-803, ISSN 0360-3016

Lassman, A. & DeAngelis, L. (2003). Brain metastases. *Neurol Clin*, Vol. 21, No. 1, pp. 1-23, vii, ISSN 0733-8619

Lee, Y.; Park, N.; Kim, J.; et al. (2008). Gamma-knife radiosurgery as an optimal treatment modality for brain metastases from epithelial ovarian cancer. *Gynecol Oncol*, Vol. 108, No. 3, pp. 505-509, ISSN 0090-8258

Lawlor, P.; Gagnon, B.; Mancini, I.; et al. (2000). Occurrence, causes, and outcome of delirium in patients with advanced cancer: a prospective study. *Arch Int Med*, Vol. 160, No. 6, pp. 786-794, ISSN 0003-9926

Leksell, L. (1951). The stereotaxic method and radiosurgery of the brain. *Acta Chir Scand*, Vol. 102, No. 14, pp. 316-319, ISSN 0001-5482

Lenz, M. & Fried, J. (1931). Metastases to the skeleton, brain and spinal cord from cancer of the breast and the effect of radiotherapy. *Ann Surg*, Vol. 93, No. 1, pp. 278-293, ISSN 0003-4932

Li, B.; Yu, J.; Suntharalingam, M.; et al. (2000). Comparison of three treatment options for single brain metastasis from lung cancer. *Int J Cancer*, Vol. 90, No. 1, pp. 37-45, ISSN 0020-7136

Li, J.; Bentzen, S.; Renschler, M.; et al. (2007). Regression after whole-brain radiation therapy for brain metastases correlates with survival and improved neurocognitive function. *J Clin Oncol*, Vol. 25, No. 10, pp. 1260-1266, ISSN 0732-183X

Linskey, M.; Andrews, D.; Asher, A.; et al. (2010). The role of stereotactic radiosurgery in the management of patients with newly diagnosed brain metastases: a systematic review and evidence-based clinical practice guideline. *J Neurooncol*, Vol. 96, No. 1, pp. 45-68, ISSN 0167-594X

Loeffler, J.; Kooy, H.; Wen, P.; et al. (1990). The treatment of brain metastases with stereotactic radiosurgery. *Journal of Clinical Oncology*, Vol. 8, No. 4, pp. 576-582, ISSN 0732-183X

Lindquist, C. (1989). Gamma knife surgery for recurrent solitary metastasis of a cerebral hypernephroma: case report. *Neurosurgery*, Vol. 25, No. 5, pp. 802-804, ISSN 0148-396X

Lorenzoni, J.; Devriendt, D.; Massager, N.; et al. (2004). Radiosurgery for treatment of brain metastases: estimation of patient eligibility using three stratification systems. *Int J Radiat Oncol Biol Phys*, Vol. 60, No. 1, pp. 218-24, ISSN 0360-3016

Mathieu, D.; Kondziolka, D.; Flickinger, J.; et al. (2008). Tumor bed radiosurgery after resection of cerebral metastases. *Neurosurgery*, Vol. 62, No. 4, pp. 817-824, ISSN 0148-396X

Mehta, M. (2011). The dandelion effect: treat the whole lawn or weed selectively? *J Clin Oncol*, Vol. 29, No. 2, pp. 121-124, ISSN 0732-183X

Meyers C. & Wefel, J. (2003). The use of the mini-mental state examination to assess cognitive functioning in cancer trials: no ifs, ands, buts, or sensitivity. *J Clin Oncol*, Vol. 21, No. 19, pp. 3557-3558, ISSN 0732-183X

Mintz, A.; Kestle, J.; Rathbone, M.; et al. (1996). A randomized trial to assess the efficacy of surgery in addition to radiotherapy in patients with a single cerebral metastasis. *Cancer*, Vol. 78, No. 7, pp. 1470-1476, ISSN 0008-543X

Muacevic, A.; Kreth, F.; Horstmann, G.; et al. (1999). Surgery and radiotherapy compared with Gamma Knife radiosurgery in the treatment of solitary cerebral metastases of small diameter. *J Neurosurg*, Vol. 91, No. 1, pp. 35-43, ISSN 0022-3085

Muacevic, A.; Wowra, B.; Siefert, A.; et al. (2008). Microsurgery plus whole brain irradiation versus Gamma Knife surgery alone for treatment of single metastases to the brain: a randomized controlled multicentre phase III trial. *J Neurooncol*, Vol. 87, No. 3, pp. 299-307, ISSN 0167-594X

Murray, K.; Scott, C.; Greenberg, H.; et al. (1997). A randomized phase III study of accelerated hyperfractionation versus standard in patients with unresected brain metastases: a report of the Radiation Therapy Oncology Group (RTOG) 9104. *Int J Radiat Oncol Biol Phys*, Vol. 39, No. 1, pp. 571-574, ISSN 0360-3016

Nam, T.; Lee, J.; Jung, Y.; et al. (2005). Gamma Knife surgery for brain metastases in patients harboring four or more lesions: survival and prognostic factors. *J Neurosurg*, Vol. 102 (Supplement), pp. 147-150, ISSN 0022-3085

Nieder, C.; Spanne, O.; Mehta, M.; et al. (2010). Presentation, patterns of care, and survival in patients with brain metastases: what has changed in the last 20 years. *Cancer*, Epub ahead of print (December 2010), ISSN 0008-543X

Noel, G.; Medioni, J.; Valery, C.; et al. (2003). Three irradiation treatment options including radiosurgery for brain metastases from primary lung cancer. *Lung Cancer*, Vol. 41, No. 3, pp. 333-343, ISSN 0169-5002

Oken, M.; Creech, R.; Tormey, D.; et al. (1982). Toxicity and response criteria of the Eastern Cooperative Oncology Group. *Am J Clin Oncol*, Vol. 5, No. 6, pp. 649-655, ISSN 0277-3732

O'Neill, B.; Iturria, N.; Link, M.; et al. (2003). A comparison of surgical resection and stereotactic radiosurgery in the treatment of solitary brain metastases. *Int J Radiat Oncol Biol Phys*, Vol. 55, No. 5, pp. 1169-1176, ISSN 0360-3016

Order, S.; Hellman, S.; Von Essen, C.; et al. (1968). Improvement in quality of survival following whole-brain irradiation for brain metastases. *Radiology*, Vol. 91, No. 1, pp. 149-153, ISSN 0033-8419

Park, S.; Hwang, S.; Kang, D.; et al. (2009). Gamma Knife radiosurgery for multiple brain metastases from lung cancer. *J Clin Neurosci*, Vol. 16, No. 5, pp. 626-629, ISSN 0967-5868

Patchell, R.; Tibbs, P.; Walsh, J.; et al. (1990). A randomized trial of surgery in the treatment of single metastases to the brain. *NEJM*, Vol. 322, No. 8, pp. 494-500, ISSN 0028-4793

Patchell, R.; Tibbs, P.; Regine, W.; et al. (1998). Postoperative radiotherapy in the treatment of single metastases to the brain: a randomized trial. *JAMA*, Vol. 280, No. 17, pp. 1485-1489, ISSN 0098-7484

Patchell, R.; Regine, W.; Loeffler, J.; et al. (2006). Radiosurgery plus whole-brain radiation therapy for brain metastases. *JAMA*, Vol. 296, No. 17, pp. 2089-90, ISSN 0098-7484

Patel, T.; McHugh, B.; Bi, W.; et al. (2011). A comprehensive review of magnetic resonance imaging changes following radiosurgery to 500 brain metastases. *AJNR Am J Neuroradiol*, in press, ISSN 0195-6108

Patel, T.; Ozturk, A.; Knisely, J.; et al. (2011). Implications of identifying additional cerebral metastases during Gamma Knife radiosurgery. *Int J Surg Oncol*, in press, ISSN 2090-1402

Pereira, J.; Hanson, J. & Bruera E. (1997). The frequency and clinical course of cognitive impairment in patients with terminal cancer. *Cancer*, Vol. 79, No. 4, pp. 835-842, ISSN 0008-543X

Pirzkall, A.; Debus, J.; Lohr, F.; et al. (1998). Radiosurgery alone or in combination with whole-brain radiotherapy for brain metastases. *J Clin Oncol*, Vol. 16, No. 11, pp. 3563-3569, ISSN 0732-183X

Posner, J. (1992). Management of brain metastases. *Revue Neurol (Paris)*, Vol. 148, No. 6-7, pp. 477-487, ISSN 0035-3787

Powell, J.; Chung, C.; Shah, H.; et al. (2008). Gamma Knife surgery in the management of radioresistant brain metastases in high-risk patients with melanoma, renal cell carcinoma, and sarcoma. *J Neurosurg*, Vol. 109 (Supplement), pp. 122-128, ISSN 0022-3085

Quigley, M.; Fuhrer, R.; Karlovits, S.; et al. (2008). Single session stereotactic radiosurgery boost to the post-operative site in lieu of whole brain radiation in metastatic brain disease. *J Neurooncol*, Vol. 87, No. 3, pp. 327-332, ISSN 0167-594X

Rades, D.; Bohlen, G.; Pluemer, A.; et al. (2007). Stereotactic radiosurgery alone versus resection plus whole-brain radiotherapy for 1 or 2 brain metastases in recursive partitioning analysis class 1 and 2 patients. *Cancer*, Vol. 109, No. 12, pp. 2515-2521, ISSN 0008-543X

Rades, D.; Pluemer, A.; Veninga, T.; et al. (2007). Whole-brain radiotherapy versus stereotactic radiosurgery for patients in recursive partitioning analysis classes 1 and 2 with 1 to 3 brain metastases. *Cancer*, Vol. 110, No. 10, pp. 2285-2292, ISSN 0008-543X

Rades, D.; Veninga, T.; Hornung, D.; et al. (2011). Single brain metastasis: whole-brain irradiation plus either radiosurgery or neurosurgical resection. *Cancer*, Epub ahead of print (July 2011), ISSN 0008-543X

Rauch, P.; Park, H.; Knisely, J.; et al. (2011). Delayed radiation-induced vasculitic leukoencephalopathy. *Int J Radiat Oncol Biol Phys*, in press, ISSN 0360-3016

Roberge, D.; Petrecca, K.; El Refae, M.; et al. (2009). Whole-brain radiotherapy and tumor bed radiosurgery following resection of solitary brain metastases. *J Neurooncol*, Vol. 95, No. 1, pp. 95-99, ISSN 0167-594X

Robert, C.; Thomas, L.; Bondarenko, I.; et al. (2011). Ipilimumab plus dacarbazine for previously untreated metastatic melanoma. *NEJM*, Vol. 364, No. 26, pp. 2517-2526, ISSN 0028-4793

Sato, N.; Bronen, R.; Sze, G.; et al. (1997). Postoperative changes in the brain: MR imaging findings in patients without neoplasms. *Radiology*, Vol. 204, No. 3, pp. 839-846, ISSN 0033-8419

Sause, W.; Crowley, J.; Morantz, R.; et al. (1990). Solitary brain metastases: results of an RTOG/SWOG protocol evaluating surgery + RT versus RT alone. *Am J Clin Oncol*, Vol. 13, No. 5, pp. 427-432, ISSN 0277-3732

Schoggl, A.; Kitz, K.; Reddy, M.; et al. (2000). Defining the role of stereotactic radiosurgery versus microsurgery in the treatment of single brain metastases. *Acta Neurochir*, Vol. 142, No. 6, ISSN 0001-6268

Serizawa, T.; Iuchi, T.; Ono, J.; et al. (2000). Gamma Knife treatment for multiple metastatic brain tumors compared with whole-brain radiation therapy. *J Neurosurg*. Vol. 93, No. 3 (Supplement), pp. 32-36, ISSN 0022-3085

Serizawa, T., Hirai, T.; Nagano, O.; et al. (2010). Gamma Knife surgery for 1-10 brain metastases without prophylactic whole-brain radiation therapy: analysis of cases meeting the Japanese prospective multi-institute study (JLGK0901) inclusion criteria. *J Neurooncol*, Vol. 98, No. 2, pp. 163-167, ISSN 0167-594X

Shehata, M.; Young, B.; Reid, B.; et al. (2004). Stereotactic radiosurgery of 468 brain metastases ≤2 cm: implications for SRS dose and whole brain radiation therapy. *Int J Radiat Oncol Biol Phys*, Vol. 59, No. 1, pp. 87-93, ISSN 0360-3016

Shinoura, N.; Yamada, R.; Okamoto, K.; et al. (2002). Local recurrence of metastatic brain tumor after stereotactic radiosurgery or surgery plus radiation. *J Neurooncol*, Vol. 60, No.1, pp. 71-77, ISSN 0167-594X

Sneed, P.; Lamborn, K.; Forstner, J.; et al. (1999). Radiosurgery for brain metastases: is whole brain radiotherapy necessary? *Int J Radiat Oncol Biol Phys*, Vol. 43, No. 3, pp. 549-558, ISSN 0360-3016

Sneed, P.; Suh, J.; Goetsch, S.; et al. (2002). A multi-institutional review of radiosurgery alone vs. radiosurgery with whole brain radiotherapy as the initial management of brain metastases. *Int J Radiat Oncol Biol Phys*, Vol. 53, No. 3, pp. 519-526, ISSN 0360-3016

Soltys, S.; Adler, J.; Lipani, J.; et al. (2008). Stereotactic radiosurgery of the postoperative resection cavity for brain metastases. *Int J Radiat Oncol Biol Phys*, Vol. 70, No. 1, pp. 187-193, ISSN 0360-3016

Son, C.; Jimenez, R.; Niemierko, A.; et al. (2011). Outcomes after whole brain reirradiation in patients with brain metastases. *Int J Radiat Oncol Biol Phys*, Epub ahead of print (May 2011), ISSN 0360-3016

Sperduto, P.; Berkey, B.; Gaspar, L.; et al. (2008). A new prognostic index and comparison to three other indices for patients with brain metastases: an analysis of 1,960 patients in the RTOG database. *Int J Radiat Oncol Biol Phys*, Vol. 70, No. 2, pp. 510-514, ISSN 0360-3016

Sperduto, P.; Chao, S.; Sneed, P.; et al. (2010). Diagnosis-specific prognostic factors, indexes, and treatment outcomes for patients with newly diagnosed brain metastases: a multi-institutional analysis of 4,259 patients. *Int J Radiat Oncol Biol Phys*, Vol. 77, No. 3, pp. 655-661, ISSN 0360-3016

Sperduto, P.; Kased, N.; Roberge, D.; et al. (2011). Effect of tumor subtype on survival and the Graded Prognostic Assessment for patients with breast cancer and brain metastases. *Int J Radiat Oncol Biol Phys*, Epub ahead of print (April 2011), ISSN 0360-3016

Sturm, V.; Kober, B.; Hover, K.; et al. (1987). Stereotactic percutaneous single dose irradiation of brain metastases with a linear accelerator. *Int J Radiat Oncol Biol Phys*, Vol. 13, No. 2, pp. 279-282, ISSN 0360-3016

Suzuki, S.; Omagari, J.; Nishio, S.; et al. (2000). Gamma Knife radiosurgery for simultaneous multiple metastatic brain tumors. *J Neurosurg*. Vol. 93, No. 3 (Supplement), pp. 30-31, ISSN 0022-3085

Varlotto, J.; Flickinger, J.; Niranjan, A.; et al. (2003). Analysis of tumor control and toxicity in patients who have survived at least one year after radiosurgery for brain metastases. *Int J Radiat Oncol Biol Phys*, Vol. 57, No. 2, pp. 452-464, ISSN 0360-3016

Varlotto, J.; Flickinger, J.; Niranjan, A.; et al. (2005). The impact of whole-brain radiation therapy on the long-term control and morbidity of patients surviving more than one year after Gamma Knife radiosurgery for brain metastases. *Int J Radiat Oncol Biol Phys*, Vol. 62, No. 4, pp. 1125-113, ISSN 0360-3016

Vecht, C.; Haaxma-Reiche, H.; Noordijk, E.; et al (1993). Treatment of single brain metastasis: radiotherapy alone or combined with neurosurgery? *Ann Neurol*, Vol. 33, No. 6, pp. 583-590, ISSN 0364-5134

Vogelbaum, M. & Suh, J. (2006). Resectable brain metastases. *J Clin Oncol*, Vol. 24, No. 8, pp. 1289-1294, ISSN 0732-183X

Wang, L.; Guo, Y.; Zhang, X.; et al. (2002). Brain metastasis: experience of the Xi-Jing hospital. *Stereotact and Funct Neurosurg*, Vol. 78, No. 2, pp. 70-83, ISSN 1011-6125

Webber, K.; Cooper, A.; Kleiven, H.; et al. (2011). Management of metastatic renal cell carcinoma in the era of targeted therapies. *Internal Medicine Journal*, Epub ahead of print (June 2011), ISSN 1444-0903.

Wegner, R.; Olson, A.; Kondziolka, D.; et al. (2011). Stereotactic radiosurgery for patients with brain metastases from small cell lung cancer. *Int J Radiat Oncol Biol Phys*, Epub ahead of print (February 2011), ISSN 0360-3016

Weltman, E.; Salvajoli, J.; Brandt, R.; et al. (2000). Radiosurgery for brain metastases: a score index for predicting prognosis. *Int J Radiat Oncol Biol Phys*, Vol. 46, No. 5, pp. 1155-1161, ISSN 0360-3016

Wong, W.; Schild, S.; Sawyer, T.; et al. (1996). Analysis of outcome in patients reirradiated for brain metastases. *Int J Radiat Oncol Biol Phys*, Vol. 34, No. 3, pp. 585-590, ISSN 0360-3016

Yamamoto, M.; Ide, M.; Nishio, S.; et al. (2002). Gamma Knife radiosurgery for numerous brain metastases: is this a safe treatment? *Int J Radiat Oncol Biol Phys*, Vol. 53, No. 5, pp. 1279-1283, ISSN 0360-3016

Yang, H.; Kano, H.; Lunsford, L.; et al. (2011). What factors predict the response of larger brain metastases to radiosurgery? *Neurosurgery*, Vol. 68, No. 3, pp. 682-690, ISSN 0148-396X

2

Gamma Knife Treatment for Patient Harboring Brain Metastases: How to Estimate Patient Eligibility and Survival?

José Lorenzoni[1,2], Adrián Zárate[1], Raúl de Ramón[2],
Leonardo Badínez[2,3], Francisco Bova[2] and Claudio Lühr[2]
[1]Department of Neurosurgery, Pontificia Universidad Católica de Chile, Santiago
[2]Centro Gamma Knife de Santiago, Santiago
[3]Department of Radiation Oncology, Fundación Arturo López Pérez, Santiago
Chile

1. Introduction

Gamma Knife radiosurgery is a well validated option for the treatment of brain metastases existing solid evidence reinforcing his role in the management of these tumors.

The result achieved with this technique in terms of tumor control and survival is comparable to results obtained with surgery plus whole brain irradiation. Radiosurgery has the advantages of lower complications; allow treatment of multiple lesions, permits treatment of lesions deeply located or in high functional zones, rapid recovery and lower cost.

Although radiosurgery could be useful for tumor control, increase survival and improved quality of life, there are some clinical situations where the treatment can be considered applicable and justified and others where radiosurgery could not be recommended.

For the estimation of survival many variables have been identified, the most important seem to be the Karnofsky performance status, control of the cancer disease either at the primary site as well as at the systemic level (dissemination) and the number of brain metastases.

Regarding the different variables studied in the present chapter, each variable was arranged in 1 of 5 powered categories according to the number of publications and the agreement of their findings.

1. **Consistent agreement:** there are clear coincidental conclusions among the publications, without controversial findings. In this category is highly possible that the conclusion is right.
2. **Reasonable agreement:** there are more coincidental conclusions among the publications, but with some controversial findings. In this category is quite possible that the conclusion is right.
3. **Some agreement with a trend:** there are less coincidental conclusions among the publications, more controversial findings but a trend is observed. In this category the conclusion could be right but more information is recommended.

4. **Scarce information with a trend:** A trend is observed, but because the small quantity of data more information is recommended for definitive conclusions.
5. **Scarce information with no clear trend or controversial findings:** In these cases more information is absolutely needed for having any conclusion.

Two plots for each variable were built. The first plot represents the number of publications (papers) supporting the prognostic value of the variable and the second plot shows the number of patients enrolled in such studies: better (variable is a positive prognostic factor), unaffected (variable is not a prognostic factor) and worse (variable is a negative prognostic factor).

Integrating these variables many stratification systems have been proposed for survival estimation: "Recursive Partitioning Analysis", "Score Index for Radiosurgery in Brain Metastases", Basic Score for Brain Metastases" and "Graded Prognostic Assessment Index". All of these stratifications systems allow estimating survival for a particular patient. In this chapter some more details will be given concerning the most used systems.

2. Prognostic factors for survival

2.1 Karnofsky performance status (KPS)

This variable represents the most powerful prognostic factor for survival. The majority of studies show significant influence of KPS in multivariate analysis (Simonová, 2000); Sneed, 2002; Petrovich, 2002; Wowra, 2002; Schoeggl, 2002; Hasegawa, 2003; Muacevic, 2004; Serizawa, 2005; Pan, 2006; Gaudy, 2006; Rades, 2007; Matuiew, 2007; Golden, 2008; Kased, 2009; Da Silva, 2009; Aba cioglu, 2010; Kondziolka 2011; Matsunaga 2011; Liew, 2011). Others authors have communicated significance in univariate studies (Chidel, 2000; Amendola, 2002; Lorenzoni, 2004; Frazier, 2010; Skeie, 2011). A few studies found no influence of KPS in survival (Vesagas, 2002; Hernandez, 2002; Flannery, 2003; Gerosa, 2005), nevertheless, three of these four studies have a small number of patients. A favorable Karnofsky performance status (≥70 or 80) influences positively the survival with "**consistent agreement**".

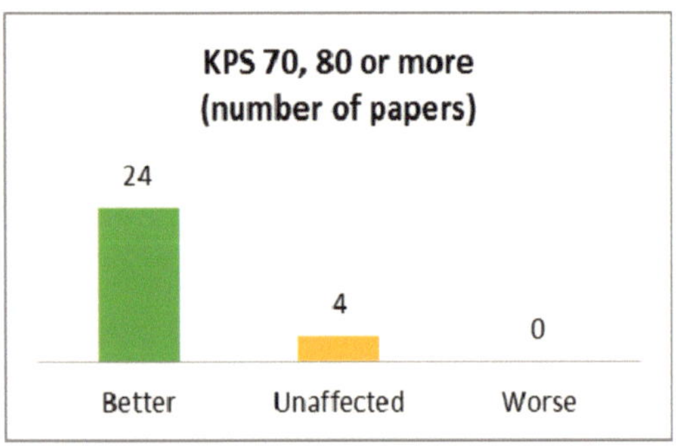

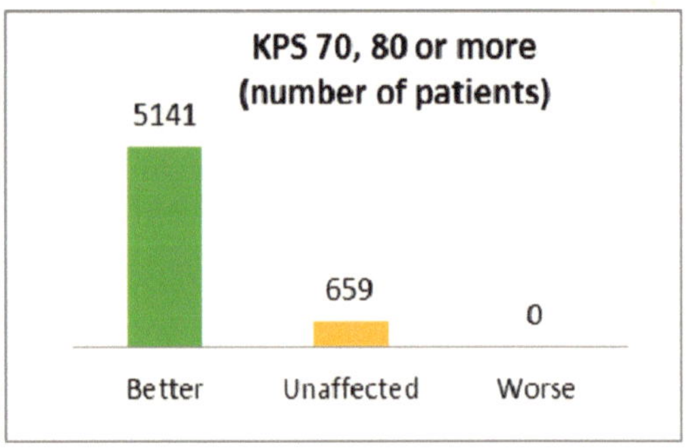

2.2 Systemic cancer control status

This variable is used for many authors as an evaluation tool for the systemic extracranial integrated situation of the cancer progression, taking into account at once the control of the primary tumor site as well as the existence of extracranial metastases. Others authors prefer to study separately the primary tumor control and the extracranial dissemination. Considering the systemic "extracranial" cancer status, there is also predominance of multivariate analysis proving its positive influence on survival (Petrovich, 2002; Serizawa, 2005; Mathiew, 2007; Kondziolka, 2011; Liew, 2011). In univariate studies 3 communications show this influence too (Hasegawa, 2003; Yu, 2005; Karlsson , 2009). Just one publication (Hernández 2002) found no influence of this variable on survival; this is a publication reporting 29 patients with renal cell carcinoma. The present study found a positive influence of Systemic cancer control status on survival with "**consistent agreement**".

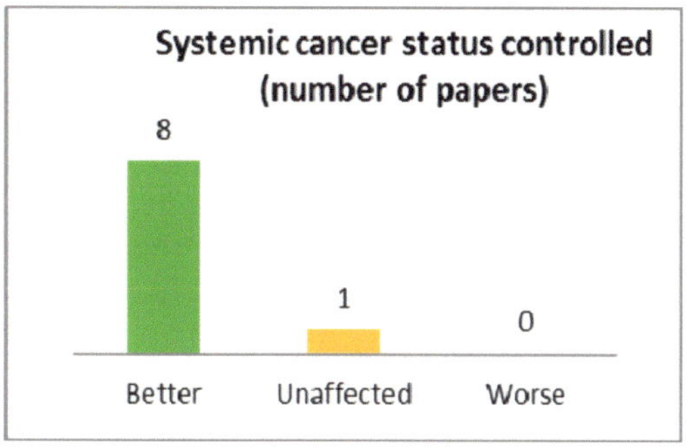

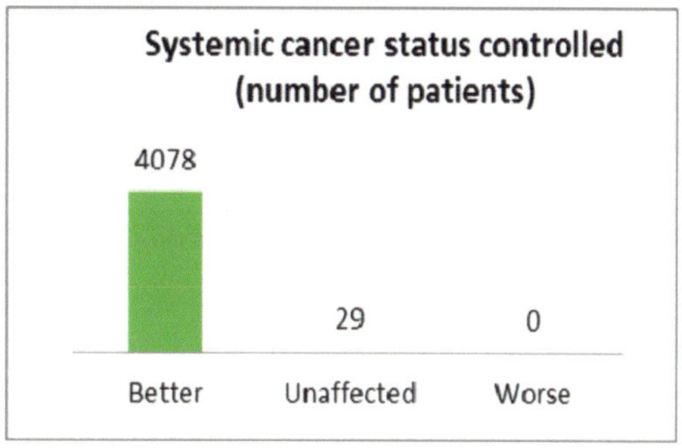

2.3 Extracranial metastases

The existence of extracranial metastatic disease has been identified as a negative prognostic factor for survival by the majority of authors either in multivariate studies (Simonová, 2000; Sneed, 2002; Rades, 2007; Golden, 2008; Matsunaga, 2011; Skeie, 2011) and in univariate studies (Chidel, 2000; Wowra, 2002; Lorenzoni, 2004; Yu, 2005; Pan, 2005). Some others manuscripts have shown no influence of this variable on survival (Hernández, 2002; Schoeggl, 2002; Jawahar, 2004; Gaudy, 2006; Kased, 2009; Da Silva, 2009; Kondziolka, 2011). Concerning the existence of extracranial metastases a negative influence on survival was found with "**reasonable agreement**".

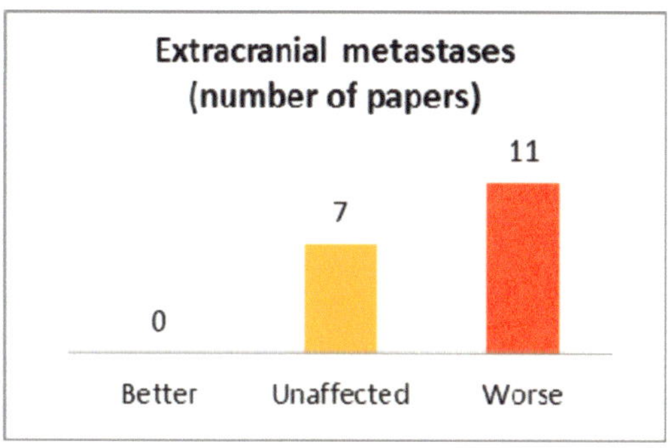

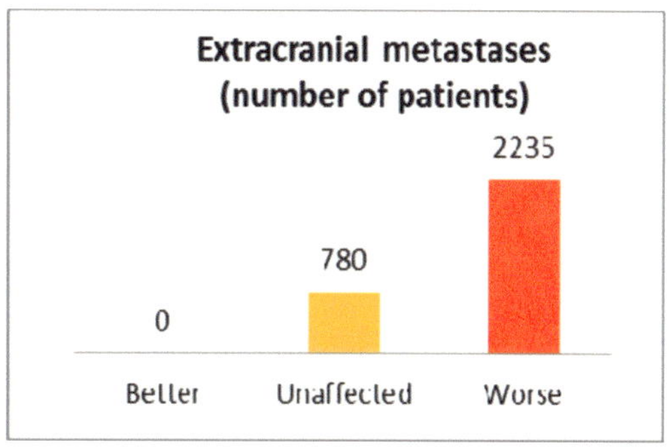

2.4 Control of the primary tumor

Positive influence of controlled primary site has been reported in multivariate study (Sneed, 2002) and in univariate studies (Lorenzoni, 2004; Jawahar, 2004; Pan, 2005; Kased, 2009). Some studies did not find significant influence (Chidel, 2000; Hernández, 2002; Golden,

2008). A positive effect on survival of the control of the primary tumor was observed with **"reasonable agreement".**

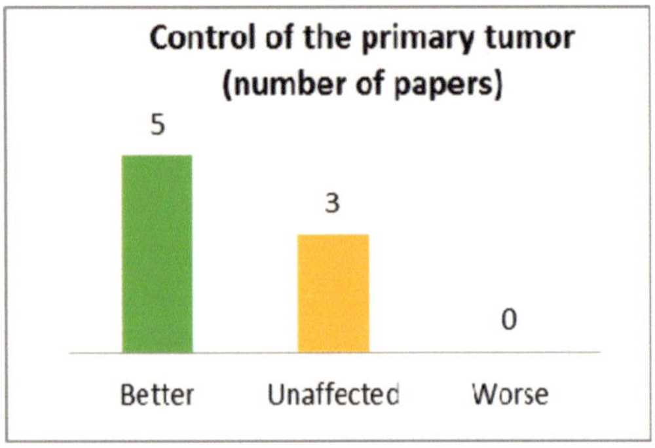

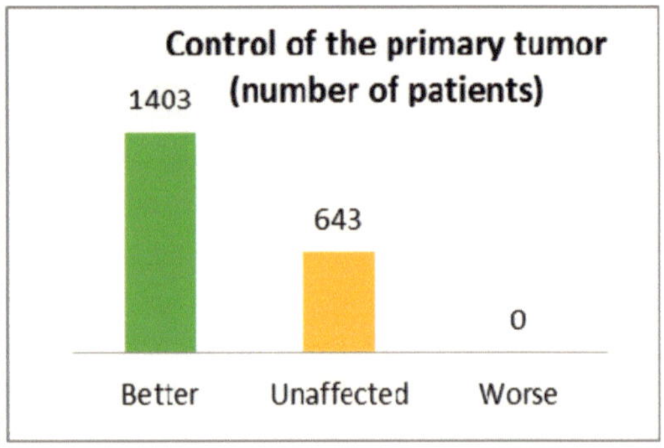

2.5 Bigger size of brain metastases

Gamma Knife radiosurgery in general indicated to patients with brain metastases with a diameter up to 3 centimeters or a volume up to 13 cubic centimeters. Some authors consider the diameter of the lesions; others consider volume and others take into account the addition of the volume of all lesions when multiple metastases are treated. An unfavorable influence of larger size of lesions have been reported in multivariate studies (Petrovich, 2002; Gaudy, 2006; Abacioglu, 2010, Kondziolka, 2011; Skeie, 2011) and in univariate studies (Simonová, 2000; Nam, 2005; Feigl, 2006; Karlsson, 2009; Kased, 2009; Frazier, 2010; Liew, 2011). No influence was communicated too (Hernández, 2002; Hasegawa, 2003; Lorenzoni, 2004; Serizawa, 2005; Yu, 2005; Gerosa, 2005; Da Silva, 2009). With regard the size of metastases a bigger size or total tumoral volume was associated with a poor survival with "**reasonable agreement**".

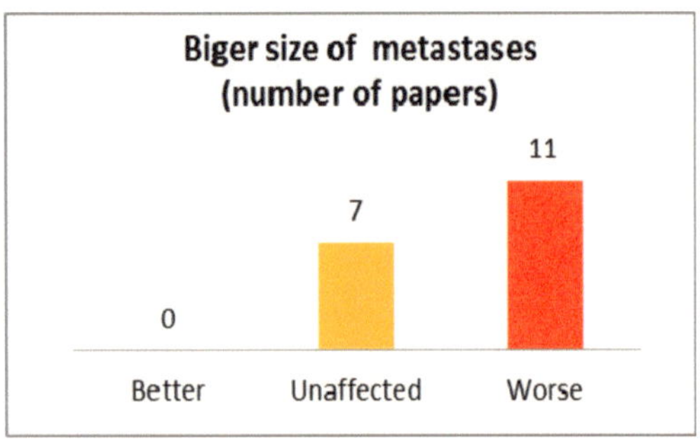

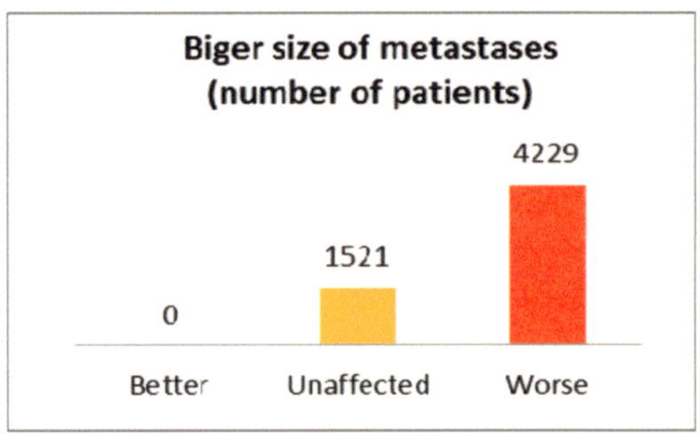

2.6 Multiple LGK treatments

After a Gamma Knife treatment for brain metastases, along the time new metastases can develop, in such situations a new Gamma Knife treatment can be offered to these patients, Pan (Pan, 2005) found a positive influence on survival the realization of a new treatments in multivariate analysis. Vesagas (Vesagas, 2002) and Yu (Yu, 2005) found benefice in univariate studies. Conversely, two authors (Hernández, 2002; Wowra, 2002) did not find any effect. Concerning new Gamma Knife treatments, a positive effect on survival has been observed with "**scarce information with a trend**".

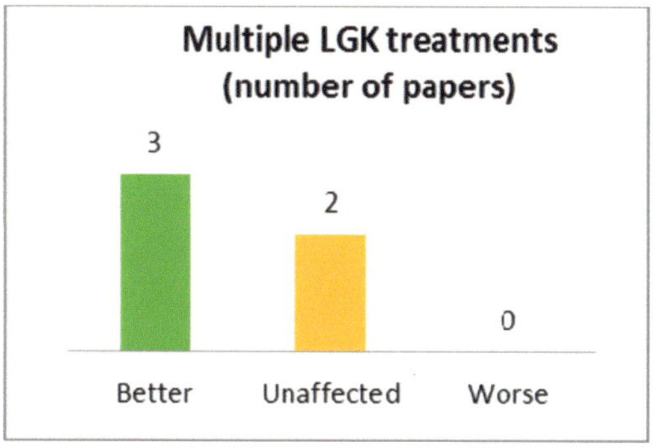

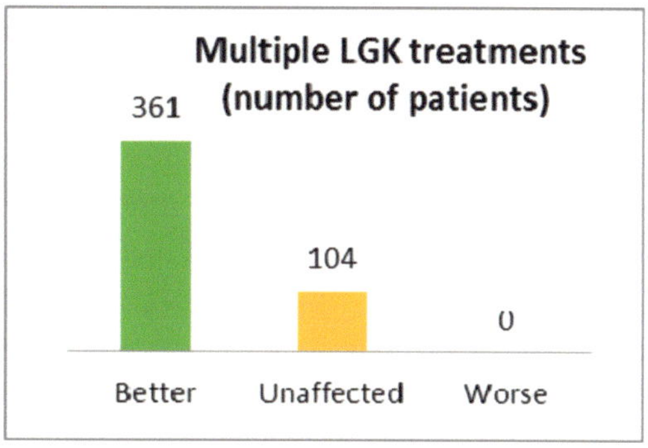

2.7 Number of brain metastases

The study of this variable is nowadays a challenge and not definitive conclusions have been stated concerning the maximal number of lesions that is reasonable to treat. A negative influence on survival of larger number of metastases have been found in multivariate analysis (Sneed, 2002; Gudy, 2006; Mathiew, 2007; Golden, 2008; Abacioglu, 2010; Liew, 2011) and in univariate ones (Vesagas, 2002; Wowra, 2002; Radbill, 2004; Nam, 2005; Serizawa, 2005; Gerosa, 2005; Feigl, 2006; Karlsson, 2009; Kondziolka, 2011; Matsunaga, 2011). Others investigators on the other hand have informed no influence of this factor on survival (Chidel, 2000; Petrivich, 2002; Hernández, 2002; Schoeggl, 2002; Hasegawa, 2003; Lorenzoni, 2004; Jawahar, 2004; Muacevic, 2004; Yu, 2005; Rades, 2007; Kased, 2009; Frazier, 2010; Skeie, 2011). When on observe the number of patients reported in the papers, it is possible to recognize that in average those manuscripts showing no influence of this variable on survival have less number of patients (put in evidence in the plot dealing with the number of patients). It seems that a higher number of brain metastases affect negatively the survival with "**reasonable agreement**".

With regard the number of brain metastases that is reasonable to treat, the higher level of evidence recommends to treat up four lesions, based in three prospective, randomized studies (Metha, 2005), nevertheless, these 3 studies included patients with a maximum of 3 or 4 lesions, then, patients with higher number of metastases were not studied.

Nam (Nam, 2005) compared a group of 84 patients with up to three brain metastases with 46 harboring 4 or more lesions. The survival of the second group (26 weeks) was significantly less than 48 weeks in the group with up to 3 metastases, Nevertheless when a multivariate analysis was done, only the RPA stratification system was the independent factor affecting survival. The author concluded that the Karnofsky performance status and the RPA stratification should be considered as the most important factors and multiplicity of the lesions alone should not be a reason for withholding Gamma Knife treatment.

Karlsson (Karlsson, 2009) in a multicentric retrospective study involving 1855 patients found no difference on survival among patients with single or multiple metastases when the the systemic status of the cancer was controlled. Moreover, there was no difference in overall survival comparing patients harboring 2 metastases, 3 to4 metastases, 5-8 metastases or ≥9 metastases.

Chang (Chang, 2010), in a series of 323 patients studied the influence on survival of the number of brain metastases. The survivals were not significantly different between patient with 1 to 5 lesions (10 months), 6 to 10 lesions (10 months), 11 to 15 lesions (13 months) and ≥15 lesions (8 months). The author concluded that Gamma Knife radiosurgery may be a good treatment option for local control of metastatic lesions and for improved survival in patients with multiple metastatic brain lesions, even those patients who harbor more than 15 brain metastases.

Serizawa (Serizawa, 2010) studied 778 patients with the following 6 inclusion criteria: newly diagnosed brain metastases, one to 10 lesions, up to 10cc of maximal volume of the larger metastasis, less than 15cc of total intracranial tumoral volume, No evidence on magnetic resonance of meningeal tumor dissemination and a KPS ≥70. There was no upfront use of whole brain irradiation. The overall survival was 8.6 months (0.72 years). There were not differences in survival between patients with single, two, 3 to 4, 5 to 6 and 7 to 10 brain metastases. The study conclusion was that the brain lesion number has no effect on survival.

Some concerns could exist in relation to the total integral dose received by the normal brain when numerous lesions are treated; Yamamoto (Yamamoto, 2002) studied the safety of this treatment situation in 80 patients with 10 or more brain lesion that underwent Gamma Knife treatment. The conclusion was that the cumulative whole brain irradiation was not exceeding the threshold level of normal brain necrosis.

With regard the number of brain metastases it seems that selecting patients with favorable Karnofsky performance status and having a controlled cancer, up to 10 or even up to 15 brain metastases could be reasonable treated, nevertheless, prospective randomized trials are desirable.

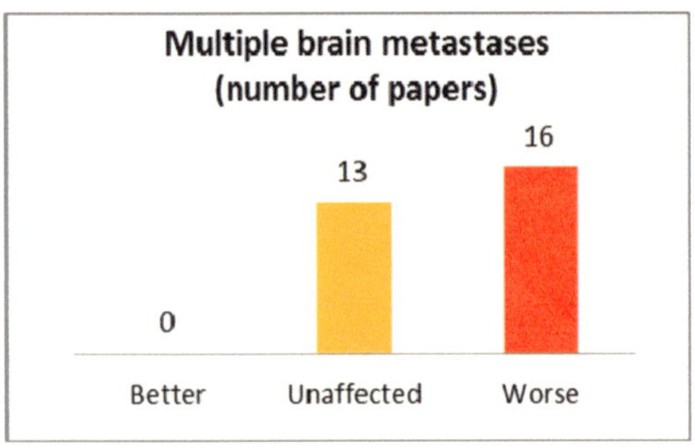

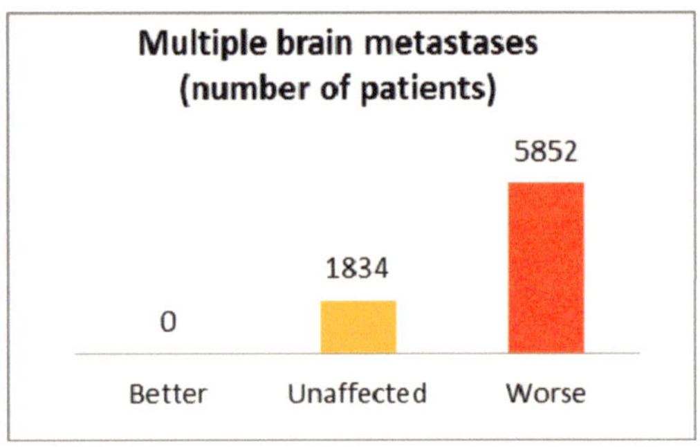

2.8 Older age

Most manuscripts show no influence of this factor on survival (Simonová, 2000; Petrovich, 2002; Hernández, 2002; Wowra, 2002; Schoeggl, 2002; Lorenzoni, 2004; Jawahar, 2004; Nam, 2005; Serizawa, 2005; Yu, 2005; Gerosa, 2005; Da Silva, 2009; Kondziolka, 2011; Matsunaga, 2011), nevertheless, when the number of patients enrolled in such studies is observed, bigger studies report a negative influence of an older age on survival in multivariate studies (Hasegawa, 2003; Pan, 2006; Gaudy, 2006; Rades, 2007; Golden 2008) as well as univariate ones (Sneed, 2002; Muacevic, 2004; Karlsson, 2009; Kased, 2009; Frazier, 2010; Liew, 2011). Older age influences negatively the survival with **"some agreement with a trend".**

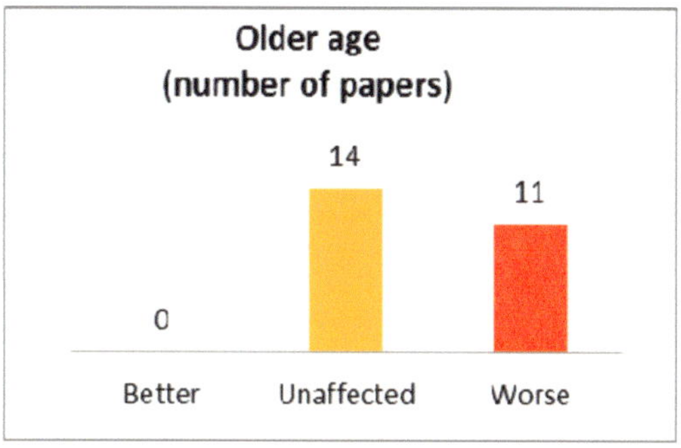

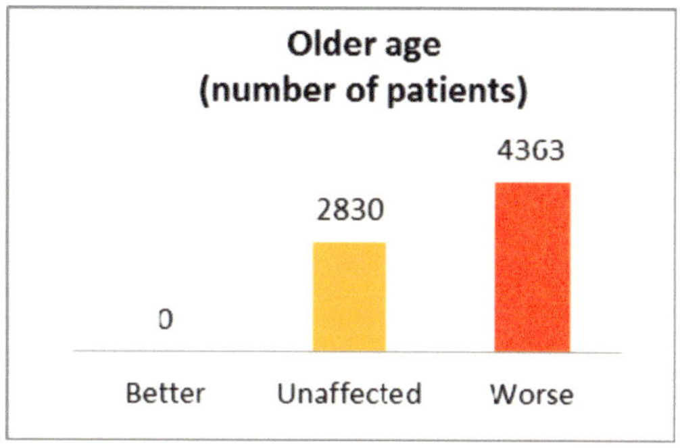

2.9 Female gender

Most studies have shown that gender is not a prognostic factor for survival (Wowra, 2002; Schoeggl, 2002; Hasegawa, 2003; Flannery, 2003; Lorenzoni, 2004; Jawahar, 2004; Nam, 2005; Rades, 2007; Mathiew, 2007; Frazier, 2010; Matsunaga, 2011), a few reports have shown positive influence of female gender on survival in multivariate analysis (Serizawa, 2005) and in univariate analysis (Amendola, 2002; Gaudy, 2006; Liew, 2011). It appears that gender do not affect survival with **"Some agreement with a trend".**

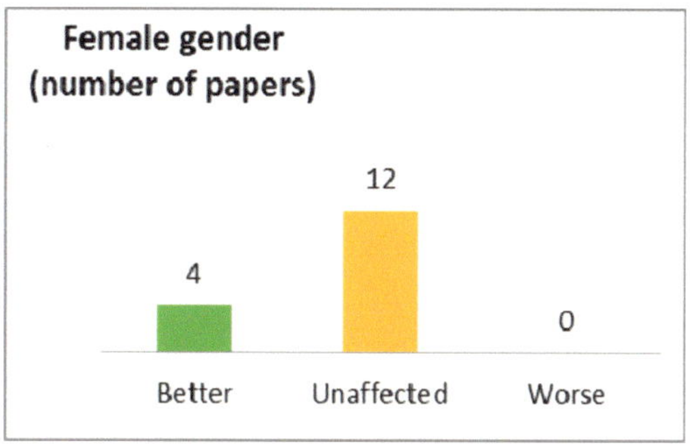

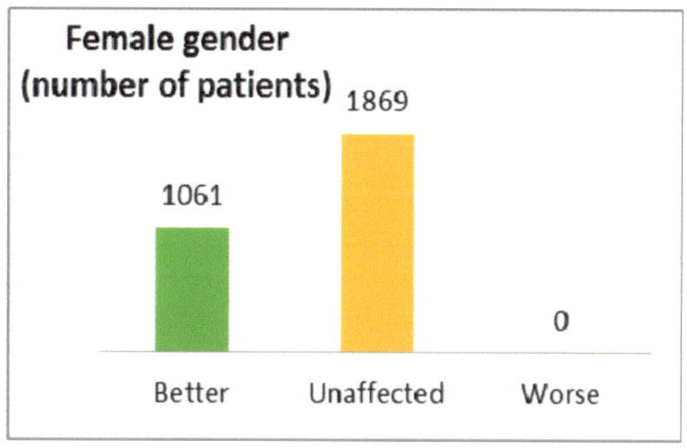

2.10 Location or histology of the primary tumor

No influence on survival of the primary tumor have been reported (Lorenzoni, 2004; Nam, 2005; Rades, 2007; Frazier, 2010), on the other hand other studies have demonstrated significant association of this variable with survival: Hasegawa (Hasegawa, 2003), in the multivariate analysis found significant lower survival in patients harboring malignant melanoma. In multivariate studies Simonová (Simonová, 2000) reported better survival in patients with breast or renal cancer, Petrovich (Petrovich, 2002) found worse survival in patients with Melanoma and colon cancer and better survival in patients with breast cancer. Vesagas (Vesagas, 2002) communicated better survival in patients with breast carcinoma. **"Scarce information with a trend"** could suggest that primary melanoma or colon cancer could be a negative prognosric factors for survival, and breast could be a positive prognostic factor.

2.11 Location of the brain metastases

Kondziolka (Kondziolka, 2011) in a series of 350 patients with breast cancer found a negative influence on survival of the brainstem location in multivariate analysis and a deep brain location of lesions in the univariate study. Gaudy-Marqueste (Gaudy-Marqueste, 2006) found worse survival in a multivariate study in patients harboring deep location of the lesions in a series of 106 patients with melanoma brain metastases. Others authors (Mathiew, 2007, Liew, 2011) have found in multivariate analysis that cerebellar tumor location was associated to poorer survival. Regarding tumor location, **"scarce information with a trend"** suggests that brainstem location, deep brain location and cerebellar location of a melanoma metastasis could be negative prognostic factors.

2.12 Latency period to brain metastases diagnose

The time elapsed between the diagnosis of the cancer and the moment of the apparition of brain metastases has been propose as a prognostic factor, two studies have shown this association on multivariate analysis (Flanery, 2003; Rades, 2007) and 3 studied on univariate analysis (Yu, 2005; Kased, 2009; Liew, 2011). Seven investigators did not found this influence (Wowra, 2002; Schoeggl, 2002; Muacevic, 2004; Serizawa, 2005; mathiew, 2007; Kondziolka, 2011; Matsunaga, 2011). **"some agreement with a trend"** could suggest that a longer latency period could be associated with longer survival.

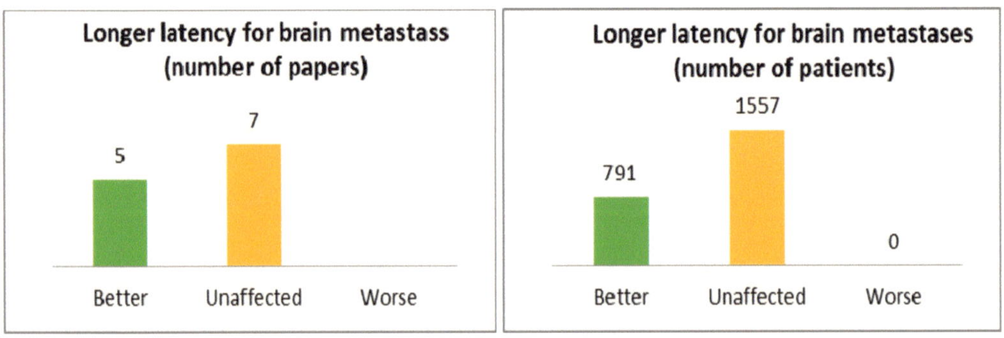

2.13 HER2/neu receptors (breast)

The two publications revised (Kassed, 2009; Kondziolka, 2011) have shown on multivariate analysis a positive association of the existence of the HER2/neu receptors with a favorable survival. In spite of the strong association, it was considered that **"scarce information with a trend"** support this finding.

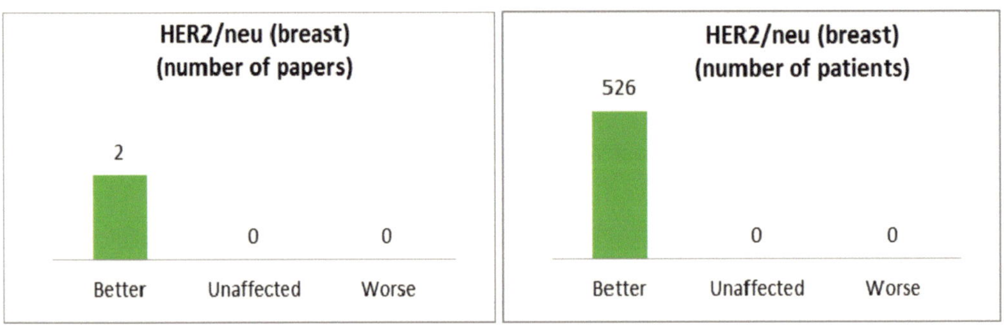

2.14 Estrogen receptors (breast)

Among two publications revised, one found positive influence of the existence of estrogen receptors on survival (Kassed, 2009). Kondziolka (Kondziolka, 2011) on the other hand, report no influence of this variable on survival. **"Scarce information with a trend"** could suggest that the presence of estrogen receptors could be associates with a longer survival.

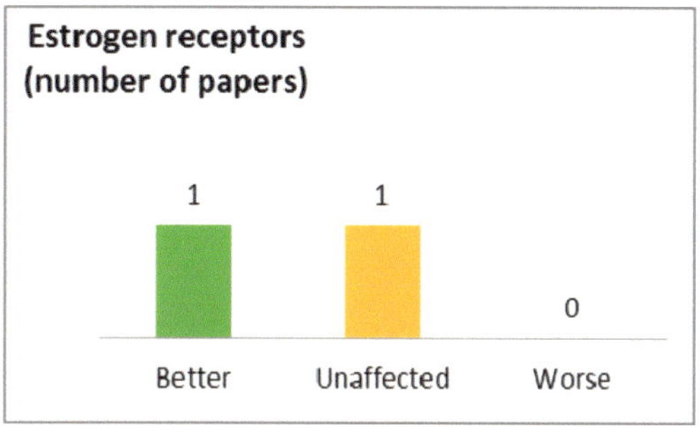

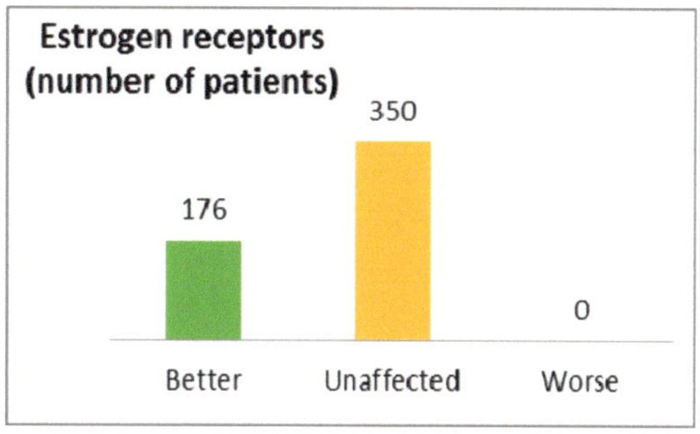

2.15 Whole brain radiotherapy

This was the only prognostic factor in the present study where after the analysis of many manuscripts absolute **"consistent agreement"** exists. All the articles revised report no benefit in terms of survival when whole brain radiotherapy is added to Gamma Knife radiosurgery (Chidel, 2000; Sneed, 2002; Petrovich, 2002; Jawahar, 2002; Vesagas, 2002; Schoeggl, 2002; Flannery, 2003; Lorenzoni, 2004; Muacevic, 2004; Nam, 2005; Gerosa, 2005; Pan, 2005; Mathiew, 2007; Da Silva, 2009; Frazier, 2010, Abacioglu, 2010; Liew, 2011; Skeie, 2011).

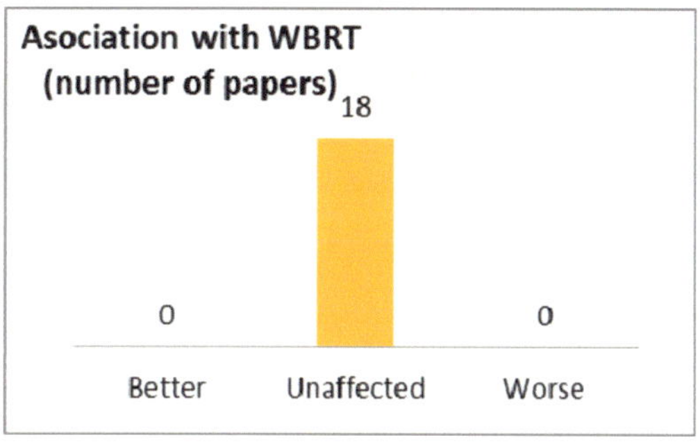

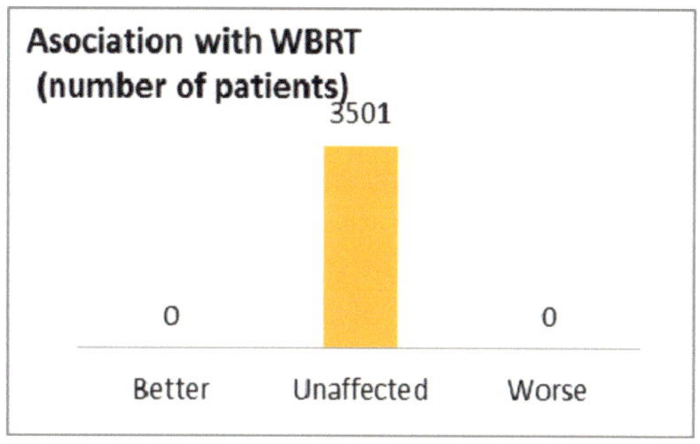

3. Stratification systems used in radiosurgery

The combination and integration of some of the strongest prognostic factors allow creating score systems or stratification systems as tools for patient survival estimation. Many of these have been proposed and all of them have shown to be reliable:

3.1 Recursive Partitioning Analysis (RPA)

This system is the most used and widely known. It was proposed initially for patients treated with whole brain radiotherapy (Gaspar, 1997; Gaspar, 2000) and subsequently tested and used for radiosurgery (Sanghavi, 2001; Lorenzoni, 2004; Nieder, 2009). It considers Karnofsky, age, the control of the primary tumor and the existence of extracranial metastases (table 1).

In the study of Sanghavi (Sanghavi, 2001) the median survival for patients in cathegories I, II and III were 16.1, 10.3 and 8.7 months respectively. Subsequently, in the study of Lorenzoni (Lorenzoni 2004) the survival were 27.6, 10.7 and 2.8 months for classes I, II and III respectively. This score system has not good specificity for detecting patients with short survival. In the study of Lorenzoni (Lorenzoni, 2004) the maximal survival reached by patients in the poorer category (RPA III) was 11 months. The advantage of RPA is to be a reliable and easy system. As a disadvantage it could be considered the heterogeneity of the category II and as it was mentioned before it´s relative reduced capacity for detecting patients with very short survival.

RPA I:	Karnofsky ≥ 70 Age less than 65 years Primary tumor controlled No extracranial metastases
RPA II:	Karnofsky ≥ 70 Do not fulfill criteria for RPA I
RPA III:	Karnofsky < 70

Table 1. RPA.

3.2 Score Index for Rradiosurgery in brain metastases (SIR)

The "Score index for radiosurgery in brain metastases" (SIR) was described by Weltman (Weltman, 2000; Weltman, 2001) and validated afterwards (Lorenzoni, 2004). It uses five prognostic factors: Age, Karnofsky, systemic disease status, the size and the number of lesions (table 2).

In the article of Weltman (Weltman, 2000), the survivals for patients with scores 8-10, 4-7 and 1-3 were 31.4, 7 and 2.9 months respectively. In the study of Lorenzoni (Lorenzoni, 2004), the survivals were 27.7, 10.8, 4.6 and 2.4 for patients with scores 8-10, 5-7, 4 and 1-3 respectively. In the study of Lorenzoni SIR was the best system according to statistic significance. This score system represents quite a good specificity for detecting patients with short survival; in the study of Lorenzoni (Lorenzoni, 2004) the maximal survival reached by patients in the poorer category was 7 months. SIR has a more complex format what could be considered a relative disadvantage.

Variable	0	1	2
Age	≥60	51-59	≤50
Karnofsky	≥50	60-70	≥80
Systemic disease status	PD	PR-SD	CR-NED
Large lesión volume (cc)	>13	5-13	<5
Number of lesions	≥3	2	1
		(Range: 0 to 10 points)	

PD: progressive disease, PR: partial remission, SD: stable disease, CR: complete remission, NED: no evidence of disease.

Table 2. SIR.

3.3 Basic Score for Brain Metastases (BSBM)

The Basic score for brain metastases was described by Lorenzoni (Lorenzoni, 2004; Lorenzoni, 2009). It was conceived as an attempt to develop a score system with a good balance between reliability and simplicity. It takes into account the three most powerful prognostic factors for survival (karnofsky, Control of the primary tumor and the existence of extracranial metastases), assigning on point for each factor (Table 3). Additionally, when associations of variables were analyzed in the original study (Lorenzoni, 2004), an "intrinsic" representation of other two linked variables (number of lesions and size of lesions) was demonstrated: 1- The number of lesions is represented by the existence of extracranial metastases (60% of patients with 3 or more brain metastases had extracranial metastases versus just 36% of patients with one or two brain metastases, p=0.04) and 2- The maximal size of lesions is represented by the Karnofsky (50% of patients with a brain metastasis volume ≥ 9 cc had an unfavorable Karnofsky index versus just 16% of patients with a maximal volume less than 9cc, p=0.01). This system does not take into account the patient age.

In the original manuscript of Lorenzoni (Lorenzoni, 2004), the survival was undefined (more than 50% of patients alive at 32 months) in patients with scores 3, 13.1 months for score 2, 3.3 months for score 1 and 1.9 months for score 0. This score system presented the best specificity for detecting patients with short survival: the maximal survival reached by any patient in the poorer category (score 0) was only 4 months. The main advantages of BSBM is it extreme simplicity and as it was mentioned, the high capacity for detecting patients with a very poor life expectancy.

Karnofsky ≥ 80	1 point
Primary tumor controlled	1 point
No extracranial metastases	1 point
	(Range: 0 to 3 points)

Table 3. BSBM.

3.4 Others score systems for radiosurgery

Some other authors have proposed systems such as GGS (Golden, 2008), and a Melanoma-specific system, MM.GKR (Gaudy-Marqueste, 2006).

4. Stratification systems tested with whole brain radiotherapy databases

Some systems have been developed recently based on databases of patients treated with fractionated whole brain irradiation but not jet tested for stereotactic radiosurgery. The graded prognostic assessment index (GPA) and some primary tumor-specific scores are the most common. All of these systems could be useful for patients treated with radiosurgery but its efficiency must be proved. Some differences could be found with regard to statistical testing, in fact, the survival of patients treated with radiosurgery could be twice compared with the survival of patients treated with whole brain radiotherapy (Sanghavi, 2001).

4.1 Graded Prognostic Assessment Index (GPA)

Proposed by Sperduto (Sperduto, 2008) using the RTOG database of 1960 patients treated with whole brain radiotherapy from five randomized prospective trials. It considers four prognostic factors: Age, Karnofsky, number of lesions and the existence of extracranial metastases (figure 4). GPA has also a more complex format that could be considered a relative disadvantage.

In the original article of Sperduto (Sperduto, 2008), in addition to the description of the GPA, the author performed a study using also others pre-existing score systems (RPA, SIR and BSBM). According to RPA, the survivals reported were 7.7, 4.5 and 2.3 months for patients in the categories I, II and III respectively.

Using SIR, the survivals were 8.8, 6 and 2.1 months for the scores 8-10, 4-7 and 1-3 respectively. With regard BSBM, the survivals were 7, 5.1, 3.4 and 2.2 months for scores 3, 2, 1, and 0 respectively.

In the GPA proposed the survivals were 11, 6.9, 3.8 and 2.6 months for patients with scores 3.5-4, 3, 1.5-2.5 and 0-1.

Nieder (Nieder, 2008) tested this score in 232 patients treated with whole brain radiotherapy. According to RPA, the survivals reported were 10.8, 3.2 and 2 months for patients in the categories I, II and III respectively. Using SIR, the survivals were 8.7, 4.1 and 1.7 months for the scores 8-10, 4-7 and 1-3 respectively. With regard BSBM, the survivals were 11.5, 3.9, 2.4 and 1.9 months for scores 3, 2, 1, and 0 respectively. In the GPA proposed the survivals were 10.3, 5.6, 3.5 and 1.9 months for patients with scores 3.5-4, 3, 1.5-2.5 and 0-1.

Concerning the capacity for detecting patients with the poorer survival, the most efficient system was the "basic score for brain metastases" (BSBM) (Nieder, 2010; Villà, 2011).

Variable	0	0.5	1
Age	≥60	51-59	≤50
Karnofsky	<70	70-80	90-100
Number of lesions	>3	2-3	1
Extracranial metastases	yes	-	No
		(Range: 0 to 4 points)	

Table 4. GPA.

4.2 Others primary tumor-specific score systems tested for whole brain radiotherapy

Other authors have proposed primary-specific systems, such as Breast cancer-specific score (Nieder, 2009), Breast-GPA (Sperduto, 2011), and Melanoma-GPA (Sperduto, 2010) among others.

5. Conclusions

Gamma Knife radiosurgery is a highly effective method for controlling brain metastases and it can be useful and safely offered to those patients that fulfill the following conditions:

1. Karnofsky performance status ≥ 70,
2. Tumors with a maximum diameter of 3 centimeters or a maximum volume of 13 cubic centimeters.
3. No significant mass effect and absence of intracranial hypertension.
4. No evidence of leptomeningeal dissemination.
5. Up to 10 to 15 brain lesions (more recent observational non randomized studies) or up to 4 brain lesions (prospective randomized trials).
6. Up to 15 cubic centimeters of total tumor mass.
7. Systemic cancer diseases well controlled (desirable but not excluding condition).

Many prognostic factors for survival have been identified, among them, Karnofsky performance status (KPS) have been considered the most powerful followed by the status of the cancer disease (overall systemic cancer status or a separate analysis of the control of the primary site and the existence of extracranial metastases).

The integration of many prognostic factors has originated score systems for survival estimation, all of these scores are reliable, and the election of one of them should be according with the best compromise with reliability and simplicity. Some scores must be proved for radiosurgery and probably in the future new or improved specific scores will be available and tested for stereotactic radiosurgery.

6. References

[1] Abacioglu, U., H. Caglar, et al. (2010). "Gamma knife radiosurgery in non small cell lung cancer patients with brain metastases: treatment results and prognostic factors." J BUON 15(2): 274-280.
[2] Amendola, B. E., A. Wolf, et al. (2002). "Radiosurgery as palliation for brain metastases: a retrospective review of 72 patients harboring multiple lesions at presentation." J Neurosurg 97(5 Suppl): 511 514.
[3] Chang, W. S., H. Y. Kim, et al. (2010). "Analysis of radiosurgical results in patients with brain metastases according to the number of brain lesions: is stereotactic radiosurgery effective for multiple brain metastases?" J Neurosurg 113 Suppl: 73-78.
[4] Chidel M, Suh J, Reddy C, Chao S, Lundbeck M, Barnett G (2000). "Application of recursive partitioning analysis and evaluation of the use of whole brain irradiation among patients treated with stereotactic radiosurgery for newly diagnosed brain metastases." Int J Radiat Oncol Phys 47: 993-9.
[5] Da Silva, A. N., K. Nagayama, et al. (2009). "Gamma Knife surgery for brain metastases from gastrointestinal cancer." J Neurosurg 111(3): 423-430.
[6] Feigl, G. C. and G. A. Horstmann (2006). "Volumetric follow up of brain metastases: a useful method to evaluate treatment outcome and predict survival after Gamma Knife surgery?" J Neurosurg 105 Suppl: 91-98.
[7] Flannery, T. W., M. Suntharalingam, et al. (2003). "Gamma knife stereotactic radiosurgery for synchronous versus metachronous solitary brain metastases from non-small cell lung cancer." Lung Cancer 42(3): 327-333.
[8] Frazier, J. L., S. Batra, et al. (2010). "Stereotactic radiosurgery in the management of brain metastases: an institutional retrospective analysis of survival." Int J Radiat Oncol Biol Phys 76(5): 1486-1492.

[9] Gaspar L, Scott Ch, Rotman M et al. (1997). "Recursive partitioning analysis (RPA) of prognostic factors in three radiation therapy oncology group (RTOG). " Int J Radiat Oncol Biol Phys 37: 745-751.

[10] Gaspar L, Scott Ch, Murray K et al. (2000). "Validation of the RTOG recursive partitioning analysis (RPA) classification for brain metastases." " Int J Radiat Oncol Biol Phys 47: 1oo1-1006".

[11] Gaudy-Marqueste, C., J. M. Regis, et al. (2006). "Gamma-Knife radiosurgery in the management of melanoma patients with brain metastases: a series of 106 patients without whole-brain radiotherapy." Int J Radiat Oncol Biol Phys 65(3): 809-816.

[12] Gerosa, M., A. Nicolato, et al. (2005). "Analysis of long-term outcomes and prognostic factors in patients with non-small cell lung cancer brain metastases treated by gamma knife radiosurgery." J Neurosurg 102 Suppl: 75-80.

[13] Golden, D. W., K. R. Lamborn, et al. (2008). "Prognostic factors and grading systems for overall survival in patients treated with radiosurgery for brain metastases: variation by primary site." J Neurosurg 109 Suppl: 77-86.

[14] Hasegawa, T., D. Kondziolka, et al. (2003). "Brain metastases treated with radiosurgery alone: an alternative to whole brain radiotherapy?" Neurosurgery 52(6): 1318-1326; discussion 1326.

[15] Hernandez, L., L. Zamorano, et al. (2002). "Gamma knife radiosurgery for renal cell carcinoma brain metastases." J Neurosurg 97(5 Suppl): 489-493.

[16] Jawahar, A., F. Ampil, et al. (2004). "Management strategies for patients with brain metastases: has radiosurgery made a difference?" South Med J 97(3): 254-258.

[17] Karlsson, B., P. Hanssens, et al. (2009). "Thirty years' experience with Gamma Knife surgery for metastases to the brain." J Neurosurg 111(3): 449-457.

[18] Kased, N., D. K. Binder, et al. (2009). "Gamma Knife radiosurgery for brain metastases from primary breast cancer." Int J Radiat Oncol Biol Phys 75(4): 1132-1140.

[19] Kondziolka, D., H. Kano, et al. (2011). "Stereotactic radiosurgery as primary and salvage treatment for brain metastases from breast cancer. Clinical article." J Neurosurg 114(3): 792-800.

[20] Liew, D. N., H. Kano, et al. (2011). "Outcome predictors of Gamma Knife surgery for melanoma brain metastases. Clinical article." J Neurosurg 114(3): 769-779.

[21] Lorenzoni, J., D. Devriendt, et al. (2004). "Radiosurgery for treatment of brain metastases: estimation of patient eligibility using three stratification systems." Int J Radiat Oncol Biol Phys 60(1): 218-224.

[22] Lorenzoni, J. G., D. Devriendt, et al. (2009). "Brain stem metastases treated with radiosurgery: prognostic factors of survival and life expectancy estimation." Surg Neurol 71(2): 188-195; discussion 195, 195-186.

[23] Mathieu, D., D. Kondziolka, et al. (2007). "Gamma knife radiosurgery in the management of malignant melanoma brain metastases." Neurosurgery 60(3): 471-481; discussion 481-472.

[24] Matsunaga, S., T. Shuto, et al. (2011). "Gamma Knife surgery for brain metastases from colorectal cancer. Clinical article." J Neurosurg 114(3): 782-789.

[25] Mehta M, Tsao M, Whelan T et al. (2005). "The American society for therapeutic radiology and oncology (ASTRO) evidence-based review of the role of radiosurgery for brain metastases." Int J Radiat Oncol Biol Phys 63: 37-46.

[26] Muacevic, A., F. W. Kreth, et al. (2004). "Stereotactic radiosurgery for multiple brain metastases from breast carcinoma." Cancer 100(8): 1705-1711.

[27] Nam, T. K., J. I. Lee, et al. (2005). "Gamma knife surgery for brain metastases in patients harboring four or more lesions: survival and prognostic factors." J Neurosurg 102 Suppl: 147-150.

[28] Nieder C, Marienhagen k, Geinitz H et al. (2008). "Validation of the graded prognostic assessment index for patients with brain metastases". "Acta oncologica 1-4, first article.

[29] Nieder C, Marienhagen k, Astner S et al. (2009). "Prognostic scores in brain metastasesfrom breast cancer". BMC cancer 9: 105.

[30] Nieder C, Pawinsky A, Molls M. (2010). "Prediction of short survival in patients with brain metastases based on three different scores: a role for 'triple-negative' status?". Clin Oncol (R Coll Radiol).22(1):65-9.

[31] Pan, H. C., J. Sheehan, et al. (2005). "Gamma knife surgery for brain metastases from lung cancer." J Neurosurg 102 Suppl: 128-133.

[32] Petrovich Z, Yu C, Giannotta S, ODay S, Apuzzo M. (2002). "Survival and pattern of failure in brain metastases treated with stereotactic Gamma Knife radiosurgery." J Neurosurg 97 (5 Suppl): 499-506.

[33] Radbill, A. E., J. F. Fiveash, et al. (2004). "Initial treatment of melanoma brain metastases using gamma knife radiosurgery: an evaluation of efficacy and toxicity." Cancer 101(4): 825-833.

[34] Rades, D., G. Bohlen, et al. (2007). "Stereotactic radiosurgery alone versus resection plus whole-brain radiotherapy for 1 or 2 brain metastases in recursive partitioning analysis class 1 and 2 patients." Cancer 109(12): 2515-2521.

[35] Sanghavi S, Saranarendra S, Miranpuri B et al. (2001). "Radiosurgery for patients with brain metastases: a multi-institutional analysis stratified by the RTOG recursive partitioning analysis method." " Int J Radiat Oncol Biol Phys 51: 426-434.

[36] Schoeggl, A., K. Kitz, et al. (2002). "Stereotactic radiosurgery for brain metastases from colorectal cancer." Int J Colorectal Dis 17(3): 150-155.

[37] Serizawa, T., N. Saeki, et al. (2005). "Gamma knife surgery for brain metastases: indications for and limitations of a local treatment protocol." Acta Neurochir (Wien) 147(7): 721-726; discussion 726.

[38] Simonová G, Liscak R, Novotny J Jr, Novotny J. (2000). " Solitary brain metastases treated with the Leksell Gamma Knife: prognostic factors for patients.

[39] Skeie, B. S., G. O. Skeie, et al. (2011). "Gamma knife surgery in brain melanomas: absence of extracranial metastases and tumor volume strongest indicators of prolonged survival." World Neurosurg 75(5-6): 684-691.

[40] Serizawa T, Hirai T, Nagano O, Higuchi Y, Matsuda S, Ono J, Saeki N (2010). "Gamma Knife surgery for 1-10 brain metastases without prophylactic whole-brain radiation therapy: analysis of casesmeeteng the Japanese prospective multi-institute study (JLGK0901) inclusion criteria." J neurooncol 98: 163-7.

[41] Sneed, P. K., J. H. Suh, et al. (2002). "A multi-institutional review of radiosurgery alone vs. radiosurgery with whole brain radiotherapy as the initial management of brain metastases." Int J Radiat Oncol Biol Phys 53(3): 519-526.

[42] Sperduto P, Berkey B, Gaspar L et al. (2008). "A new prognostic index and comparison to three other indices for patients with brain metastases: an analysis of 1960 patients in the RTOG database". " Int J Radiat Oncol Biol Phys 70: 510-514".
[43] Sperduto P, Kased N, Xu R et al. (2011). "Effect of Tumor Subtype on Survival and the Graded Prognostic Assessment for Patients With Breast Cancer and Brain Metastases". Int J Radiat Oncol Biol Phys April 14, (epub ahead of print).
[44] Vesagas, T. S., J. A. Aguilar, et al. (2002). "Gamma knife radiosurgery and brain metastases: local control, survival, and quality of life." J Neurosurg 97(5 Suppl): 507-510.
[45] Villà S, Weber DC, Moretones C, Mañes A et al. (2011). "Validation of the new Graded Prognostic Assessment scale for brain metastases: a multicenter prospective study." Radiat Oncol. Mar 2; 6:23.
[46] Weltman E, Salvajoli J, Brandt R et al. (2000). "Radiosurgery for brain metastases: a score index for predicting prognosis." " Int J Radiat Oncol Biol Phys 46: 1155-1161".
[47] Weltman E, Salvajoli J, Brandt R et al. (2001) "Radiosurgery for brain metastases: Who may not benefit?." " Int J Radiat Oncol Biol Phys 51: 1320-1327".
[48] Wowra, B., M. Siebels, et al. (2002). "Repeated gamma knife surgery for multiple brain metastases from renal cell carcinoma." J Neurosurg 97(4): 785-793.
[49] Yamamoto, M., M. Ide, et al. (2002). "Gamma Knife radiosurgery for numerous brain metastases: is this a safe treatment?" Int J Radiat Oncol Biol Phys 53(5): 1279-1283.
[50] Yu, C. P., J. Y. Cheung, et al. (2005). "Prolonged survival in a subgroup of patients with brain metastases treated by gamma knife surgery." J Neurosurg 102 Suppl: 262-265.

3

Radiosurgical Treatment of Intracranial Meningiomas: Update 2011.

M. Gerosa et al.*
Multidisciplinary Neuro-Oncologic Group of Verona,
Department of Neurosurgery,
University Hospital (AOUI) of Verona, Verona,
Italy

1. Introduction

Meningiomas account for 16%-25% of all intracranial tumors, and quite often they rank amongst the most frequent neuro-oncological diagnostic subgroups in European or American registries (4, 5, 8, 54) As regards their natural history, (23, 29, 46, 55, 56, 59, 61) the few reported series of conservatively managed symptomatic meningiomas–bearing adequate FU- have documented a consistent progression in approximately one-third of patients, although in a wide spectrum of variability (TABLE 1).

The average annual incidence is 5-6 new cases per 100,000 (F/M ratio roughly 3:1) and it is lower in pediatrics, even though younger patients may show quite malignant oncotypes (4, 5, 8, 24, 43, 46, 59, 61, 64, 71, 73, 81). However, younger patients may show quite aggressive oncotypes (64, 71, 73). Growing human, sanitary and social costs are more pronounced in females because of the quoted demographic data.

At uni-multivariate analysis, the main factors putatively associated with more- or-less pronounced aggressiveness seem to be represented by younger age and T2-hyperintensity, or by presence of calcifications, respectively (TABLE 1). As expected, grade 2 and 3 meningiomas entail a more severe prognosis (30, 39, 40, 48, 51, 56, 62), thereby justifying the advocated multidisciplinary treatments in such instances (30, 54 62, 84,85).

* R. Foroni[1], M. Longhi[1], A. De Simone[1], F. Alessandrini[2], P. Meneghelli[1], B. Bonetti[3], C. Ghimenton[4], T. Sava[5], S. Dall'Oglio[6], A. Talacchi[1], C. Cavedon[7], F. Sala[1], R. Damante[1], F. Pioli[6], S. Maluta[6] and A. Nicolato[1]
[1]*Department of Neurosurgery,*
[2]*Department of Neuroradiology,*
[3]*Department of Neurology,*
[4]*Department of Neuropathology,*
[5]*Department of Medical Oncology,*
[6]*Department of Radiation Oncology,*
[7]*Department of Medical Physics,*
Multidisciplinary Neuro-Oncologic Group of Verona, University Hospital (AOUI) of Verona, Verona, Italy

2. Treatment options

Surgery still represents the mainstay in the specific neurosurgical armamentarium. Indeed, whenever feasible, a Simpson grade 1 resection of the tumor should be considered the golden therapeutic standard, reducing immediately any mass effect, and alleviating clinical signs and symptoms (2, 10, 11, 33, 41, 45, 52- 54 , 75, 80).

Author (year) (Reference)	No. of patients	Mean follow-up (mo)	No. (%) showing growth	Average growth rate	Factors commonly associated with an aggressive cell kinetic	Factors commonly observed in resting tumors
Olivero et al. (1995) (61)	45	32	10 (22.2)	2.4 mm/year		
Go et al. (1998) (23)]	35	74	4 (11.4)	3.2 mm/year		Calcification
Kuratsu et al. (2000) (43)	63	27.8	20 (31.7)		T2 hyperintensity	Calcification
Niiro et al. (2000) (59)	40	41.8	14 (35)		Larger size, T2 hyperintensity, male sex	Calcification
Yoneoka et al. (2000) (81)	37	50.4	9 (24.3)	1.36 cm3/year	Younger age, larger tumors	
Nakamura et al. (2003) (55)	41	43	14 (34)	0.796 cm3/year	Younger age, T2 hyperintensity	Calcification
Herscovici et al. (2004) (29)	43	67	16 (37)	4 mm/year	Younger age, sphenoid ridge	Calcification, smaller tumors
Yano and Karatsu (2006) (80)	67	>60	25 (37.3)	1.9 mm/year	T2 hyperintensity	Calcification

Table 1. Natural history of meningiomas. Reported growth rates in conservatively treated series.

In facts, local recurrence rates at 10 year-follow up are **directly related** to Simpson's grade of radicality, with 10-33% after complete resection (Simpson 1-2), and 55-75% after partial-to-minimal removal (i.e. Simpson 3-6) (33, 45, 48, 52, 53, 75, 80). This seems particularly true in the vast majority of convexity meningiomas, whereas results are less warranted in critical locations, like in skull base tumors.

Indeed, despite surgical advances, whenever these tumors are infiltrating the skull base, cranial nerves, or vascular structures, complete resection may not be feasible without unacceptable morbidity and sometimes mortality rates. Considering some of the largest published series, gross total removal of basal meningiomas sounds achievable in 60%-87.5% of the patients with 30%-56% of severe complications - particularly frequent in grade 2-3 histotypes - and a median postoperative mortality rate of 3.6 % (0%-9%) (11, 12, 45, 48, 75, 76, 79, 80). The main factors conditioning the extent of removal in skull base locations have been extensively analyzed in the literature, thereby creating the "resectability grading" where the final score represents the sum of each of the most relevant limiting factors: from cranial nerve involvement to vessel encasement, from extrafossa invasion to previous radiation treatments (45, 63, 74, 78, 82, 86).

Three large single-institution series with 10 to 15 years' follow-up, documenting rates of recurrence following GTR alone

		Local Recurrence Rate (%)		
Authors & Year	No. of Patients	5-yr	10-yr	15-yr
Mirimanoff et al., 1985	145	7	20	32
Condra et al., 1997	175	7	20	24
Stafford et al., 1998	465	12	25	—

Table 2a. (53, 10, 77)

Four single-institution series with 10- to 20-year follow-up, assessing rates of recurrence following STR alone

		Local Progression Rate (%)			
Authors & Year	No. of Patients	5-yr	10-yr	15-yr	20-yr
Wara et al., 1975	58	47	62	—	74
Mirimanoff et al., 1985	80	37	55	91	—
Condra et al., 1997	55	47	60	70	—
Stafford et al., 1998	116	39	61	—	—

Table 2b. (83, 53, 10, 77)

Table 2. Meningiomas: analysis of recurrence rate after gross total removal (GTR: TABLE 2a) compared to subtotal removal (STR: TABLE 2b)

The observed wide spectrum of recurrence rates (from 0 to 17%), is seemingly linked not only to the pre-existing W.H.O.'s and Simpson's grade, but also to the duration of follow up periods, although the latter is an often disregarded/underestimated parameter in the literature (10, 53, 69, 70, 75, 76, 79).

The non negligible problems with surgical radicality in crucial sites, may be further complicated by the presence of „aggressive" cytotypes, most often responsible for early recurrences shortening patients' survival (TABLE 2&3).

Author (ref)	Period	N.Pts	Mal. Definition	Survival
Harris (27)	1987-2001	12	WHO 2000	59% 5yr
				0% 10 yr
Perry (64-65)	1970-1997	27	Frank anaplasia	32% 5yr
Hug (30)	1973-1995	16	WHO 1993	51% 5yr
Palma (62)	1951-1986	29	WHO 1993	64% 5yr
				35% 10 yr
Ware (84)	1988-2002	17	WHO 1993	59% 5 yr
				15% 10 yr
Ojemann (60)	1991-1999	22	WHO 1993	40% 5 yr
Goldsmith (24)	1967-1990	23	Unique grading scheme	58% 5 yr.

Table 3. Recently published series of malignant meningiomas: 5- 10 yr survival.

Finally, also the tackling issues of meningiomatosis, contribute to explain the special momentum of combined, multidisciplinary approaches including Gamma Knife Radio Surgery (GKR).

3. Gamma knife radiosurgery

The fundamental reasons for the growing role of this technique, particularly in highly critical intracranial meningiomas, may be briefly summarized as follows:

1. fine tuning of the dosimetry planning. With the advent of hardware and software stereotactic sophistication, the process of 3D recognition of the tumor - as well as to spare the adjacent critical structures has gradually become more and more refined. A major role to this regard has been played by image co-registration, morpho-functional integration (functional MRI / spectroscopy, specific metabolic PET scan mapping etc.) on one side, and by the use of "hybrid shots" with the new "Perfexion" whenever dealing with crucial targeting (7, 36, 50, 57, 58, 66).
2. the introduction of dedicated algorhitms accurately "driving" the dose planning system, with probabilistic models including stockastic monitoring, quadrature-sum analysis (20) and linear-quadratic formalisms (32). These techniques, and the concomitant diffusion of phantom studies, have repeatedly confirmed the reliability of such referrals, consistently improving the main conformity indexes. To date, the recommended "surface- or "peripheral "doses" for meningiomas range from 11 - to - 15 Gy (16, 36, 37, 41, 47, 49, 54, 72).

The "ideal" - i.e. the most biologically justified - targeting dose- volume in these peculiar lesions, is still a matter of debate, with a spectrum of options: from including "only" the gross, T1 contrast enhancing tumor, plus a supposedly infiltrated margin of a few mm (39,40,50), up to the controversial inclusion either of the "dural tail", or of the hyperostotic bone. However, the former - according to extremely refined studies - has been shown to be essentially composed by hypervascular dura with surprisingly none of the expected tumor colonies (34). The latter - according to Pieper- should be almost constantly (25/26 cases) infiltrated, even in presence of negative imaging (67). In these cases, ablative radiosurgery on the hyperostotic bone might have the same meaning of Simpson's grade 1 in surgical approaches (67).

3. a deeper radiobiological experience. Radiosurgery, like most radiation treatments, hitting the biological target, results in the formation of free radicals as electrons are freed from their atoms. Their main in vivo effect is closely related to a variety of local conditions: first of all the particular oncotype and its cellular peculiarities ("alpha-beta ratio" (35), superoxide-enzyme characterization, sister-chromatide exchange potential etc.) defining the radio-sensitivity; then the quality and quantity of radiation dosimetry, the targeted volume etc., up to the microscopic model of energy deposition. On the basis of these features, meningiomas mostly belong to relatively radiosensitive, "late responding tissues" (LRT) frequently exploiting local hypoxic shields (3, 13, 30, 49), particularly in the elderly (59).

As a consequence effective dosages are in the lower range, not far from normal cell radiosensitivity thresholds, whilst the time-interval for the effect is close to maximum in vivo doubling time (3, 7, 16, 31, 68, 69, 70, 71, 72).

- At present, over half a million people have been treated by GKR all over the world, at a continuously increasing annual rate (in 2010 roughly 50,000 patients), with intracranial meningiomas actually representing approximately one third of these patients.

It is generally accepted that the putative mechanism of action of SRS is intimately dependent not only upon the mentioned technical variables (dose-volume integral, timing, target cytology), but as well as upon the goal we are pursuing ("tumor growth control", necrotic evolution, "ephaptic block" etc.) (38, 39, 40). As regards meningiomas, routine protocols are focused on "Tumor Growth Control" (TGC) probably obtained through a combined mechanism: 1. Direct cytotoxicity, presumably promoting apoptosis; 2. Damage to the neoplastic vascular supply, mediated by inhibited growth factors (VEGF, EGF, Factor 8th etc.) 3. Inactivation/destruction of hormonal receptors (e.g. Octreotide- r) (57, 58). **Moreover, it should be stressed that meningiomas located in highly vascularized-oxygenated regions of the brain (cavernous sinus, sagittal sinus etc), due to still poorly known mechanisms (e.g. mutilation of the the superoxide dismutase chain etc.)** usually exibit a more pronounced radiosensitivity, with sometimes spectacular results (Fig. 1).

If we examine clinical and radiological results in the largest published series of intracranial meningiomas treated during the last decade with different radiosurgical techniques (TABLE 4), some qualifying tenets of these therapeutic approaches appear certainly significant and reliable.

A. The overall neuro-radiological results are rewarding and stable. Unfortunately, the available literature is of poor statistical quality, also because of the difficulties in performing prospective randomized, adequately stratified clinical trials. Therefore most comparative analyses are based on EBM Class III Data, with only a few studies presenting Class II informations. However, given the definition of "Local Tumor Control" as a post-treatment computerized target volume equal-to or smaller than the original, the 5yr actuarial Tumor Control Rates after GKRS range from 86.2% to 97.9%.

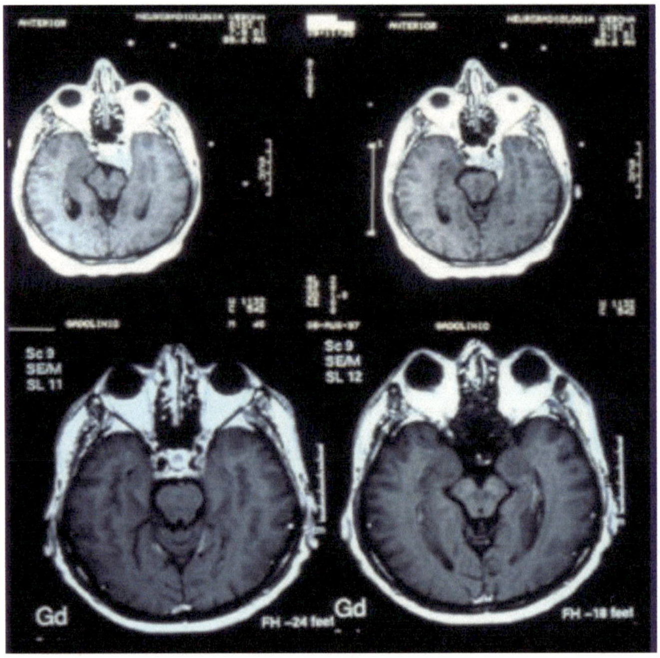

Fig. 1. Left cavernous sinus meningioma before (top) and two years after GKRS. Note the drastic shrinkage of the tumor, not unusual in these locations.

Furthermore, in GKR treated patients, primary or "imaging diagnosed" meningiomas share a significantly higher 5yr-PFS (87%-95%) than recurrences (34%-97%).

B. Clinical outcome usually matches these observations, also in our experience (122). Adopting the concept of clinical improvement as the resolution of neurological symptoms, and/or increased pre-operative performances, the vast majority of cases shows stable or improved KPS and neurological gradings at 5-7 years or longer FU. A recent review published by the Pittsburgh Gamma Knife Center (39, 40) confirms in a cohort of 972 patients, with a long term follow up (for some of them up to 20 years) an overall tumor control rate up to 97% a definitively low overall morbidity rate (7.7%) slightly higher for crucial locations such as the cavernous sinus and petroclival region.

As a rule, the cytological grading is the main determinant of the radiosurgical effectiveness. Malignant meningiomas maybe extremely aggressive (Fig. 2) - as mentioned above, with marked endovascular infiltration and neoangiogenesis, requiring multimodality management that include resection, fractionated radiation therapy, brachytherapy, and proton-photon therapy (84, 85, 86).

Similarly, patients with benign histotypes (gr. 1) are usually characterized by 5yr actuarial tumor control rates (87%-96%) much higher than those with atypic (49%-77%) or anaplastic (0%-19%) lesions (21, 24, 37, 49, 63, 73, 77). As shown in (TABLE 4), the still limited number of reports with a mean follow up period of 7-10 years have consistently confirmed these differential LTC levels (3, 15, 41, 63, 70)

Pubblication Year	Authors	Group	No. Pts.	SRS technique	LTC % (5 yr)
1994	Goldsmith et al (24)	San Francisco (USA)	140 (117 benign, 23 malignant)	Proton Beam	89 (ben), 48 (mal)
1998	Hakim et al (26)	Boston (USA)	127 (155 tumors, of which 106 benign)	LINAC	89.3 for the benign tumors
2001	Pendl et al [63]	Graz (Austria)	197 (198 tumors)	GK	98 (for 164 patients)
2001	Stafford et al [77]	Rochester (USA)	190 (206 tumors)	GK	93 for the benign, 68 for the atypical and 0 for the malignant tumors at 5 years
2002	Eustacchio et al[18]	Graz (Austria)	121	GK	98.3
2002	Nicolato et al [58]	Verona (Italy)	122	GK	96.5 at 5yr
2003	Chang et al[16]	Seoul (Korea)	179 (194 tumors)	GK	97.1
2003	Pollock et al [69-70]	Rochester (USA)	330 (356 tumors)	GK	94
2004	DiBiase et al [13]	Camden (USA)	137	GK	86.2 at 5 yr
2005	Friedman et al.[21]	Gainesville (USA)	210	LINAC	96 for benign, 77 for atypical and 19 for malignant tumors at 5 yr
2005	Kreil et al[41]	Graz (Austria)	200	GK	98.5 at 5yr
2005	Malik et al[49]	Sheffield (United Kingdom)	277 (309 tumors)	GK	87 (typ), 49 (atyp), 0 (mal) at 5 yr
2007	Feigl et al[19]	Hannover (Germany)	211 (243 tumors)	GK	86.3 at 4yr
2007	Hasegawa et al[128]	Komaki, (Japan)	115	GK	87 at 5 yr
2007	Kollová et al[37]	Prague (Czech Republic)	368 (400 tumors)	GK	98 at 5 yr
2008	Iwai et al[31]	Osaka (Japan)	108	GK	93 at 5 yr
2008	Kondziolka et al[139-40]	Pittsburgh (USA)	972 (1,045 tumors)	GK	97 (ben) at 5yr
2009	Colombo et al[19]	Vicenza (Italy)	199	CyberKnife	93.6 at 5yr
2009	Takanashi et al[178]	Sapporo (Japan)	101	GK	95.5% in cav.sin. 98.4% in post.fossa

Table 4. GKR-, PROTON BEAMLINAC- and Cyberknife-based stereotactic radiosurgery in meningiomas. Synopsis of the largest published series of the last two decades comparing local tumor control rates.

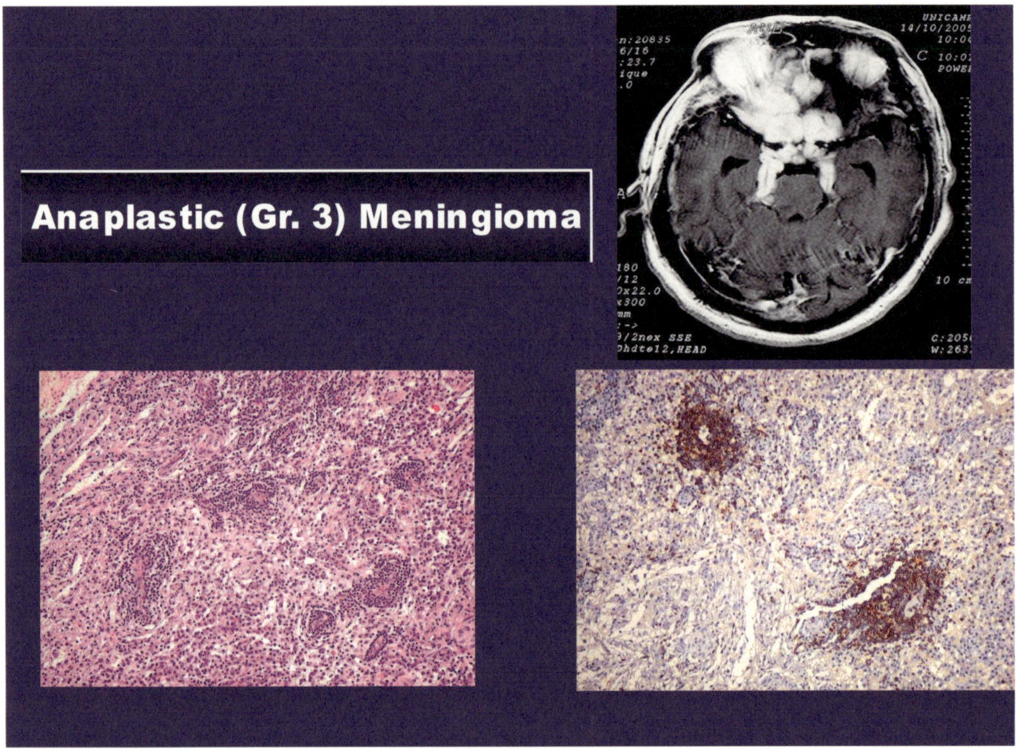

Fig. 2. Anaplastic (gr.3) meningioma. Note the pronounced endo-perivascular tumor cell coating.

Furthermore, it is worth stressing that - even treating larger volumes - either with reduced dosages or with fractionated schedules, the literature shows no evidence of significantly increased "Adverse Radiation Effects" ("ARE"). Probably because the risk of "ARE" gradually subsides with lower prescription doses (3, 18, 19, 22, 31, 38, 47, 49, 64, 65, 70).

C. Nonetheless, also in meningioma radiosurgical treatments, several limits, pitfalls and risks remain to be tackled. Quoting some of the most intriguing:
   a. The satellite edema, particularly pronounced in the convexity regions or in parasagittal locations and rarely documented in skull base tumors, probably represent the dominant figure in the early stages of the "Peritumoral Imaging Changes". The main conditioning factors that may heavily influence the severity of these processes, are essentially related to the specific radiosurgical parameters: e.g. dose volume integral, conformity index etc. (6, 20, 22, 56, 72, 83, 86) However, recent reports have emphasized the extremely high chances to maintain adequate LTC rates - without increasing side effects- by treating larger meningiomas with either fractionated schedules or reduced dosages (3, 13, 18, 19, 22, 24, 31, 32).
   b. the controversial or disappointing results obtained in atypic and anaplastic lesions (17, 25, 27, 30, 51, 73), sometimes characterized by intra- or extraneuraxis metastatization (17) or by enhanced growth after radiosurgery (6, 14, 42);
   c. the still pronounced morbidity rate of this technique on sensory nerves (6, 14, 77).

d. finally, potential problems with undue hotspots on strategic vessels within the dosimetry area (1, 15).

D. A comparative analysis of Cyberknife-based (9,44) radiosurgical experiences in meningiomas versus GKR experiences clearly shows that follow up period is longer for GKR - several reports reaching 8-10 years mean FU vs. 5-6 years for Linac series. Targeted tumor volumes are extremely variable with both approaches, whereas the relative marginal dosages (12-15 Gy) as well as the tumor control rates (usually over 90%) are quite similar. The incidence of sequelae with both techniques is quantitatively (3-13%) and qualitatively reasonable, severe neurological worsening is extremely rare, with no reported mortality.

E. **Oncogenicity**. The relative risk of carcinogenesis after radiosurgery in the central nervous system has been calculated by means of probabilistic methods, and varies from 1.57 to 8.75 for a dose of 1 Gy, increasing in time up to 18.4 between 20 and 25 years (7, 55). The long-term (30 year) risk of newer radiation induced tumors in meningioma patients has been estimated in 1 per 1,000 treated patients (4, 5, 24, 42, 55). The natural incidence of new gliomas in the population (1/10,000 every year), and the number of meningiomas treated over 3 decades with SRS worldwide (75,000) must be the basic reference for any reliable statistical evaluation. As a consequence, the so far extremely rare (4 cases) reported instances of malignant brain tumors diagnosed in SRS - treated meningioma patients are probably an underestimation of the real incidence, that, however, does not seem to defray further development of this technique.

4. References

[1] Abeloos L, Levivier M, Devriendt D, et al: Internal carotid occlusion following gamma knife radiosurgery for cavernous sinus meningioma. Stereotact Funct Neurosurg 85:303-306, 2007.

[2] Bambakidis NC, Kakarla UK, Kim LJ, et al: Evolution of surgical approaches in the treatment of petroclival meningiomas: a retrospective review. Neurosurgery 62(Suppl 3):1182-1191, 2008

[3] Bledsoe JM, Link MJ, Stafford SL, et al: Radiosurgery for large-volume (> 10 cm^3) benign meningiomas. J Neurosurg Sept 18, 2009

[4] Central Brain Tumor Registry in the United States: Statistical report: primary brain tumors in the Unites States, 1992-1997. Hinsdale, Il: CBTRUS, 2001.

[5] Central Brain Tumor Registry of the United States: Statistical report: primary brain tumors in the United States, 1998-2002. Hinsdale, Il: CBTRUS, 2005.

[6] Chang JH, Chang JW, Choi JY, et al: Complications after gamma knife radiosurgery for benign meningiomas. J Neurol Neurosurg Psychiatry 74:226-230, 2003.

[7] Clark BG, Candish C, Vollans E, et al: Optimization of stereotactic radiotherapy treatment delivery technique for base-of-skull meningiomas. Med Dosim 33:239-247, 2008

[8] Claus EB, Bondy ML, Schildkraut JM, et al: Epidemiology of intracranial meningioma. Neurosurgery 57:1088-1095, 2005.

[9] Colombo F, Casentini L, Cavedon C, et al: Cyberknife radiosurgery for benign meningiomas: short-term results in 199 patients. Neurosurgery 64:A7-13, 2009.

[10] Condra KS, Buatti JM, Mendenhall WM, et al: Benign meningiomas: primary treatment selection affects survival. Int J Radiat Oncol Biol Phys 39:427-436, 1997.
[11] Couldwell WT, Fukushima T, Giannotta SL, et al: Petroclival meningiomas: surgical experience in 109 cases. J Neurosurg 84:20-28, 1996.
[12] DeMonte F, Smith HK, al-Mefty O: Outcome of aggressive removal of cavernous sinus meningiomas. J Neurosurg 81:245-251,1994
[13] DiBiase SJ, Kwok Y, Yovino S, et al: Factors predicting local tumor control after gamma knife stereotactic radiosurgery for benign intracranial meningiomas. Int J Radiat Oncol Biol Phys 60:1515-1519, 2004.
[14] Dropcho EJ: Neurotoxicity of radiation therapy. Neurol Clin 28:217-234, 2010.
[15] Dufour H, Muracciole X, Metellus P, et al: Long-term tumor control and functional outcome in patients with cavernous sinus meningiomas treated by radiotherapy with or without previous surgery: is there an alternative to aggressive tumor removal? Neurosurgery 48:285-294, 2001.
[16] Elia AE, Shih HA, Loeffler JS: Stereotactic radiation treatment for benign meningiomas. Neurosurg Focus 23:E5, 2007
[17] Eom KS, Kim DW, Kim TY: Diffuse craniospinal metastases of intraventricular rhabdoid papillary meningioma with glial fibrillary acidic protein expression: a case report. Clin Neurol Neurosurg 111:619-623, 2009
[18] Eustacchio S, Trummer M, Fuchs I, et al: Preservation of cranial nerve function following Gamma Knife radiosurgery for benign skull base meningiomas: experience in 121 patients with follow-up of 5 to 9.8 years. Acta Neurochir 84(Suppl):71-76, 2002.
[19] Feigl GC, Bundschuh O, Gharabaghi A, et al: Volume reduction in meningiomas after gamma knife surgery. J Neurosurg 102(Suppl):189-194, 2005.
[20] Fowler JF: Sensitivity analysis of parameters in linear-quadratic radiobiologic modeling. Int J Radiat Oncol Biol Phys 73:1532-1537, 2009
[21] Friedman WA, Murad GJ, Bradshaw P, et al: Linear accelerator surgery for meningiomas. J Neurosurg 103:206-209, 2005.
[22] Ganz JC, Reda WA, Abdelkarim K: Adverse radiation effects after Gamma Knife Surgery in relation to dose and volume. Acta Neurochir 151:9-19, 2009
[23] Go RS, Taylor BV, Kimmel DW: The natural history of asymptomatic meningiomas in Olmsted County, Minnesota. Neurology 51:1718-1720, 1998.
[24] Goldsmith B: Meningioma. In: Leibel S, Phillips T (eds): Textbook of Radiation Oncology. Philadelphia: WB Saunders, 1998.
[25] Goyal LK, Suh JH, Mohan DS, et al: Local control and overall survival in atypical meningioma: a retrospective study. Int J Radiat Oncol Biol Phys 46:57-61, 2000
[26] Hakim R, Alexander E, 3rd, Loeffler JS, et al: Results of linear accelerator-based radiosurgery for intracranial meningiomas. Neurosurgery 42:446-453, 1998.
[27] Harris AE, Lee JY, Omalu B, et al: The effect of radiosurgery during management of aggressive meningiomas. Surg Neurol 60:298-305, 2003.
[28] Hasegawa T, Kida Y, Yoshimoto M, et al: Long-term outcomes of Gamma Knife surgery for cavernous sinus meningioma. J Neurosurg 107:745-751, 2007.

[29] Herscovici Z, Rappaport Z, Sulkes J, et al: Natural history of conservatively treated meningiomas. Neurology 63:1133-1134, 2004.

[30] Hug EB, Devries A, Thornton AF, et al: Management of atypical and malignant meningiomas: role of high-dose, 3D-conformal radiation therapy. J Neurooncol 48:151-160, 2000

[31] Iwai Y, Yamanaka K, Yasui T, et al: Gamma knife surgery for skull base meningiomas. The effectiveness of low-dose treatment. Surg Neurol 52:40-44, 1999.

[32] Iwata H, Shibamoto Y, Murata R, et al: Estimation of errors associated with use of linear-quadratic formalism for evaluation of biologic equivalence between single and hypofractionated radiation doses: an in vitro study. Int J Radiat Oncol Biol Phys 75:482-488, 2009.

[33] Jung HW, Yoo H, Paek SH, et al: Long-term outcome and growth rate of subtotally resected petroclival meningiomas: experience with 38 cases. Neurosurgery 46:567-574, 2000.

[34] Kawahara Y, Niiro M, Yokoyama S, et al: Dural congestion accompanying meningioma invasion into vessels: the dural tail sign. Neuroradiology 43:462-465, 2001

[35] Kocher M, Wilms M, Makoski HB, et al: Alpha/beta ratio for arteriovenous malformations estimated from obliteration rates after fractionated and single-dose irradiation. Radiother Oncol 71:109-114, 2004.

[36] Koga T, Maruyama K., Igaki H., et al. The value of image co-registration during stereotactic radiosurgery. Acta Neurochir. (Wien) 151: 465-471, 2009

[37] Kollova A, Liscak R, Novotny J Jr, et al: Gamma Knife surgery for benign meningioma. J Neurosurg 107:325-336, 2007.

[38] Kondziolka D, Kano H, Kanaan H, et al: Stereotactic radiosurgery for radiation-induced meningiomas. Neurosurgery 64:463-469, 2009

[39] Kondziolka D, Madhok R, Lunsford LD, et al: Stereotactic radiosurgery for convexity meningiomas. J Neurosurg 111:458-463, 2009

[40] Kondziolka D, Mathieu D, Lunsford LD, et al: Radiosurgery as definitive management of intracranial meningiomas. Neurosurgery 62:53 58, 2008

[41] Kreil W, Luggin J, Fuchs I, et al: Long term experience of gamma knife radiosurgery for benign skull base meningiomas. J Neurol Neurosurg Psychiatry 76:1425-1430, 2005

[42] Kunert P, Matyja E, Janowski M, et al: Rapid growth of small, asymptomatic meningioma following radiosurgery. Br J Neurosurg 23:206-208, 2009

[43] Kuratsu J, Kochi M, Ushio Y: Incidence and clinical features of asymptomatic meningiomas. J Neurosurg 92:766-770, 2000.

[44] Lartigau E, Mirabel X, Prevost B, et al: Extracranial stereotactic radiotherapy: preliminary results with the CyberKnife. Onkologie 32:209-215, 2009.//

[45] Levine ZT, Buchanan RI, Sekhar LN et al.Proposed grading system to predict the extent of resection and outcome for cranial base meningiomas. Neurosurgery 45: 221-230, 1999.

[46] Longstreth WT, Jr., Dennis LK, McGuire VM, et al: Epidemiology of intracranial meningioma. Cancer 72:639-648, 1993

[47] Ma L, Chuang C, Descovich M, et al: Whole-procedure clinical accuracy of gamma knife treatments of large lesions. Med Phys 35:5110-5114, 2008.

[48] Mahmood A, Qureshi NH, Malik GM: Intracranial meningiomas: analysis of recurrence after surgical treatment. Acta Neurochir 126:53-58, 1994.

[49] Malik I, Rowe JG, Walton L, et al: The use of stereotactic radiosurgery in the management of meningiomas. Br J Neurosurg 19:13-20, 2005.

[50] Maruyama K, Kamada K, Shin M et al Integration of three dimensional corticospinal tractography into treatment planning for gamma knife surgery. J Neurosurg 102 673-677, 2005

[51] Mathiesen T, Lindquist C, Kihlstrom L, et al: Recurrence of cranial base meningiomas. Neurosurgery 39:2-7, 1996.

[52] McDermott MW, Quiñones-Hinojosa A, Fuller GN, et al: Meningiomas. In: Levin VA (ed): Cancer in the Nervous System, 2nd ed. New York: Oxford University, 2002.

[53] Mirimanoff RO, Dosoretz DE, Linggood RM et al. Meningioma: analysis of recurrence and progression following neurosurgical resection. J. Neurosurg. 62: 18-24, 1985.

[54] Modha A, Gutin PH: Diagnosis and treatment of atypical and anaplastic meningiomas: a review. Neurosurgery 57:538-550, 2005

[55] Muracciole X, Regis J. : Radiosurgery amd carcinogenesis risk. Progr. Neurol. Surg. 21: 207-213, 2008.

[56] Nakamura M, Roser F, Michel J, et al: The natural history of incidental meningiomas. Neurosurgery 53:62-70, 2003.

[57] Nicolato A, Foroni R, Grigolato D et al.: 111 Indium-octreotide brain scintigraphy: a prognostic factor in skull base meningiomas treated with Gamma Knife Radiosurgery. Q J Nucl Med 48:26-32, 2004.

[58] Nicolato A, Giorgetti P, Foroni R et al.: Gamma Knife radiosurgery in skull base meningiomas: a possibile relationship between somatostatin receptor decrease and early neurological improvement without tumor shrinkage at short-term imaging follow-up. Acta Neurochir 147:367-375, 2005.

[59] Niiro M, Yatsushiro K, Nakamura K, et al: Natural history of elderly patients with asymptomatic meningiomas. J Neurol Neurosurg Psychiatry 68:25-28, 2000.

[60] Ojemann SG, Sneed PK, Larson DA, et al: Radiosurgery for malignant meningioma: results in 22 patients. J Neurosurg 93(Suppl 3):62-67, 2000.

[61] Olivero WC, Lister JR, Elwood PW: The natural history and growth rate of asymptomatic meningiomas: a review of 60 patients. J Neurosurg 83:222-224, 1995.

[62] Palma L, Celli P, Franco C, et al: Long-term prognosis for atypical and malignant meningiomas: a study of 71 surgical cases. J Neurosurg 86:793-800, 1997.

[63] Pendl G, Eustacchio S, Unger F: Radiosurgery as alternative treatment for skull base meningiomas. J Clin Neurosci 8(Suppl 1):12-14, 2001.

[64] Perry A, Dehner LP: Meningeal tumors of childhood and infancy. An update and literature review. Brain Pathol 13:386-408, 2003

[65] Perry A, Louis DN, Scheithauer BW, et al.: Meningeal tumors. In: Louis DN, Ohgaki H, Wiestler OD, Cavenee WK (eds): World Health Organization Classification of Tumours of the Central Nervous System. Lyon: IARC, 2007.

[66] Petti PL, Larson DA, Kunwar S: Use of hybrid shots in planning Perfexion Gamma Knife treatments for lesions close to critical structures. J Neurosurg 109(Suppl):34-40, 2008

[67] Pieper DR, Al-Mefty O, Hanada Y, et al: Hyperostosis associated with meningioma of the cranial base: secondary changes or tumor invasion. Neurosurgery 44:742-746, 1999

[68] Pollock BE, Stafford SL, Utter A, et al: Stereotactic radiosurgery provides equivalent tumor control to Simpson Grade 1 resection for patients with small- to medium-size meningiomas. Int J Radiat Oncol Biol Phys 55:1000-1005, 2003

[69] Pollock BE: Stereotactic radiosurgery for intracranial meningiomas: indications and results. Neurosurg Focus 14:e4, 2003

[70] Pollock BE: Stereotactic radiosurgery of benign intracranial tumors. J. Neurooncol. 92:337-343, 2009

[71] Riemenschneider MJ, Perry A., Reifenberger G: Histological classification and molecular genetics of meningiomas. Lancet Neurol. 5 : 1045-1054, 2006

[72] Rogers L, Mehta M: Role of radiation therapy in treating intracranial meningiomas. Neurosurg Focus 23:E4, 2007.

[73] Rosenberg LA, Prayson RA, Lee J, et al: Long-term experience with World Health Organization grade III (malignant) meningiomas at a single institution. Int J Radiat Oncol Biol Phys 74:427-432, 2009

[74] Saberi K., Meybodi AT, Rezai AS. Levine-Sekhar grading system for prediction of the extent of resection of cranial base meningiomas revisited: study of 124 cases. Neurosurg. Rev. April 29 (2) :138-144, 2006

[75] Samii M, Klekamp J, Carvalho G: Surgical results for meningiomas of the craniocervical junction. Neurosurgery 39:1086-1094,1996

[76] Sekhar LN, Swamy NK, Jaiswal V, et al: Surgical excision of meningiomas involving the clivus: preoperative and intraoperative features as predictors of postoperative functional deterioration. J Neurosurg 81:860-868, 1994

[77] Stafford SL, Pollock BE, Leavitt JA, et al: A study on the radiation tolerance of the optic nerves and chiasm after stereotactic radiosurgery. Int J Radiat Oncol Biol Phys 55:1177-1181, 2003.

[78] Takanashi M, Fukuoka S, Hojyo A, et al: Gamma knife radiosurgery for skull-base meningiomas. Prog Neurol Surg 22:96-111, 2009.

[79] Thomas NW, King TT: Meningiomas of the cerebellopontine angle. A report of 41 cases. Br J Neurosurg 10:59-68, 1996.

[80] Yano S, Kuratsu J: Indications for surgery in patients with asymptomatic meningiomas based on an extensive experience. J Neurosurg 105:538-543, 2006.

[81] Yoneoka Y, Fujii Y, Tanaka R: Growth of incidental meningiomas. Acta Neurochir 142:507-511, 2000.

[82] Walsh MT, Couldwell WT: Management options for cavernous sinus meningiomas. J Neurooncol 92:307-316, 2009

[83] Wara WM, Sheline GE, Newmann H, et al : Radiation therapy of meningiomas. Am. J. Roentgenology, Radium Ther., Nucl. Med 123: 453-458, 1975.

[84] Ware ML, Larson DA, Sneed PK, et al: Surgical resection and permanent brachytherapy for recurrent atypical and malignant meningioma. Neurosurgery 54:55-63, 2004
[85] Wenkel E, Thornton AF, Finkelstein D, et al: Benign meningioma: partially resected, biopsied, and recurrent intracranial tumors treated with combined proton and photon radiotherapy. Int J Radiat Oncol Biol Phys 48:1363-1370, 2000
[86] Whittle IR, Smith C, Navoo P, et al: Meningiomas. Lancet 363:1535-1543, 2004

4

Gamma Knife Radiosurgery for the Vestibular Schwannomas, Technical Considerations and Hydrocephalus as a Complication

Sung Kyoo Hwang, Kisoo Park, Dong Hyun Lee,
Seong Hyun Park, Jaechan Park and Jeong Hyun Hwang
Department of Neurosurgery, Kyungpook National University Hospital
Korea

1. Introduction

Vestibular schwannomas are slow-growing, benign tumours. Microsurgery has been the standard treatment for vestibular schwannoma over the past 30 years. Following the introduction of stereotactic radiosurgery for the treatment of vestibular schwannoma in 1969, its increasing use worldwide had led to its acceptance by many as a safe and efficient alternative to microsurgery. The primary advantages of stereotactic radiosurgery are its safety in terms of morbidity and its high tumour control rate.

Because the cerebello-pontine angle is composed of many important cranial nerves and vessels, planning quality is expressed as various indices such as conformity or homogeneity that are regarded as being related to the development of complications. Improved technology and the development of the new gamma knife radiosurgery units—such as the automatic positioning system and the fusion technique in the gamma plan—increase the planning accuracy of the irradiated target area. However, the relationship with the course of the response of the tumour and the complication rate remains poorly understood. In this chapter, we will review how the high conformity indices contribute to the post-radiosurgery course of the disease by analysing the literature.

With regard to the complications of stereotactic radiosurgery (despite the many benefits that allow it replace microsurgery as a primary treatment modality), additional research is needed to reduce the complications that are associated with stereotactic radiosurgery in order to improve patient quality of life. Complications that are associated with stereotactic radiosurgery for vestibular schwannoma include hearing deficits, facial palsy, hydrocephalus, and brain stem damage, although the incidence of some of these conditions is much lower than with microscopic open surgery. We reviewed complications and their risk factors (with a particular emphasis on hydrocephalus) from our experience of gamma knife radiosurgery for the treatment of vestibular schwannoma.

Regarding hydrocephalus, this complication can occur at various stages during the natural course of a vestibular schwannoma. The reported incidence ranges from 3.7% to 15% of cases (Atlas et al., 1996; Litvack et al., 2003). Large vestibular schwannomas sometimes cause obstructive hydrocephalus; however, CSF malabsorption may be the cause of communicating-type hydrocephalus. The hydrocephalus can develop as a complication of treatment using either gamma knife radiosurgery or microsurgery. However, the incidence, aetiological factors, mechanisms, and management of hydrocephalus following stereotactic radiosurgery and microsurgery are not well understood. We present a review of the incidence, characteristics and management experience of hydrocephalus in patients with vestibular schwannoma who were treated using gamma knife radiosurgery and compare these findings with those of patients who received microsurgery as the primary treatment.

2. Technical consideration of gamma knife radiosurgery for treating vestibular schwannoma

2.1 Conformity

Vestibular schwannomas are located in the cerebello-pontine angle, and in most cases, they extend into the internal acoustic foramen. Many functionally important structures such as the trigeminal, facial and acoustic nerves, arteries, and the brainstem are located around the tumour. Many of the hazards of microsurgery for vestibular schwannoma are related to the tumour's location. Damaging these structures during microsurgery is the most common cause of morbidity and mortality. Gamma knife radiosurgery should also take these structures into consideration. The principle underlying gamma knife radiosurgery is the concentration of high energy into the localised area of the lesion while sparing surrounding functional structures. Accumulated data have justified the use of gamma knife radiosurgery as the primary treatment of vestibular schwannoma without causing significant complications related to the damage of the important surrounding structures. Historically, many experts in this field have reduced the radiation dose without compromising the tumour control rate. A marginal dose of 12 or 13Gy is now accepted as the standard dose for controlling a tumour using gamma knife radiosurgery. However, although the intended marginal dose is similar, the planned radiation field can differ in its conformity and distribution of radiation. Several parameters have been proposed to describe the quality of the radiation plan. Aside from these parameters, one should consider that some specific structures are more vulnerable to even relatively low doses of radiation. Special somatic sensation fibres are regarded to be more vulnerable to external damage, including radiation, than are other cranial nerves. In this regard, hearing loss is a high concern when using gamma knife radiosurgery for treating a vestibular schwannoma.

To achieve maximum effectiveness, radiosurgery should deliver the highest permissible radiation to the target whilst reducing the surrounding radiation dose as rapidly as possible. To quantify this quality of planning, various conformity and sensitivity indices are used. Advances in the gamma knife radiosurgery unit—including the automatic positioning system, gamma plan, and (more recently) the new Perfexion system—provide higher accuracy and improved patient convenience and comfort. Hayashi et al. (Hayashi et al., 2006) introduced the concept of robotic micro-radiosurgery and demonstrated high accuracy in the planning of gamma knife radiosurgery.

A dose-volume histogram of the gamma plan that represents the three-dimensional dose distribution provides a measure of the quality of planning. The neurosurgeon or radiation oncologist who is responsible for the radiosurgery uses this dose-volume histogram to compare the conformity of the dose plan to concentrate the radiation dose at the target. However, there are no established standard parameters, and even the role for such parameters in the control of the disease with gamma knife radiosurgery has not been clarified. The most commonly used parameter to quantify the dose distribution of the tumour and normal tissue is conformity. Various conformity indices have been proposed by many authors. The Radiation Therapy Oncology Group proposed several routine evaluation parameters for stereotactic radiotherapy plans, including the quality of coverage, the homogeneity index, and the conformity index (Feuvret et al., 2006; Nedzi et al., 1993). Paddick (Paddick, 2000) proposed an index based on the dose-volume histogram and volume analysis tools of the GammaPlan criticizing existing indices. Figure 1 shows the basic concept of the planning during radiosurgery, and Figue 2 typical dose-volume histogram with volume measurement in the GammaPlan. Here, we present several examples of parameters that are used in gamma knife radiosurgery in Table 1.

The role of these quality parameters in the complication and tumour control rates is not clear and may differ based on the disease. With regard to metastatic tumours, Woo et al. (Woo et al., 2010) reported that a high conformity dose plan was related with a poor tumour control rate. Nakamura et al. (Nakamura et al., 2001) studied 1,338 available artriovenous malformation patients who were treated with gamma knife radiosurgery and found that the conformity index was higher than in the linac surgery series, and the complication rate was not related to the conformity index. Beegle et al. (Beegle et al., 2007) studied 390 patients with regard to the issue of conformity and dose gradient in treating vestibular schwannoma and found no significant effect of these dosimetric parameters on cranial neuropathy. These authors found that tumour volume and dose were associated with an increased risk of facial weakness and facial sensory change (Beegle, et al., 2007). These disparate findings indicate that a standard index does not exist (Feuvret, et al., 2006).

It is interesting to note that the gradient index (which represents radiation dispersion outside of the target) is not related with the adverse radiation effect (Hayhurst et al., 2011). It is assumed that a marginal radiosurgery dose for treating vestibular schwannoma is sufficiently low to spare the surrounding cranial nerve and brain stem. The tumour control rate and hearing outcome are not significantly related to conformity indices of dose distribution within and surrounding the target volume (Massager et al., 2011). The outcome seems to be influenced more by the local radiation dose that is delivered to specific structures or volumes than by the global dose gradient (Massager, et al., 2011).

Although the complication rate is related to tumour size (but not to the conformity index), the relationship between the tumour control rate and the conformity index is not known. This is due to several factors. First, tumour size decreases during the prolonged times following gamma knife radiation therapy, and the response of a vestibular schwannoma following gamma knife radiosurgery in terms of genetic and pathological alterations is poorly understood. Secondly, most responsible neurosurgeons and radiation oncologists always apply the maximum effort to achieve a higher available conformity. Planning priority could differ according to various indications. Dose planning for treating vestibular schwannoma places high priority on the dose conformity whilst sparing the neighbouring facial nerves and brain stem, despite a slightly reduced coverage of the tumour. On the other hand, with regard to metastatic tumours, target coverage receives the highest priority (Lomax & Scheib, 2003). Lamax and Scheib (Lomax & Scheib, 2003) reported a median conformity index for vestibular schwannoma of 0.85 and a median target coverage of 92%, whereas for metastasis, these values were 0.67 and 100%, respectively.

Thus, it is difficult to evaluate the role of conformity in radiosurgery for treating vestibular schwannoma. Accumulated data from long-term follow-up studies are clearly needed. The effect regarding small vascular injuries due to radiosurgery remains poorly understood. There is general agreement that the size of the tumour is related to complications that are associated with the treatment. Hayhurst et al. (Hayhurst, et al., 2011) reported that adverse radiation effects were increased with target volumes that were greater than 2.1 cc; in addition, they reported a second peak at 5 cc. However, several authors reported positive treatment results even for large tumours (Iwai et al., 2003; Rowe et al., 2003a). In selecting a candidate for radiosurgery, tumour size should be a primary consideration. To prevent complications (in particular, facial nerve palsy), some authors recommend using a partial or subtotal microsurgical removal approach while applying special care to preserve the facial nerve, and this should then be followed by a secondary gamma knife radiosurgery (Fuentes et al., 2008; C. K. Park et al., 2006).

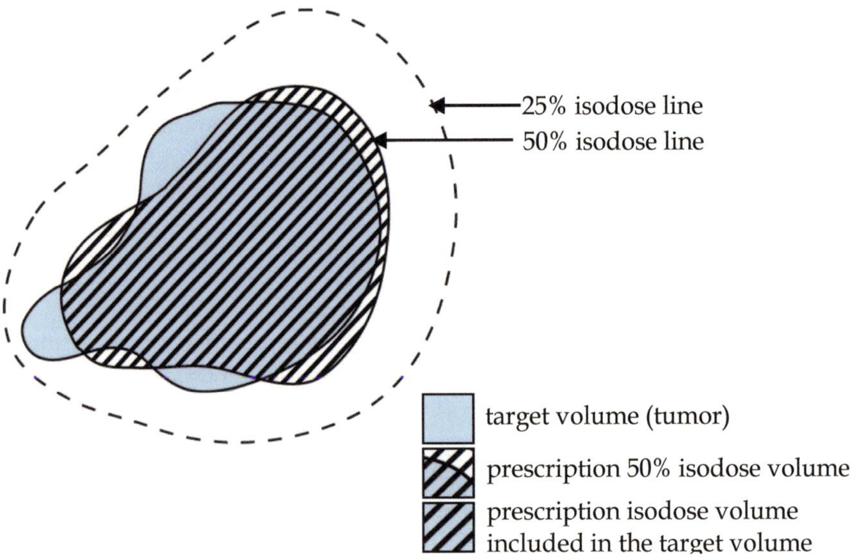

Fig. 1. Schematic drawing of planning of gamma knife radiosurgery of the tumour.

Conformity index of Paddick (Paddick, 2000): $\frac{(TV_{PIV})^2}{TV \times PIV}$

CI_{RTOG} (Shaw et al., 1993) = PIV/TV

Gradient index (Paddick & Lippitz, 2006) = $\frac{PIV_{25\%}}{PIV_{50\%}}$

CI_{RTOG}: conformity index of Radiation Treatment Oncology Group
TV: target volume
PIV: prescription isodose volume
TV_{PIV}: prescription isodose volume included in the target volume
$PIV_{25\%}$: prescription 25% isodose volume
$PIV_{50\%}$: prescription 50% isodose volume

Table 1. Examples of quality indices of radiosurgery.

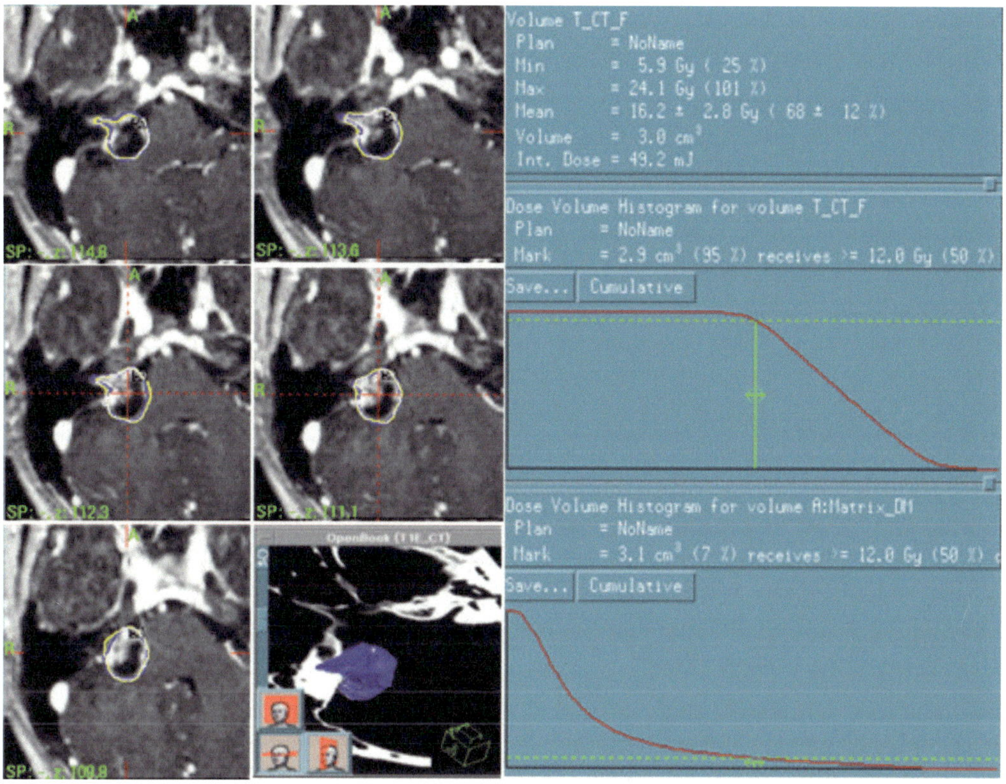

Fig. 2. Typical plan of gamma knife radiosurgery for treating vestibular schwannoma and the dose-volume curve. The prescription 50% isodose is 12 Gy. In this 53-year-old female patient, the target volume (tumour volume) was 2.9 cc, and 95% of this volume received more than 12 Gy. The total volume that received more than 12 Gy in the brain was 3.1 cc. The volume outside of the target area that received more than 12 Gy was 0.2 cc.

2.2 Hearing preservation

Hearing preservation is another important issue to consider in the treatment of vestibular schwannoma with either microsurgery or radiosurgery. The hearing preservation rate following microsurgery was reported to be 40-70% in patients with serviceable hearing (Betchen et al., 2005; Briggs et al., 2000; Samii et al., 2008; Samii & Matthies, 1997a, 1997b; Samii et al., 1997; Staecker et al., 2000). Hearing preservation is an important issue in gamma knife radiosurgery as well. As the experience with gamma knife radiosurgery has grown, the radiation dose has decreased. Currently, a marginal dose of 12 or 13 Gy is the standard dose for treating vestibular schwannoma. Regis et al. (Regis et al., 2008) reported a 60% hearing preservation rate in patients in a large study with a mean follow-up of 7 (minimum 3) years. These authors also mentioned that patients who were not treated using gamma knife radiosurgery lost an average of 9-39 dB compared with an average loss of 2 dB at 3 years following radiosurgery, which corresponds with a preservation of hearing functionality of 60-75%. Tamura et al. (Tamura et al., 2009) reported a 78.4% hearing preservation rate in Gardner-Robertson Class 1 patients. The probability of preserving functional hearing was higher in patients who had initial symptoms that were other than a decrease in hearing, in patients who were younger than 50 years, and in those patients whose cochlea received a dose of less than 4 Gy during treatment. (Tamura, et al., 2009).

The mechanism that underlies hearing deterioration following gamma knife radiosurgery is not fully understood. Some of the mechanisms that have been proposed include a temporary expansion of the tumour in the canal, vascular insufficiency of the auditory system, the toxic dispersion of free radicals, among others (Chang et al., 1998; Regis, et al., 2008; Timmer et al., 2009; Wackym et al., 2010).

A tolerable dose for the cochlea has not been clearly established. However, several studies have proposed a threshold of 4 Gy for radiosurgery (Anker & Shrieve, 2009; Regis, et al., 2008; Timmer, et al., 2009; Wackym, et al., 2010). Keeping the cochlear dose below this threshold is therefore recommended. Combined imaging using a CT scan and MRI is helpful for identifying the intracanalicular boundary between the tumour and the cochlear structure. Plugging or sector occlusion strategies provide the steep drop out of the radiation dose that is applied to these structures. The potential for improved hearing following radiosurgery has also been reported. Narajan et al. (Niranjan et al., 1999) reported improved hearing in 21 of 487 consecutive radiosurgery patients. Although this may not represent the actual potential for hearing improvement, it provides evidence that hearing improvement is at least possible following radiosurgery (Niranjan, et al., 1999).

2.3 Non-auditory complications

Hayhurst et al. (Hayhurst, et al., 2011) reviewed the non-auditory complications that were associated with gamma knife radiosurgery in 80 patients who were followed for more than 2 years. Twenty-seven (33.8%) of their patients developed non-auditory adverse radiation effects, and patients with a target volume that exceeded a threshold of 5 cc were more likely to develop complications. Treatment plan dosimetric characteristics are not associated with adverse radiation effects. Applying the maximum dose to the 5th cranial nerve is a reliable predictor of trigeminal dysfunction with a threshold of 9 Gy. However, the dose that is tolerated by the cranial nerves is not clear, and reports vary among authors. Anker and Shrieve (Anker & Shrieve, 2009) reviewed the literature and reported the recommended normal structure dose constraints in which one could avoid complications when using a single fraction. According to their study, the maximum doses for sparing trigeminal and facial function are below than 12.5-13 and 12.5-15 Gy, respectively.

3. Hydrocephalus as a complication of gamma knife radiosurgery and risk factors

3.1 Hydrocephalus and gamma knife radiosurgery

Hydrocephalus can occur at various stages during the natural course of a vestibular schwannoma (K. Park et al., 2009), and the reported incidence ranges from 3.7 to 15% of cases (Atlas, et al., 1996; Pirouzmand et al., 2001; Rogg et al., 2005). Occasionally, a large vestibular schwannoma can cause obstructive hydrocephalus, and CSF mal-absorption may be the cause of the communicating hydrocephalus (Gardner et al., 1954; Prasad, 2001; Rogg, et al., 2005). It has been proposed that protein molecules clog the pores of the semi-permeable membrane that forms the barrier in the arachnoid granulations, thereby leading to impaired absorption of CSF. Among 157 patients who were reported by Rogg et al. (Rogg, et al., 2005), 28 (18%) had a pre-existing hydrocephalus before receiving treatment; 39% of these patients had a non-communicating hydrocephalus, and 61% had a communicating type, and no significant association with tumour size was observed.

We reviewed experiences of hydrocephalus in patients with vestibular schwannomas who were treated in our institute using gamma knife radiosurgery and compared these findings with those patients who received microsurgery as the primary treatment.

3.2 Materials and methods

We conducted a retrospective review of 51 patients who were treated with gamma knife radiosurgery for a vestibular schwannoma (group 1) from January 2005 through December 2010 and 19 consecutive patients who were treated with microsurgery as the primary treatment (group 2) from January 2003 through May 2008. The diagnoses of vestibular schwannoma and hydrocephalus and the measurement of the tumour size were based on the results of the CT scan and MRI results. Hydrocephalus was diagnosed using the age-adjusted bicaudate index (van der Jagt et al., 2009). The size of tumour was calculated on the basis of the largest diameter of the tumour on the MRI scan.

Radiosurgery was performed using a Leksell Gamma Knife Model C (Elekta Instrument AB, Stockholm, Sweden) with Gamma Plan ver. 5.34 (Elekta Instrument). The marginal doses were 12 and 13 Gy in 39 and 12, respectively; the maximum doses were 24 and 26 Gy. Microsurgeries were performed with the retrosigmoid or translabyrinthine approach according to the preference of the surgeon preferences and the hearing status of the patient. The CSF diversion procedure that was used for the hydrocephalus was either an endoscopic third ventriculostomy or a ventriculo-peritoneal shunt.

Before and after the radiosurgery or microsurgery, the development of hydrocephalus with regard to the patient's age, tumour size, and radiation dose were evaluated, and the management of hydrocephalus was discussed. The statistical analysis was performed using the chi square or Fisher's exact test. Differences with a p-value of less than 0.05 were considered to be statistically significant.

3.3 Results

In group 1, all of the patients were followed for more than 6 months, and the mean follow-up duration was 37.9 months (range, 7-76 months). The mean age of the patients was 54.7 years (range, 13-74 years). The mean maximum tumour diameter was 1.6 cm (range, 0.4 - 3.7 cm). In group 2, nineteen patients were followed for more than 6 months, and the mean follow-up was 21.2 months (range, 6 - 54 months). The mean age of the patients was 50 years (range, 23 - 67 years). The mean maximum tumour diameter was 3.1 cm (range, 1 - 5.5 cm) (Table 2).

In group 1, five patients had hydrocephalus before undergoing gamma knife radiosurgery. None of the patients with a tumour diameter of less than 1 cm had hydrocephalus. Three patients had a tumour that was between 1- 3 cm, and two had a tumour that was larger than 3 cm. The hydrocephalus in the one out of three patients with a tumour diameter of less than 3 cm was improved progressively following gamma knife radiosurgery. After gamma knife radiosurgery, a newly developed (*de novo*) hydrocephalus was noted in six of the patients. In two of the patients with pre-gamma knife radiosurgery hydrocephalus and with a tumour that was larger than 3 cm, the hydrocephalus was worse following treatment. Among the 46 patients with a tumour diameter less than 3 cm, three developed *de novo* hydrocephalus after gamma knife radiosurgery. Three of the five patients with the tumour size larger than 3 cm developed hydrocephalus after gamma knife radiosurgery. The size of the tumour was significantly related with the *de novo* development of hydrocephalus ($p<0.05$). The patient characteristics are presented in Table 3 and 4. A marginal dose of radiosurgery and patient age were not significantly associated with hydrocephalus.

	Group 1(n=51) (GKRS)	Group 2 (n=19) (Microsurgery)
Mean age, years (range)	54.7 (13-74)	50 (23-67)
Sex (M:F)	15:36	3:16
Mean follow-up, months (range)	37.9 (7-76)	21.2 (6-54)
Mean tumour diameter, cm (range)	1.6(0.4-3.7)	3.2 (1-5.5)
MaximumTumour diameter, cm		
<1	5	0
1-3	41	7
≥3	5	12

Table 2. Demographic and clinical parameters of the patients who underwent gamma knife radiosurgery (GKRS) or microsurgery.

	Total Patients (n=51)	Hydrocephalus before GKRS (n=5)	Hydrocephalus after GKRS (n=11)	*p*-value
Age				
<50 years	14	2	1	NS
≥50 years	37	3	10	
Maximum tumour diameter, cm (see Table 4 for detailed data)			total (*de novo*)	See Table 3
<1	5	0	0 (0)	
1-3	41	3	6 (3)	
≥3	5	2	5 (3)	
Prescription dose (50%)				
12 Gy	39	5	7	NS
13 Gy	12	0	4	

NS: not significant

Table 3. Characteristics of the patients who underwent gamma knife radiosurgery (GKRS).

Among the 11 patients who were diagnosed with hydrocephalus, three underwent a CSF diversion procedure due to clinical deterioration or increasing ventricle size. Two of these patients initially underwent an endoscopic third ventriculostomy because their hydrocephalus was radiologically considered to be an obstructive type (such as a poorly visualised aqueduct of Sylvius and a small fourth ventricle). However, these two patients ultimately needed to receive a ventriculo-peritoneal shunt due to endoscopic third ventriculostomy failure. One patient underwent a ventriculo-peritoneal shunt as the primary treatment for hydrocephalus. The protein levels in the CSF of the patients with hydrocephalus were not routinely evaluated. However, two of the three patients who

Size of tumour	Number of patients	Pre-GKRS hydrocephalus		Post-GKRS hydrocephalus	
		No	Yes	total number	*de novo*
<1	5	5	0	0	0
1-3	41	38^{*}	3	6	3^{*}
≥3	5	$3^{§}$	2	5	$3^{§}$

1. GKRS: gamma knife radiosurgery
2. * and §: The *p*-value was less than 0.05, representing *de novo* development of post-gamma knife radiosurgery and was significantly related to the tumour size.

Table 4. Development of hydrocephalus according to tumour size.

underwent a CSF shunting procedure had elevated ventricular CSF protein levels of 147 and 150 mg/dl. Three of the five patients who developed hydrocephalus with a tumour that was larger than 3 cm underwent surgery using the translabyrinthine approach due to persistent symptoms or an enlarged tumour.

In group 2, seven of the patients had hydrocephalus before microsurgery, and all of these patients had a maximum tumour diameter that was larger than 3 cm. After microsurgery, all of the cases of hydrocephalus improved (Table 5). Tumour size, patient age, and surgical procedure were not significantly related to hydrocephalus and microsurgery.

	Total Patients (n=19)	Hydrocephalus before microsurgery (n=7)	Hydrocephalus after microsurgery (n=0)	*p*-value
Age				
<50 years	8	2	0	NS
≥50 years	11	5	0	
Maximum tumour diameter, cm				NS
1-3	7	0	0	
>3	12	7	0	
Surgical approach				
Retrosigmoid	15	3	0	NS
Translabyrinthine	4	4	0	

NS: Not significant (*p*>0.05)

Table 5. Characteristics of the patients who underwent microsurgery.

3.4 Discussion regarding the development of hydrocephalus in patients with vestibular schwannoma and their management

It has been reported that both gamma knife radiosurgery and microsurgery can contribute to the development or aggravation of hydrocephalus (Fukuda et al., 2007; Roche et al., 2008). However, the mechanism that is associated with the development of hydrocephalus following gamma knife radiosurgery is not known. Obstructive cases are not common, particularly if care is taken to avoid treating large tumours with a significant mass effect (Roche, et al., 2008). Sawamura et al. (Sawamura et al., 2003) studied a group of patients who underwent stereotactic radiation therapy and suggested that radiation-induced modifications of the tumour resulted in an accumulation of cellular and protein-laden material from the degradation and necrosis of the tumour. Although we did not analysed the CSF protein content in all patients, two of the patients who underwent a CSF shunting procedure had elevated ventricular CSF protein levels of 147 and 150 mg/dl. A systematic analysis of the biochemical components in the CSF in vestibular schwannoma has not been reported. In addition, the mechanism of hydrocephalus that is associated with microsurgery remains to be clarified. One likely explanation is that after microsurgery, the local inflammatory processes might impair circulation. Following the direct manipulation of the tumour capsule, the delivery of intracisternal haemoglobin and protein-laden material have been observed (Nassar & Correll, 1968; Samii & Matthies, 1997b). In our series, however, we found no *de novo* development or aggravation of hydrocephalus following microsurgery.

The incidence of hydrocephalus—including non-obstructive hydrocephalus—was higher in patients with larger tumours, and 3 cm is typically considered to be the maximum size for gamma knife radiosurgery. Four of the five patients with a tumour diameter that was larger than 3 cm had hydrocephalus that was believed to be the obstructive type radiologically due to a narrowing of the aqueduct of Sylvius and a normal or collapsed 4th ventricle, despite having enlarged lateral and third ventricles. Therefore, we initially performed an endoscopic third ventriculostomy in two of these patients. However, the patients' symptoms and ventricle size did not improve, and a ventriculo-peritoneal shunt was ultimately placed. In our cases, there was a weak correlation between the size of the tumour and obstructive type hydrocephalus. Hayhurst et al. (Hayhurst et al., 2006) reported a role of endoscopic third ventriculostomy in hydrocephalus after treating vestibular schwannomas. When successful, endoscopic third ventriculostomy has several benefits over placing a ventriculo-peritoneal shunt. We therefore recommend carefully selecting patients for the indication of undergoing an endoscopic third ventriculostomy.

Several authors have reported treatment strategies for hydrocephalus before microsurgery or gamma knife radiosurgery (Atlas, et al., 1996; Fukuda, et al., 2007; Roche, et al., 2008). With respect to microsurgery, several investigators preferred a wait-and-see-approach and therefore focused only on the surgery for the tumour. In most cases, the hydrocephalus resolved, and there was no need for additional shunt surgery. Atlas et al. (Atlas, et al., 1996) reported 14 patients with hydrocephalus in a series of 104 consecutive cases of vestibular schwannoma. In nine of these cases, the treatment consisted only of tumour removal, and there were no cases that required ventricular drainage or a shunting procedure following microsurgery. In a larger series of 1,000 cases of vestibular schwannoma, Samii and Matthies (Samii & Matthies, 1997b) reported that pre-existing hydrocephalus required CSF shunt insertion in nine of the cases (1%) before removal of the tumour.

The decision of whether to perform a shunt procedure for hydrocephalus before gamma knife radiosurgery remains challenging. Noren (Noren, 1998) reported that treatment-related peritumour reactions were sufficient to block CSF circulation and required shunt insertion in 1.4% of vestibular schwannoma cases that were treated using gamma knife radiosurgery. According to other reported studies of gamma knife radiosurgery, shunt surgery was needed in 0 to 3% of cases (Chopra et al., 2007; Pollock et al., 1995). In our series, 1 out of 46 (2.1%) patients with a tumour diameter that was less than 3 cm required a shunting procedure, whereas two out of five patients with a large tumour underwent a shunting procedure (and another two patients underwent microsurgery after gamma knife radiosurgery). Two of the patients with pre-gamma knife radiosurgery hydrocephalus and a tumour diameter that was larger than 3 cm worsened during the initial follow-up after gamma knife radiosurgery. In addition, two of the patients with pre-gamma knife radiosurgery hydrocephalus and a tumour diameter that was less than 3 cm improved after gamma knife radiosurgery. These findings support a wait-and see-policy when pre-gamma knife radiosurgery hydrocephalus or newly developed hydrocephalus occurs in patients with a small or medium size vestibular schwannoma. The progression of hydrocephalus must be followed closely, and patients with a large vestibular schwannoma must be monitored more intensely.

4. Conclusions

The vestibular schwannomas are located in the cerebello-pontine angle, in which many functionally important structures are included. Radiosurgery has become a reliable alternative treatment to the microsurgery for vestibular schwannoma. High conformity and sensitivity in the planning of radiosurgery are required to prevent the complication. However, most of the reports emphasize that the tumour size is the most important factor to reduce the complication. Keeping the cochlear dose below 4Gy is recommended for hearing preservation.

The development or worsening of hydrocephalus is a major complication of both gamma knife radiosurgery and microsurgery. In our experience, it can be assumed that in some patients, gamma knife radiosurgery plays a direct role in the occurrence of hydrocephalus but has no relationship to tumour growth or treatment failure. The presence of a large tumour was a significant factor that was associated with the development of both communicating and non-communicating hydrocephalus. The course and symptoms of hydrocephalus that develops following gamma knife radiosurgery differ from those in patients who are treated with microsurgery. Most microsurgery patients can be managed conservatively; however, many of the hydrocephalus patients who were treated with gamma knife radiosurgery required shunt surgery. Patients should be closely monitored for the development of hydrocephalus following gamma knife radiosurgery. Endoscopic third ventriculostomy was not effective in the management of hydrocephalus.

5. Acknowledgments

As the senior author (SKH), I sincerely appreciate the commitment of the entire medical and technical staff, in particular Byung Mok Kim M.S., medical physicist, and Ms. Ji Yeon Kim of the Gamma Knife Centre of Kyungpook National University Hospital. I would like to express that this manuscript could not have been completed without the great help of Eun Young Kang, M.S., and our secretary, Miss Mi Jin Kim, to whom I am grateful. I would like to dedicate this manuscript to my late son, Jong Won Hwang, M.D., who passed away leaving me a bitter grief.

6. References

Anker, C. J., & Shrieve, D. C. (2009). Basic principles of radiobiology applied to radiosurgery and radiotherapy of benign skull base tumors. *Otolaryngol Clin North Am, 42*(4), 601-621

Atlas, M. D., Perez de Tagle, J. R., Cook, J. A., Sheehy, J. P., & Fagan, P. A. (1996). Evolution of the management of hydrocephalus associated with acoustic neuroma. *Laryngoscope, 106*(2 Pt 1), 204-206

Beegle, R. D., Friedman, W. A., & Bova, F. J. (2007). Effect of treatment plan quality on outcomes after radiosurgery for vestibular schwannoma. *J Neurosurg, 107*(5), 913-916

Betchen, S. A., Walsh, J., & Post, K. D. (2005). Long-term hearing preservation after surgery for vestibular schwannoma. *J Neurosurg, 102*(1), 6-9

Briggs, R. J., Fabinyi, G., & Kaye, A. H. (2000). Current management of acoustic neuromas: review of surgical approaches and outcomes. *J Clin Neurosci, 7*(6), 521-526

Chang, S. D., Poen, J., Hancock, S. L., Martin, D. P., & Adler, J. R., Jr. (1998). Acute hearing loss following fractionated stereotactic radiosurgery for acoustic neuroma. Report of two cases. *J Neurosurg, 89*(2), 321-325

Chopra, R., Kondziolka, D., Niranjan, A., Lunsford, L. D., & Flickinger, J. C. (2007). Long-term follow-up of acoustic schwannoma radiosurgery with marginal tumor doses of 12 to 13 Gy. *Int J Radiat Oncol Biol Phys, 68*(3), 845-851

Feuvret, L., Noel, G., Mazeron, J. J., & Bey, P. (2006). Conformity index: a review. *Int J Radiat Oncol Biol Phys, 64*(2), 333-342

Fuentes, S., Arkha, Y., Pech-Gourg, G., Grisoli, F., Dufour, H., & Regis, J. (2008). Management of large vestibular schwannomas by combined surgical resection and gamma knife radiosurgery. *Prog Neurol Surg, 21*, 79-82

Fukuda, M., Oishi, M., Kawaguchi, T., Watanabe, M., Takao, T., Tanaka, R., & Fujii, Y. (2007). Etiopathological factors related to hydrocephalus associated with vestibular schwannoma. *Neurosurgery, 61*(6), 1186-1192; discussion 1192-1183

Gardner, W. J., Spitler, D. K., & Whitten, C. (1954). Increased intracranial pressure caused by increased protein content in the cerebrospinal fluid; an explanation of papilledema in certain cases of small intracranial and intraspinal tumors, and in the Guillain-Barre syndrome. *N Engl J Med, 250*(22), 932-936

Hasegawa, T., Fujitani, S., Katsumata, S., Kida, Y., Yoshimoto, M., & Koike, J. (2005). Stereotactic radiosurgery for vestibular schwannomas: analysis of 317 patients followed more than 5 years. [Clinical Trial Comparative Study]. *Neurosurgery, 57*(2), 257-265; discussion 257-265

Hayashi, M., Ochiai, T., Nakaya, K., Chernov, M., Tamura, N., Maruyama, T., Yomo, S., Izawa, M., Hori, T., Takakura, K., & Regis, J. (2006). Current treatment strategy for vestibular schwannoma: image-guided robotic microradiosurgery. *J Neurosurg, 105 Suppl*, 5-11

Hayhurst, C., Javadpour, M., O'Brien, D. F., & Mallucci, C. L. (2006). The role of endoscopic third ventriculostomy in the management of hydrocephalus associated with cerebellopontine angle tumours. *Acta Neurochir (Wien), 148*(11), 1147-1150; discussion 1150

Hayhurst, C., Monsalves, E., Bernstein, M., Gentili, F., Heydarian, M., Tsao, M., Schwartz, M., van Prooijen, M., Millar, B. A., Menard, C., Kulkarni, A. V., Laperriere, N., & Zadeh, G. (2011). Predicting Nonauditory Adverse Radiation Effects Following Radiosurgery for Vestibular Schwannoma: A Volume and Dosimetric Analysis. *Int J Radiat Oncol Biol Phys 2011 April 28 [Epub ahead of print]*

Iwai, Y., Yamanaka, K., & Ishiguro, T. (2003). Surgery combined with radiosurgery of large acoustic neuromas. *Surg Neurol, 59*(4), 283-289; discussion 289-291

Litvack, Z. N., Noren, G., Chougule, P. B., & Zheng, Z. (2003). Preservation of functional hearing after gamma knife surgery for vestibular schwannoma. *Neurosurgical focus, 14*(5), e3

Lomax, N. J., & Scheib, S. G. (2003). Quantifying the degree of conformity in radiosurgery treatment planning. *Int J Radiat Oncol Biol Phys, 55*(5), 1409-1419

Massager, N., Lonneville, S., Delbrouck, C., Benmebarek, N., Desmedt, F., & Devriendt, D. (2011). Dosimetric and Clinical Analysis of Spatial Distribution of the Radiation Dose in Gamma Knife Radiosurgery for Vestibular Schwannoma. *Int J Radiat Oncol Biol Phys 2011 May 27 [Epub ahead of print]*

Nakamura, J. L., Verhey, L. J., Smith, V., Petti, P. L., Lamborn, K. R., Larson, D. A., Wara, W. M., McDermott, M. W., & Sneed, P. K. (2001). Dose conformity of gamma knife radiosurgery and risk factors for complications. *Int J Radiat Oncol Biol Phys, 51*(5), 1313-1319

Nassar, S. I., & Correll, J. W. (1968). Subarachnoid hemorrhage due to spinal cord tumors. *Neurology, 18*(1 Pt 1), 87-94

Nedzi, L. A., Kooy, H. M., Alexander, E., 3rd, Svensson, G. K., & Loeffler, J. S. (1993). Dynamic field shaping for stereotactic radiosurgery: a modeling study. *Int J Radiat Oncol Biol Phys, 25*(5), 859-869

Niranjan, A., Lunsford, L. D., Flickinger, J. C., Maitz, A., & Kondziolka, D. (1999). Can hearing improve after acoustic tumor radiosurgery? *Neurosurg Clin N Am, 10*(2), 305-315

Noren, G. (1998). Long-term complications following gamma knife radiosurgery of vestibular schwannomas. *Stereotact Funct Neurosurg, 70 Suppl 1*, 65-73

Paddick, I. (2000). A simple scoring ratio to index the conformity of radiosurgical treatment plans. Technical note. *Journal of neurosurgery, 93 Suppl 3*, 219-222

Paddick, I., & Lippitz, B. (2006). A simple dose gradient measurement tool to complement the conformity index. *J Neurosurg, 105 Suppl*, 194-201

Park, C. K., Jung, H. W., Kim, J. E., Son, Y. J., Paek, S. H., & Kim, D. G. (2006). Therapeutic strategy for large vestibular schwannomas. *J Neurooncol, 77*(2), 167-171

Park, K., Hwang, S. K., Park, S. H., Park, J., Hwang, J. H., & Park, Y. M. (2009). Changes of hydrocephalus after gamma knife radiosurgery in patients with vestibular schwannoma: A comparison with microsurgery. *J Korean Brain Tumor Soc, 8*(2), 126-130

Pirouzmand, F., Tator, C. H., & Rutka, J. (2001). Management of hydrocephalus associated with vestibular schwannoma and other cerebellopontine angle tumors. *Neurosurgery, 48*(6), 1246-1253; discussion 1253-1244

Pollock, B. E., Lunsford, L. D., Kondziolka, D., Flickinger, J. C., Bissonette, D. J., Kelsey, S. F., & Jannetta, P. J. (1995). Outcome analysis of acoustic neuroma management: a comparison of microsurgery and stereotactic radiosurgery. *Neurosurgery, 36*(1), 215-224; discussion 224-219

Prasad, D. (2001). Vestibular schwannomas: radiosurgery. *J Neurosurg, 94*(1), 141-142

Regis, J., Tamura, M., Delsanti, C., Roche, P. H., Pellet, W., & Thomassin, J. M. (2008). Hearing preservation in patients with unilateral vestibular schwannoma after gamma knife surgery. *Prog Neurol Surg, 21*, 142-151

Roche, P. H., Khalil, M., Soumare, O., & Regis, J. (2008). Hydrocephalus and vestibular schwannomas: considerations about the impact of gamma knife radiosurgery. *Prog Neurol Surg, 21*, 200-206

Rogg, J. M., Ahn, S. H., Tung, G. A., Reinert, S. E., & Noren, G. (2005). Prevalence of hydrocephalus in 157 patients with vestibular schwannoma. *Neuroradiology, 47*(5), 344-351

Rowe, J. G., Radatz, M. W., Walton, L., Hampshire, A., Seaman, S., & Kemeny, A. A. (2003a). Gamma knife stereotactic radiosurgery for unilateral acoustic neuromas. *J Neurol Neurosurg Psychiatry, 74*(11), 1536-1542

Rowe, J. G., Radatz, M. W., Walton, L., Hampshire, A., Seaman, S., & Kemeny, A. A. (2003b). Gamma knife stereotactic radiosurgery for unilateral acoustic neuromas. *Journal of neurology, neurosurgery, and psychiatry, 74*(11), 1536-1542

Samii, M., Gerganov, V., & Samii, A. (2008). Hearing preservation after complete microsurgical removal in vestibular schwannomas. *Prog Neurol Surg, 21*, 136-141

Samii, M., & Matthies, C. (1997a). Management of 1000 vestibular schwannomas (acoustic neuromas): hearing function in 1000 tumor resections. *Neurosurgery, 40*(2), 248-260; discussion 260-242

Samii, M., & Matthies, C. (1997b). Management of 1000 vestibular schwannomas (acoustic neuromas): surgical management and results with an emphasis on complications and how to avoid them. *Neurosurgery, 40*(1), 11-21; discussion 21-13

Samii, M., Matthies, C., & Tatagiba, M. (1997). Management of vestibular schwannomas (acoustic neuromas): auditory and facial nerve function after resection of 120 vestibular schwannomas in patients with neurofibromatosis 2. *Neurosurgery, 40*(4), 696-705; discussion 705-696

Sawamura, Y., Shirato, H., Sakamoto, T., Aoyama, H., Suzuki, K., Onimaru, R., Isu, T., Fukuda, S., & Miyasaka, K. (2003). Management of vestibular schwannoma by fractionated stereotactic radiotherapy and associated cerebrospinal fluid malabsorption. *J Neurosurg, 99*(4), 685-692

Shaw, E., Kline, R., Gillin, M., Souhami, L., Hirschfeld, A., Dinapoli, R., & Martin, L. (1993). Radiation Therapy Oncology Group: radiosurgery quality assurance guidelines. *Int J Radiat Oncol Biol Phys, 27*(5), 1231-1239

Staecker, H., Nadol, J. B., Jr., Ojeman, R., Ronner, S., & McKenna, M. J. (2000). Hearing preservation in acoustic neuroma surgery: middle fossa versus retrosigmoid approach. *Am J Otol, 21*(3), 399-404

Tamura, M., Carron, R., Yomo, S., Arkha, Y., Muraciolle, X., Porcheron, D., Thomassin, J. M., Roche, P. H., & Regis, J. (2009). Hearing preservation after gamma knife radiosurgery for vestibular schwannomas presenting with high-level hearing. *Neurosurgery, 64*(2), 289-296; discussion 296

Timmer, F. C., Hanssens, P. E., van Haren, A. E., Mulder, J. J., Cremers, C. W., Beynon, A. J., van Overbeeke, J. J., & Graamans, K. (2009). Gamma knife radiosurgery for vestibular schwannomas: results of hearing preservation in relation to the cochlear radiation dose. *Laryngoscope, 119*(6), 1076-1081

van der Jagt, M., Hasan, D., Dippel, D. W., van Dijk, E. J., Avezaat, C. J., & Koudstaal, P. J. (2009). Impact of early surgery after aneurysmal subarachnoid haemorrhage. *Acta Neurol Scand, 119*(2), 100-106

Wackym, P. A., Runge-Samuelson, C. L., Nash, J. J., Poetker, D. M., Albano, K., Bovi, J., Michel, M. A., Friedland, D. R., Zhu, Y. R., & Hannley, M. T. (2010). Gamma knife surgery of vestibular schwannomas: volumetric dosimetry correlations to hearing loss suggest stria vascularis devascularization as the mechanism of early hearing loss. *Otol Neurotol, 31*(9), 1480-1487

Woo, H. J., Hwang, S. K., Park, S. H., Hwang, J. H., & Hamm, I. S. (2010). Factors related to the local treatment failure of gamma knife surgery for metastatic brain tumors. *Acta neurochirurgica, 152*(11), 1909-1914

5

Gamma Knife Radiosurgery in the Management of Unusual Grade I/II Primitive Neuroepithelial Tumours of the Brain

A. Nicolato[1], M. Longhi[1], R. Foroni[2], F. Alessandrini[2], A. De Simone[1], C. Ghimenton[2], A. De Carlo[1], P. Mirtuono[3] and M. Gerosa[1]

Multidisciplinary Neurooncologic Group of Verona,
[1]Department of Neurological Sciences
[2]Department of Pathology and Diagnosis
[3]Department of Neurological, Neuropsychological, Morphological and Movement Sciences
Section Anatomy, University Hospital (AOUI) of Verona, Italy

1. Introduction

Now, Gamma Knife radiosurgery (GKRS) is considered a first choice therapeutic option in a wide setting of malignant and benign intracranial diseases. Particularly, the application of GKRS in pilocytic (GI) and diffuse (GII) astrcytomas, which currently represent the most frequent brain neoplasms in children and young adults, has been often described. In the different series, the reported overall tumor growth control (TGC) varies between 50%-100%, the Overal Survival (OS) is 78.6%-100% with a 5-year local progression free survival (PFS) comprised between 88.9% and 97.4%. The GKRS-related permanent neurologic morbidity is generally less then 5% (0%-7%) (Kano et al., 2009a; Kano et al., 2009b; Boethius et al., 2002; Hadjipanayis et al., 2002a; Hadjipanayis et al., 2002b; Kida et al., 2000; Simonova et al., 2005; Heppner et al., 2005). Therefore, GKRS is considered an effective and safe therapeutic tool in the multidisciplinary treatment of pilocytic and diffuse astrcytomas, as well. Nevertheless, the effectiveness of GKRS is much less known as concerns other unusual Low-Grade Primitive Neuroepithelial Tumors (LGPNTs) of the brain because data regarding the long-term efficacy of GKRS on a large series of patients with such tumors is lacking. The aim of this chapter is to assess the value of GKRS in the management of such cerebral tumors. The interest of this study is founded on several observations: 1) unusual LGPNTs are rare tumours; there are a few series with at least ten reported cases, only (Hasegawa et al., 2002; Kim et al., 2007); 2) these tumors are frequently deep-seated in the brain or located in functional cerebral regions, thus gross total surgical removal may often be highly risky or impossible sometimes; 3) unusual LGPNTs are more frequent in children and young adult patients (Reyns et al., 2006; Yen et al., 2007). Furthermore, the management of residual, recurrent or unresectable tumours represent a challenge for neurosurgeons and neurooncologists due to: 1) histotypes with frequently high radio- and chemo-resistance; 2) high risk of permanent delayed brain tissue radiation damage in often very young patients and with long life expectancy. The reason behind the increased use of GKRS in unusual LGPNTs, also, is that the highly conformal treatment planning possible with this technique allows delivery of citotoxic dose of radiation to the target field while minimazing the dose delivered to neighboring vital structures. Hence, radiosurgery may be a less morbid alternative for treating deep-seated or functional-located lesions surrounded by eloquent structures. It therefore becomes possible to avoid toxic systemic side effects due to less effective antiblastic drugs, to preserve neurological function, to prevent further tumor growth and/or reinterventions in residual or recurrent tumors with remarkably low risks of acute radiation injury or delayed radiation therapy (RT)-related sequelae. In this chapter, the results of a retrospective study on 30 unusual LGPNTs of the brain treated with GKRS and followed up for at least 2 years will be presented and discussed. The end-points of this study will regard the OS, overall local TGC, actuarial Survival and local PFS (on the whole series and evaluated on different histologies) rates, and GKRS-related permanent side effects. Furthermore, a statistical analysis concerning the identification of potential prognostic factors influencing post-GKRS OS and local PFS among some selected independent variables will be performed, as well.

2. Materials and methods

2.1 Overall series

Between February 1993 and February 2009, GKRS was performed on 30 patients (Table 1) with unusual LGPNTs of the brain (Grade I-II according to the WHO classification) (Louis et al., 2007). Inclusion criteria for GKRS included: lesions deep-seated in the brain or located in eloquent regions, histology confirmation, residual or recurrent tumors, tumor volume (TV) less than 15 cc, conditions of high operative risk, and patient refusal of microsurgery or reoperation.

Histology	N° Pt M/F	Age yr Mean (Range)	Surgery /Biopsy	TV cc Mean (Range)	Pre-GK Treats.
Overall series	16/14	38.4 (7-70)	20/10	4.9 (0.7-14.5)	2 RT 1 RT+Ch
Pineocytoma	5/5	31.5 (7-58)	6/4	5.0 (0.8-11.7)	1 RT
CPP	6/2	44.2 (22-70)	5/3	3.7 (0.7-9.9)	1 RT
CN	1/3	33.2 (21-43)	4/0	6.5 (3.7-9.0)	None
PXA	1/2	48.0 (28-64)	2/1	7.3 (2.3-14.5)	None
Miscellaneous: Ganglioglioma Subependymoma Oligoastrocytoma Papillary Gl. Tum.	2/3	19,2 (11-24)	3/2	3.7 (0.7-11.3)	1 RT+Ch

N° Pt = number of treated patients; yr = year; TV = tumor volume; cc = cubic cm; Pre-GK Treats. = pre-gamma knife treatments; M = male; F = female; RT = radiotherapy; Ch = chemotherapy; Papillary Gl. Tum. = papillary glioneuronal tumor.

Table 1. Summary of clinical characteristics of 30 unusual LGPNTs treated with GKRS at University Hospital of Verona from February 1993 to February 2009.

The histologic types and grading were as follows: 10 pineocytomas (Grade I), 8 choroid plexus papillomas (CPP) (Grade I), 4 central neurocytomas (CN) (Grade II), 3 pleomorphic xanthoastrocytomas (PXA) (Grade II), 2 gangliogliomas (Grade I), 1 subependymoma (Grade I), 1 papillary glioneuronal tumor (Grade I), and 1 mixed oligoastrocytoma (Grade II). All tumors were histologically verified: 20/30 (67%) were surgical residuals or post-operative recurrences, while biopsy confirmed the diagnosis in the remaining 10/30 cases: 4 (13%) during neuroendoscopy approach and 6 (20%) with stereotactic brain intervention. There were 16 males and 14 females; the mean age of the clinical series was 34.7 years (7-70 years). Further pre-GKRS treatments were as follows: RT alone, 2/30 patients (7%), and RT followed by chemotherapy, 1/30 (3%). The TV was always less than 15 cc. In 24/30 patients, pre-GKRS neurologic deficits were documented. The mean and range values of the radiosurgical dose planning parameters are summarized in Table 2.

Histology		Dose Plan Mean	Parameters (Range)	
	PD Gy	PI %	ID mJ	# Shots
Overall series	16.5 (12-22.4)	50.2 (40-70)	104 (11.4-257.4)	9.6 (1-25)
Pineocytoma	16.7 (13-20)	50.5 (50-55)	110.1 (18.9-257.4)	13.9 (5-25)
CPP	15.1 (12-20.2)	48.7 (45-50)	72.9 (11.4.189.7)	7.1 (3-11)
CN	16.4 (14-18)	47.5 (40-50)	151.6 (84.2-185.4)	7.0 (5-10)
PXA	17.0 (13-20)	50.0 (50-50)	152.1 (69.6-248.5)	10.3 (2-25)
Miscellaneous: Ganglioglioma Subependymoma Oligoastrocytoma Papillary Gl.Tum.	18.2 (12.5-22.4)	54.0 (50-70)	74.4 (19.8-191.09	6.8 (1-16)

PD = prescription dose; Gy = gray; PI = prescription isodose; ID = integral dose; mJ = milli Joule;
# Shots = number of isocenters.

Table 2. Summary of radiosurgical parameters of 30 unusual LGPNTs treated with GKRS at University Hospital of Verona from February 1993 to February 2009.

The mean prescription dose (PD) was 16.5 Gy while the mean prescription isodose (PI) corresponded to 50.2%. The average value of integral dose (ID), parameter which describes the relationship between treated TV and delivered dose appropriately, was 104 mJ. The mean number of shots needed for dose planning was 9.6. Follow-up data, including causes of death, were obtained from hospital notes, imaging studies, and contact with relatives and family physicians. Medical records and MRI scans for all patients were carefully reviewed by neurosurgeons and neuroradiologists. This retrospective study was approved by the Ethical Commetee of our University Hospital. All patients identifiers were removed before data analysis.

2.1.1 Pineocytoma

In the group of pineocytoma, 7 out of 10 patients were young adults, under 40-year-old. Diagnosis was confirmed by bioptic samples harvest during a neuroendoscopic procedure in 4 cases. In the other histologic groups, there were no patients in whom the histologic diagnosis was achieved following a neuroendoscopic intervention. The treated TV was always inferiour to 12 cc (mean, 5.0 cc). Only a 58-year-old woman, operated on in another institution, underwent RT following incomplete surgical removal. Neurologic deficits were present in 9/10 patients at the moment of GKRS. The 10 pineocytoma tumors were administered a radiosurgical dose comprised between 13 and 20 Gy with a mean PI of 50.5% and a mean ID of 110.1 mJ. The dose plannings for pineocytoma were particularly conformal as documented by the higher mean number of utilized isocenters (13.9) compared to the mean number of shots employed in the other histologic groups.

2.1.2 Choroid plexus papilloma (CPP)

The mean age in this group of patients was 44.2 years and most cases were males. The tumors were located in the following sites: 2 cerebellum, 2 ponto-cerebellar angle, 1 basal ganglia, 1 brain stem, 1 pineal region, and 1 skull base. Diagnosis was achieved by surgical intervention in 5 out of 8 cases. The TV treated with GKRS was always small, mean 3.7 cc, inferiour to the means of all the other histologic types of our series. In a 25-year-old man, two operations where performed before GKRS: the last histological examination confirmed a grade I CPP. Only in one case, RT was performed after partial surgical resection and before GKRS. All the patients complaint neurologic symptoms at last evaluation prior to GKRS. From the radiosurgical point of view, the mean PD and ID were lower than those of all the other histologic groups of our series, probably due to the highly critical brain location of most of these tumors.

2.1.3 Central neurocytoma (CN)

The mean age was 33.2 years. The tumor location was in the lateral ventricles in 2 cases, and one case in the basal ganglia and in the occipital lobe, respectively. Histologic diagnosis was defined by means of surgical intervention in all neoplasms. In 2 out of 4 patients, the pre-GKRS neurologic evaluation was negative. The mean TV treated with radiosurgery was 6.5 cc. None of the patients underwent to other treatments prior to GKRS. The mean PD and ID were 16.4 Gy and 151.6 mJ, respectively.

2.1.4 Pleomorphic xanthoastrocyroma (PXA)

Mean age and TV treated with GKRS (48.0 years and 7.3 cc, respectively) in this group of patients were higher than in the other groups of our series. Tumor lacations were as follows: 1 brain stem, 1 temporal, and 1 temporo-occipital. In 2 cases, diagnosis was achieved by surgical intervention. In a 28-year old man affected with cystic right temporo-occipital PXA, a double stereotactic procedure was performed in the same neurosurgical session (Figure 1): first, an Ommaya reservoir was inserted for cyst aspiration; secondly, a biopsy of the tumor solid nodule for histopathological diagnosis definition was performed preceeded by changing of stereotactic coordinates and trajectory. All patients were symptomatic at the time of radiosurgery. No other treatment before GKRS was performed. Mean PD and ID delivered were higher than in the other groups of our series (17.0 Gy and 152.1 mJ, respectively).

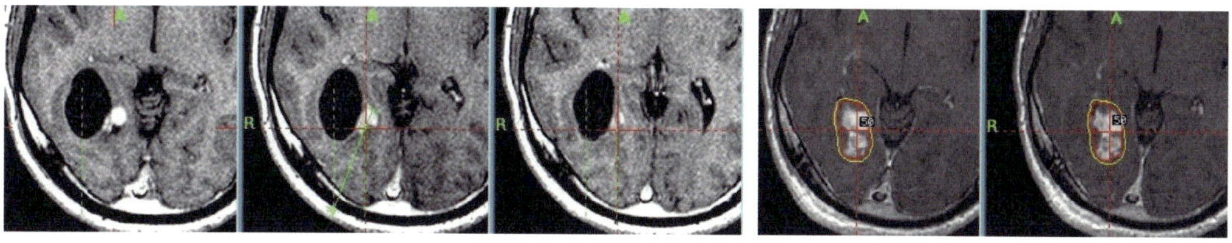

A B

Fig. 1. A) 28-year old man with cystic temporo-occipital PXA. Calculation of stereotactic coordinates and trajectory for Ommaya reservoir insertion and tumor nodule biopsy. B) GKRS dose planning performed on shrinkaged tumor 10 days after double stereotactic intervention.

2.1.5 Others (Miscellaneous)

This group of patients included 2 gangliogliomas (Grade I), 1 subependymoma (Grade I), 1 papillary glioneuronal tumor (Grade I), and 1 mixed oligoastrocytoma (Grade II). The mean age (19.2 years) was lower than in all the other groups. There were 2 males and 3 females. The tumor sites were as follows: 2 deep frontal, 1 basal ganglia, 1 occipital, and 1 third ventricle. There were 3 pre-GKRS surgical interventions and 2 stereotactic brain biopsies. In 3 out of 5 patients, neurologic examination resulted negative on the day of radiosurgery. The mean TV treated with GKRS was 3.7 cc. A 24-year-old woman underwent stereotactic brain biopsy for a left frontal deep-seated tumor in another institution. Histologic diagnosis was grade II mixed oligoastrocytoma and a treatment protocol of RT and chemo-therapy was performed successively. In this group, the mean selected PI (54%) was higher than in all the other patient of our series.

2.2 Radiosurgical technique and procedure

Our radiosurgical technique was already described in detail in previous reports (Lunsford et al., 1989, Nicolato et al., 1997). In brief, after the application of the magnetic resonance imaging (MRI) compatible Leksell Model G stereotactic frame (Elekta Instruments AB, Stockholm, Sweden) to the patient's head, high resolution 1.0 Tesla MRI was performed in all cases. Millimetric volumetric images in axial and coronal orthogonal planes after gadolinium enhancement were used. First a sagittal MRI localizer or a 3-D scout survey (which included axial, coronal and sagittal images) were performed. Contrast enhanced Spoiled Gradient Recalled Acquisition in Steady State (SPGR) sequence was then used to image the tumor and surrounding brain. T2 weighted MR images using Fast Spin Echo technique also were acquired to assess the infiltrative tumor volume. The target volume included enhanced and non-enhanced tumor regions. Three-dimensional dose plans were developed by using commercially available software, i.e., Kula (Elekta Instruments) from February 1993 to February 1998 and Leksell Gamma Plan (versions 4.12, 5.34 and 8.3, Elekta Instruments) after February 1998. The neurological surgeon, radiation oncologist, and medical physicist created a highly conformal dose planning using multiple collimators and performed the dose selection. In all patients, the radiosurgery dose was prescribed to the entire tumor volume as defined using contrast enhanced imaging. GKRS was performed with either Model B, C 201-source Co60, or Perfexion Leksell Gamma Knife (Elekta Instruments). The procedure was performed under local anesthesia in 28/30 patients;

general anesthesia was administered in the two children younger than 14. All patients were discharged from the hospital within 24 hours after treatment, and they were evaluated clinically and with serial contrast-enhanced imaging using MRI at intervals of 6 months. The neurological status of the patient during the follow-up period was defined as no deficit pre-GKRS, if the patient were without deficits before radiosurgery and remained clinically negative, improved, in case of complaint amelioration, stable or worsened. For the evaluation of TV, the mass lesion was measured by using the Gamma Plan software or the OsiriX medical imaging program (version 4.19) developed at the University Hospital of Geneva, Switzerland. Local TGC was defined as complete disappearance of enhancing and nonenhancing neoformation, lesion shrinkage or stable disease.

2.3 Statistical analysis

Survival and local PFS curves were calculated using the life-table system and the Kaplan-Meier method (Kaplan & Meier, 1958). Length of survival and local PFS were evaluated on an actuarial basis from the day of GKRS treatment to the time of patient death or tumor progression and/or last follow-up, respectively. Survival and local PFS curves were compared and evaluated using Breslaw's test (Breslaw,1974). We performed an univariate analysis using the log-rank test to detect variables that might influence the length of survival and local PFS. We matched the survival with four different variables, age, sex (male vs. female), histologic type (pineocytoma vs. choroid plexus papilloma vs. central neurocytoma vs. pleomorphic xanthoastrocytoma vs. miscellaneuos), prior surgical resection vs. biopsy, and the local PFS with seven different parameters, age, sex (male vs. female), histologic type (pineocytoma vs. choroid plexus papilloma vs. central neurocytoma vs. pleomorphic xanthoastrocytoma vs. miscellaneuos), prior surgical resection vs. biopsy, prescription dose, integral dose and length of follow-up. In Table 5, the statistical comparison between parameters in the different groups of patients were based on the Welch Modified Two-Sample t-Test. On the basis of internationally accepted criteria, values of $P \leq 0.05$ were considered statistically significant. Statistical analysis was effected using the Stata version 8.2 (StataCorp, College Station, Texas) and MATLAB for graphics.

3. Results

3.1 Overall series

The results of our series are summarized in Tables 3 and 4. The median duration of follow-up was 66.8 months (range, 24.7-195.97 months). At the end of the study, February 28th, 2009, the neurologic examination remained negative or showed an improvement of previous deficits in 16 patients, in 8 cases the complaints were stable and in the other 6 a worsening due to tumor progression was observed. Among these last patients, four were deceased. The cause of death was related to distant tumour progression in 2 cases and both to local and distant disease diffusion in the other 2 cases. The overall survival was 87%, and the actuarial survival rate at 5 and 10 years was 90% and 87%, respectively (Figure 2A). The median survival in the 4 patients who died was 50 months (range, 24.7-73 months) from GKRS. The local TGC was achieved in 27/30 (90%) tumors with a 91% local actuarial PFS both at 5 and 10 years (Figure 2B). The median time to progression for the three patients with uncontrolled tumor was 18.5 months (range, 9.8-26.7 months). No GKRS-related permanent side-effect was observed on the whole series. To date, neither malignant tumor

Histology	N° Pt	Me/Med FU mos.	Clinical Results No def./Impr	Stable	Wors.	Alive/ Dead (OS%)
Overall series	30	85.7/66.8	16/30	8/30	6‡/30	26/4¶ (87.0)
Pineocytoma	10	66.7/54.6	6/10	3/10	1/10	9/1 (90.0)
CPP	8	92.6/71.8	2/8	2/8	4/8	6/2 (75.0)
CN	4	172.0/180.6	4/4	-	-	4/0 (100.0)
PXA	3	45.6/43.7	1/3	1/3	1/3	2/1 (66.7)
Miscellaneous	5	68.0/68.3	3/5	2/5	-	5/0 (100.0)

N° Pt = number of treated patients with al least 2-year-follow-up; Me = Mean; Med = Median; mos. = months; No def./Impr = No pre-GK neurological deficit/Neurological improvement; Wors. = Neurological worsening; OS = Overall survival.
‡: due to tumor distant progression in 4 cases and both to local and distant tumor diffusion in the other 2 patients.
¶: the cause of death was tumor distant progression in 2 cases and both local and distant tumor diffusion in the other 2 patients.

Table 3. Summary of clinical results concerning 30 LGPNTs treated with GKRS at University Hospital of Verona from February 1993 to February 2009.

Histology	Act. Surv. % At 5y	At 10y	Ov. TGC%	Act. Local PFS% At 5y	At 10y	GK-related sequelae Mort.	Perm Compl	Post-GK treats.
Overall series	90.0	87.0	90.0	91.0	91.0	0.0	0.0	3 surg.int. 1 VPS 3 RT
Pineocytoma	92.0	92.0	100.0	100.0	100.0	0.0	0.0	1 RT
CPP	90.0	80.0	87.5	90.0	90.0	0.0	0.0	1 surg.int. 1 RT
CN	100.0	100.0	75.0	83.0	83.0	0.0	0.0	1 surg.int. 1 RT
PXA	80.0	80.0	66.7	80.0	80.0	0.0	0.0	1 VPS
Miscellaneous	100.0	100.0	100.0	100.0	100.0	0.0	0.0	1 surg.int.

Act. Surv. = Actuarial survival; Ov. TGC = Overall tumor growth control; Act. Local PFS = Actuarial local progression-free survival; Mort. = Mortality; Perm. Compl = Permanent Complications; Post-GK treats. = Post-GK treatments; surg.int. = surgical intervention; VPS = Ventricolo-peritoneal shunt; RT = Radiation therapy.

Table 4. Summary of outcome results concerning 30 LGPNTs treated with GKRS at University Hospital of Verona from February 1993 to February 2009.

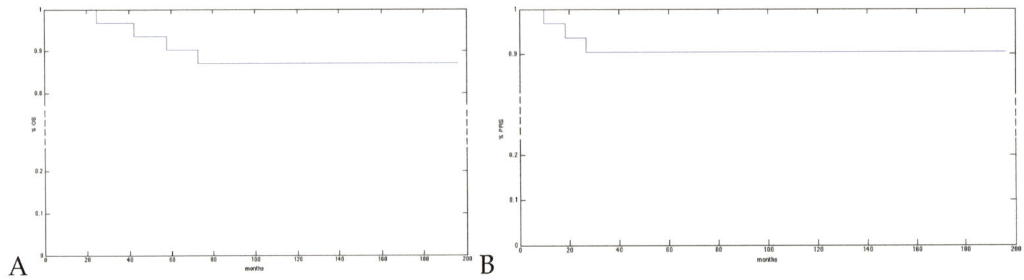

Fig. 2. Kaplan-Meier estimate of A) overall survival and B) local PFS curves in 30 LGPNTs.

transformation nor GKRS-related mortality were registered. Post-GKRS treatments were represented by: 3 surgical removals, 1 ventriculo-peritoneal shunt and 3 fractionated irradiations. No chemotherapy treatment was performed on the whole series after GKRS. All variables tested at univariate analysis on the whole series did not show a statistically significant influence either as concerns survival or local PFS rates. In particular, the different histological type analized did not seem to have prognostic significance, as well (Figures 3A and 3B). Therefore, multivariate analysis was not performed. Nevertheless, a positive trend for PD and ID seems to emerge from statistical analysis (Table 5): in the 3 patients with local progression, the mean dose delivered to the periphery of the neoplasms was lower

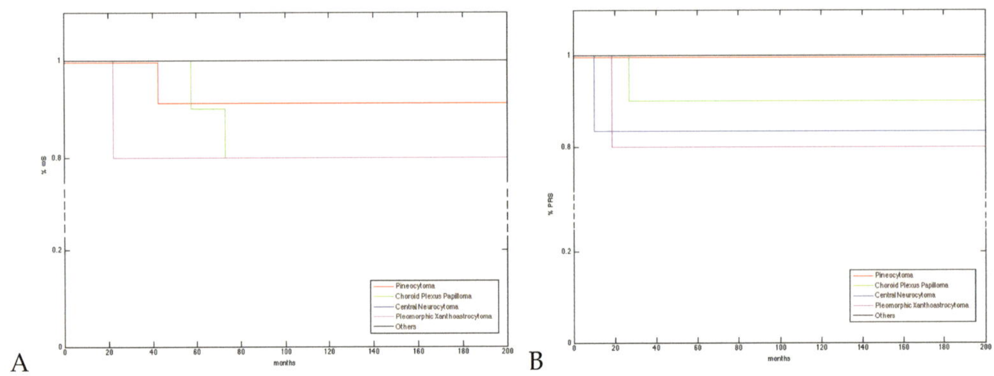

Fig. 3. Kaplan-Meier estimate of A) overall survival and B) local PFS curves after GKRS for histologic types (P = NS).

GKRS outcome	N° Pt	Mean TV (cc)	P value	Mean PD (Gy)	P value	Mean ID (mJ)	P value
Local TGC	27	4.61		16.8		98.74	
			<0.55		= 0.138		= 0.141
Local Progr.	3	7.30		14.0		151.1	

N° Pt = number of treated patients; TV = tumor volume; cc = cubic cm; PD = prescription dose; Gy = gray; ID = integral dose; mJ = milli Joule.

Table 5. statistical comparison between radiosurgical outcome and TV, PD, and ID in 30 LGPNTs treated with GKRS.

(14.0 Gy) than that of the 27 tumors with local TGC (16.8 Gy), and the mean ID was higher (151.1 mJ) compared to that of the group under control (98.74 mJ). Because the ID is the result of volume multiplied by average dose, we evaluated the mean TV between the groups of patients with under control vs. progressed neoplasms, as well. The 3 patients with tumor progression presented a mean TV of 7.3 cc versus 4.6 cc of the tumors with favourable response. Even though the statistical analysis did not shaw significant results, the considerable difference of the two mean TV values authorizes to think that a possible correlation between TV and local TGC after GKRS could be proposed. Finally, it must be considered that the small number of observations might represent a bias for the statistical analysis.

3.2 Pineocytoma

In this group of patients, the median observation time was 54.6 months (range, 25.3-130.0 months). On last follow-up day, 9 out of 10 patients were neurologically stable or improved (Table 3); only a 16-year-old boy worsened because of distant tumor progression and underwent post-GKRS RT, but unfortunately he died at 42 months from radiosurgery (OS, 90%). All the other patients did not needed further treatments following GKRS. In the whole ten pineocytomas of our series, local TGC was achieved (overall TGC, 100%) (Figure 4). The 5 and 10 year actuarial survival and local TGC were 92% and 100%, respectively (Table 4).

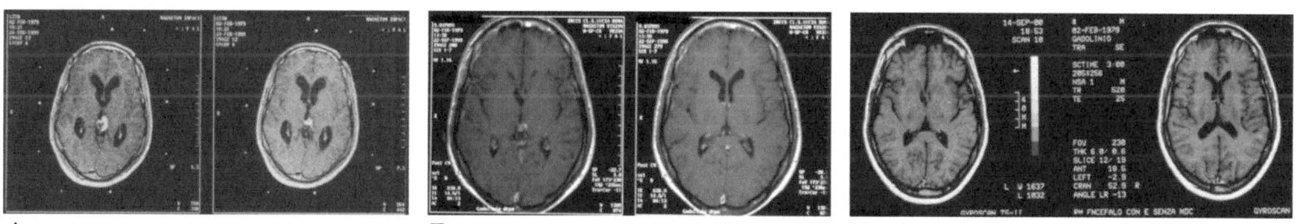

A B C

Fig. 4. A) Posterior III ventricle pineocytoma on GKRS day. The diagnosis was achieved by means of stereotactic neuroendoscopy biopsy. B) MR imaging follow-up at 3 months and C) at 18 months from GKRS showing the gradual disappearance of the tumor.

3.3 Choroid plexus papilloma (CPP)

The 8 patients of this group were followed-up for 71.8-month median time. A neurologic deterioration was observed in 4 patients: in 3 cases, due to tumor distant progression, and in 1 both to local and distant progression. During the follow-up period, 2 of these last patients died: 1 because of tumor distant progression and 1 due to local and distant progression (OS, 75%). The 5- and 10-year actuarial survival rates were 90% and 80%, respectively. Local TGC was reported in 7 patients (87.5%), with an actuarial local TGC of 90% both at 5- and 10-years. The 2 patients with distant progression refused further treatments: one of them is died at 57.7 months from GKRS, and the other is still alive with mild neurologic deficits 181.7 months after radiosurgery. The treatments performed after GKRS were surgical intervention for local tumor progression in one case and RT in another patient with distant progression.

3.4 Central neurocytoma (CN)

The median follow-up period was 180.6 months (range, 142.7-183.9 months). At last observation, all patients were neurologically intact or clinically improved. The OS and the 5-

and 10-year actuarial survival rates were 100% (Table 4). The local TGC was achieved in 3 out of 4 cases (75%) and the actuarial local TGC was 83% both at 5- and 10-years. In a 26-year-old woman with a TV at radiosurgery of 9.0 cc was decided to associate RT after GKRS. She is alive and well at 177.3 months from radiosurgery. A surgical intervention was needed in a 21-year-old man because of local progression of an intraventricular residual tumor at 9.8 months after GKRS. He underwent radiosurgery for a 5.9 cc neoplasm and the administered PD was 14.0 Gy, the lowest value than in all the other patients treated for central neurocytoma.

3.5 Pleomorphic xanthoastrocyroma (PXA)

The median follow-up time in this group of patients was 43.7 months (range, 25.1-70.9 months). At the end of the study, one patient showed an improvement of the neulogic complaints, the second was clinically stable and the third presented a gradual deterioration due to a brain stem tumor progression and died 25.1 months after GKRS. This patient was already operated prior to radiosurgery. She refused further RT and the only possible treatment was VPS. In this group, the OS and the local TGC rates were 66.7% and the actuarial survival and local TGC rates were 80% both at 5- and 10-years (Figure 5).

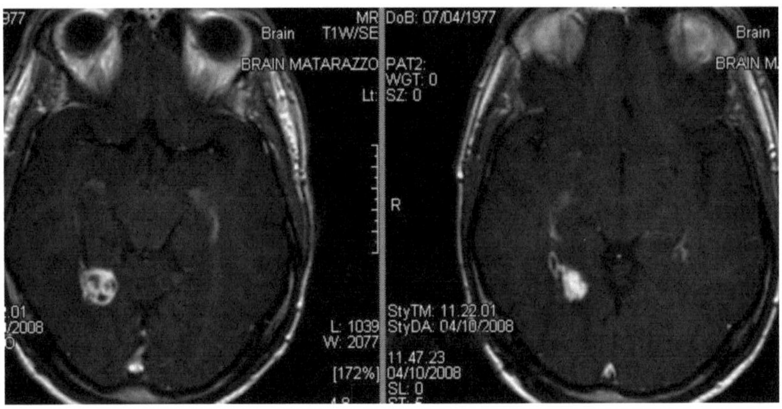

Fig. 5. Same case than in figures 1. MRI follow up at 32 months from GKRS showing a significant tumor reduction.

3.6 Others (Miscellaneous)

The median period of follow-up was 68.3 months (range, 27.5-109 months). All patients in this heterogeneous group of unusual LGPNTs showed a negative, improved or stable neurological status at last observation (OS 100%), with an actuarial survival rate at 5- and 10-years of 100% and 100%, respectively. All tumors treated with GKRS were under control (Table 4). A 24-year-old woman affected with a grade II mixed oligoastrocytoma and treated prior to radiosurgery with RT and chemotharapy elsewhere developed an expansive lesion with mass effect in left frontal region, far from the target volume treated with GKRS. Surgical removal was needed and histologic examination showed that it deals with radionecrosis, secondary to the previous RT. Now, she is well at 68.3 months from radiosurgery. She was the only patient in this group who needed a further treatment after GKRS.

4. Discussion

4.1 Overall series

Several series describing the results of stereotactic radiosurgery on LGPNTs of the brain including a large number of patients have been reported. However, they always dealt with low-grade gliomas. Kida (Kida et al., 2000) and Heppner (Heppner et al., 2005) presented their experience with GKRS on 51 and 49 patients with grade I and II astrocytomas, respectively. Hadjipanayis (Hadjipanayis et al., 2002a) treated 37 pilocytic astrocytomas of every age, and, more recently, Kano (Kano et al., 2009b) described the outcome following GKRS in 50 pilocytic astrocytomas in pediatric age, exclusively. Simonova (Simonova et al., 2005) reported a series of 70 cases including different types of grade I and II gliomas in whom stereotactic radiosurgery was applied. Sarkar (Sarkar et al., 2002) and Kano (Kano et al., 2009c) reported two GKRS studies on 18 and 30 patients affected with oligodendrogliomas and mixed oligodendroastrocytomas, respectively, but both series included low- and high-grade tumors. As concerns the unusual primitive neuroepithelial tumors of the brain, the largest published series always comprised low- and high-grade tumors (Kano et al., 2009d, Mori et al., 2009, Lekovic et al., 2007, Hasegawa et al., 2002, Kobayashi et al., 2001), while the studies with exclusively unusual LGPNTs were always represented by a few cases (usually, less than 15). To our knowledge, the work of our team represent the largest series of unusual LGPNTs treated with stereotactic radiosurgery. In a study performed on 10 patients (8 pineocytoamas, 1 CPP, and 1 CN), Lekovic (Lekovic et al., 2007) reported an overall survival of 90%, a 100% local TGC, with neither GKRS-related mortality nor permanent morbidity. But, the patients were observed for a median period of less than 2 years (20.5 months). Our results obtained on 30 patients followed up for at least 2 years (median, 66.8 months; range, 24.7-195.97 months) confirmed this excellent outcome. In brief, the 5- and 10-year actuarial survival rates were 90% and 87%, respectively, with a 91% actuarial local PFS both at 5- and 10-year. The median time to progression for the three patients with uncontrolled tumor was 18.5 months and the median survival in the 4 patients who died was 50 months. In 2 of them, the cause of death was exclusively due to tumor distant progression. Also in our series, no complications were attributable to GKRS. The only study on a series of LGPNTs in which was performed an analysis of potential prognostic factors influencing GKRS outcome is referred to Sarkar (Sarkar et al., 2002). The authors studied a series of 18 patients with 21 tumors - 10 oligodendrogliomas and 11 mixed oligoastrocytomas - and found that factors associated with an improved survival rate included younger age and smaller tumors. In our series, univariate analysis on selected independent variables did not show any factors of significance. Nevertheless, we observed that patients with local TGC presented a smaller mean TV (4.61 cc vs. 7.0 cc), a higher mean PD (16.8 Gy vs. 14.0 Gy), and a lower mean ID (98.74 mJ vs. 151.1 mJ) than those with tumor progression. This trend could suggest that multisession GKRS with the Extend System (Elekta Instrument) should be better in those patients affected with larger tumors, thus achieving an increased dose delivery to the target volume maintaining a negligible risk of permanent side effects on the surrounding normal brain tissue. Some authors (Kobayashi et al., 2001, Kim et al., 2007) propose GKRS as primary treatment without histological diagnosis when a deep-seated or critically located brain tumor showing the imaging characteristics of an unusual LGPNTs is identified. On the contrary, other collegues state that obtaining a histological diagnosis remains the main aim for rational treatment planning (Matsunaga et al., 2010; Martin et al., 2003; Yen et al., 2007;

Tyler-Kabara et al., 2001; Kano et al., 2009d; Lekovic et al., 2007; Reyns et al., 2007; Dershmukh et al., 2004). In our series,all tumors were histologically verified before GKRS. We do not believe that empirical treatment of brain tumors with radiosurgery is justified, as the treatment paradigm is critically dependent upon tumor histological grade. Therefore, it is of paramount importance to achieve the histological diagnosis for decision making prior to GKRS. We suggest the use of radiosurgery as a primary treatment modality for those patients in whom an adeguate tissue diagnosis of an unusual LGPNTs has been obtained with endoscopy or stereotactic biopsy.

4.2 Pineocytoma

Pineal region tumors are rare and account for 0.4 to 1% of intracranial tumors in Western countries and for 2.2 to 8% of intracranial tumors in northeastern Asian countries (Deshmukh et al., 2004). They are 10 times more common in children than in adults. According to the statistics of the Brain Tumor Registry of Japan, pineal parenchimal tumors such as pineocytoma or pineoblastoma account for 7% of all pineal region tumors (Kobayashi et al., 2001). Individual clinical experience of these tumors is thus limited. Pineocytoma is tipically localized to the pineal area and compresses adjacent structures, including the cerebral acqueduct, brain stem and cerebellum. Their growth may extend into the third ventricle. The majority of patients exhibit neuro-ophtalmologic findings, particularly Parinaud syndromes (Grimoldi et al., 1998). MRI findings such as enhancement, calcification, and welldefined margins are suggestive of a pineocytoma but are by no means diagnostic (Chiechi et al., 1995). Therefore, tissue diagnosis is imperative. Pineocytoma is a slowly growing tumor with a relatively favorable prognosis in most cases. According to the 2007 classification, pineocytomas correspond histologically to WHO grade I. From the pathological point of view, pineocytomas tend to recapitulate the normal pineal gland (Shild et al., 1996) (Figure 6). Despite improved microsurgical technique, resection of pineocytoma

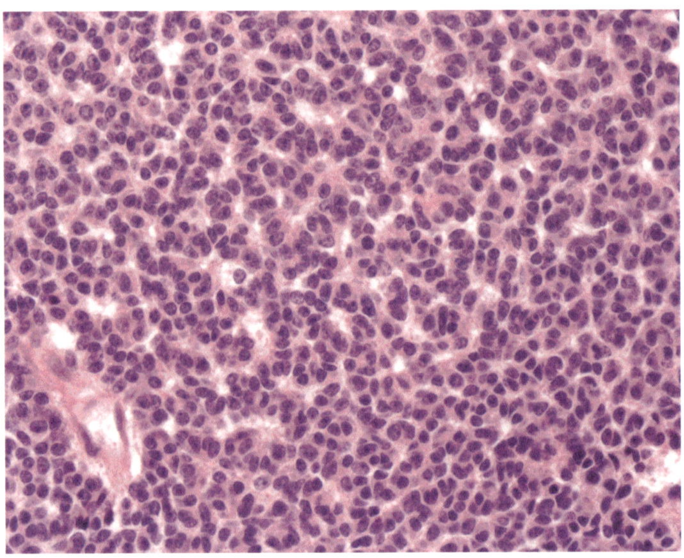

Fig. 6. Pineocytoma. X200 H-E. Classical morphological appearance of uniform cells with rosette and trabeculae.

remains a challange because of their deep location and associated critical structures. The surgical major morbidity rate associated with pineocytomas is comprised between 3% and 6.8%, and permanent minor morbidity rate was 3-28%. The risk of surgical mortality associated with pineocytoma removal has been reduced in these last 20 years, but it remains less than 2% (Friedman et al., 2001, Bruce & Ogden, 2004). The role of adjuvant RT has not been clearly delineated. Furthermore, pineacytomas are traditionally considered radioresistant tumors. For all these reasons, the use of radiosurgery in the treatment of pineocytoma is more and more growing and diffusing worldwide and studies reporting the experience of different institutions are now available (Table 6). The first and more relevant published series always regard treatment performed with GK device. The median follow-up period varies between 11.0 and 73.5 months. Neither neurological worsening nor GKRS-related permanent complications were reported. In our studies, 10 patients were followed up for a median period of 54.6 months; we observed a clinical worsening in 1 case, only, due to distant tumor progression. As concerns outcome results (Table 7), the overall survival

Author	RS dev	N° Pt	Me/Med FU mos.	Clinical Results			Sympt. Compl.	
				No def. /Impr	Stable	Wors.	Trans. %	Perm. %
Kano 2009†	GK	13	54.1 Me	66.7	-	-	23.0	0.0
Mori 2009*	GK	5	49.0/33.5	-	-	-	0.0	0.0
Lekovic 2007¶	GK	8	17.4/11.0	-	-	-	0.0	0.0
Reyns 2006	GK	7	31.7/37.0	-	-	-	-	-
Desmukh 2004¶	GK	3	19.3/12.0	-	-	-	-	-
Hasegawa 2002†	GK	10	69.1/73.5	-	-	-	10.0	0.0
Kobayashi 2001*	GK	3	21.7 Me	-	-	-	-	-
Subach 1998†	GK	8	-	-	-	-	-	-
Backlund 1974	GK	2	-	-	-	-	-	-
Present series	GK	10	66.7/54.6	6/10	3/10	1/10‡	10.0	0.0

RS dev = Radiosurgical device; N° Pt = number of treated patients; Me = Mean; Med = Median; mos. = months; No def./Impr = No pre-GK neurological deficit/Neurological improvement; Wors. = neurological worsening; Sympt. Compl. = Symptomatic complications; Trans. = transient; Perm. = Permanent; GK = Gamma Knife.

†: Departments of Neurological Surgery and Radiation Oncology, The University of Pittsburgh, and Center for Image-Guided Neurosurgery, University of Pittsburgh Medical Center, Pittsburgh, Pa., USA.

*: Nagoya Radiosurgery Center, Nagoya Kioritsu Hospital, and Gamma Knife Center, Komaki City Hospital, Komaki, Japan.

¶: Division of Neurological Surgery, Barrow Neurological Institute, St. Joseph's Hospital and Medical Center, Phoenix, Arizona, USA.

‡: due to tumor distant progression.

Table 6. Clinical data in previous and present series of pineocytomas treated with GKRS.

Author	N° Pt	Ov. Surv. %	Act. Surv. % At 5y	Act. Surv. % At 10y	Ov. Local TGC%	Act. Local PFS% At 3y	Act. Local PFS% At 5y	Act. Local PFS% At 10y
Kano 2009†	13	-	92.3	-	100.0	100.0	100.0	-
Mori 2009*	5	-	100.0	67.0	80.0	-	85.0	-
Lekovic 07¶	8	87.5	-	-	100.0	-	-	-
Reyns 2006	7	100.0	-	-	100.0	-	-	-
Desmukh 04¶	3	-	-	-	100.0	-	-	-
Hasegawa 2002†	10	90.0	-	-	100.0	-	-	-
Kobayashi 2001*	3	100.0	-	-	100.0	-	-	-
Subach 1998†	8	-	-	-	100.0	-	-	-
Backlund 1974	2	-	-	-	100.0	-	-	-
Present series	10	90.0	92.0	92.0	100.0	-	100.0	100.0

N° Pt = number of treated patients; Ov. Surv. = Overall survival; Act. Surv. = Actuarial survival; y = years; Ov. Local TGC = Overall local tumor growth control; Act. Local PFS = Actuarial local progression-free survival.
†: Departments of Neurological Surgery and Radiation Oncology, The University of Pittsburgh, and Center for Image-Guided Neurosurgery, University of Pittsburgh Medical Center, Pittsburgh, Pa., USA.
*: Nagoya Radiosurgery Center, Nagoya Kioritsu Hospital, and Gamma Knife Center, Komaki City Hospital, Komaki, Japan.
¶: Division of Neurological Surgery, Barrow Neurological Institute, St. Joseph's Hospital and Medical Center, Phoenix, Arizona, USA.

Table 7. Radiosurgical outcome in previous and present series of pineocytomas.

ranged between 87.5% and 100%. Mori (Mori et al., 2009) is the only author who reported a 10-year actuarial survival rate of 67%. In our series, the 10-year actuarial survival rate was 92%. The local TGC and PFS were excellent in all published studies. Among 5 cases with a median follow-up of 33.5 months, Mori (Mori et al., 2009) reported that the tumors were controlled in 4 cases. Only one patient developed cerebrospinal fluid dissemination after GKRS. Lekovic (Lekovic et al., 2007) described only 1 death in a series of 8 pineocytomas. The patient died 2 months after GKRS; however, MR images obtained immediately before the patient's death showed a 75% reduction in the size of the lesion. Kano (Kano et al., 2009d) reported a 5-year local PFS rate of 100% in 13 pineocytomas observed for a median period of 54.1 months. Reyns (Reyns et al., 2006) treated 8 pineocytomas and in 7 of them a follow-up period was available (median, 37.0 months). The author reported a 100% rate of overall survival and local TGC and he suggested that GKRS may represent a useful therapeutic modality in selected cases of pineal parenchymal tumours as part of a multidisciplinary approach. Our data achieved on a series with long term observation period strengthen the extremely encouraging results already published. Hence, GKRS has showed to be a valid, effective and safe treatment modality in benign tumors with critical surgical approach and considered relatively radioresistant to conventional fractionated RT, such as the pineocytoma. The excellent radiosurgical outcome is still present in long-term studies, as well. Therefore, we conclude that GKRS must be taken into account when considering the treatment management of pineocytoma, also as a primary choice in selected patients providing that a previous histopathological diagnosis is assured.

4.3 Choroid plexus papilloma (CPP)

CPPs are epithelial tumors of the choroid plexus that account for <1% of adult brain tumors (Kim et al., 2008). The majority occur within the ventricular system, the lateral ventricle being the most frequent location in children and the IVth ventricle in adults. The usual MRI findings are characterized by large, circumscribed, contrast-enhanced intraventricular tumor with occasional cyst formation and associated hydrocephalus. Tumoral calcification may be seen on plain radiographs. CPPs are slow-growing, epithelial tumors of the choroid plexus defined as grade I according to the WHO classifacation. Microsurgical resection is the preferred management for these tumors. Gross total resection is expected to be curative, with infrequent recurrence (Krishnan et al., 2004). However, complete resection is not always possible because CPPs have a deep-seated location, close proximity to critical structures (e.g. brain-stem), florid vascularity, and capacity for local invasion into underlying brain parenchyma (Krishnan et al., 2004). Furthermore, microsurgery-related permanent complications are not negligible with morbidity and mortality rates up to 25% and 16.7%, respectively (Talacchi et al., 1999). Acute postoperative complications were frequent, most notably a 22% incidence of temporary swallowing dysfunction. This condition often led to placement of a percutaneous endoscopic gastrostomy tube or tracheostomy for aspiration, or both (Krishnan et al., 2004). Therefore, additional options for treatment resistant residual or recurrent tumors are needed. Additional management options in grade I CPP include repeat surgery and RT. Krishman (Krishman et al., 2004) noted that irradiation after subtotal resection was associated with a failure of local tumor control in one half of patients. They concluded that conventional fractionated RT after initial subtotal resection did not improve outcomes. The use of stereotactic radiosurgery for CPP has been described rarely. To date, there are 9 cases reported, only (Tables 8 and 9). Duke (Duke et al., 1997) published the first case of a third-ventricle CPP who underwent radiosurgery with an excellent neurologic and imaging result. Eder (Eder et al., 2001) reported one case of CPP in pediatric age with TV shrinkage following GKRS. Also Lekovic (Lekovic et al., 2007) reported one case with partial response at 95 months from radiosurgery. To date, the most numerous published series goes back to Kim (Kim et al., 2008), who treated with GKRS 11 locally or distant recurrent intracranial CPPs in 6 patients. He described rates of overall survival and local TGC of 66.7% and 36.4%, respectively, but the study included some aggressive tumors, also. To our knownledge, the present is the largest series ever reported before regarding 8 patients affected with intracranial CPP and treated with radiosurgery. They were followed up for a median period of 71.8 months; the 5-year actuarial survival and local PFS rates were 90% and 90%, respectively. Even though the number of reported patients is limited, the long lasting TGC in most cases without GKRS-related permanent side effects strongly suggests that radiosurgery could represent a valid alternative for the treatment of intracranial CPP, especially in resistant tumors, thus avoiding invasive and high risk repeated microsurgery and the potential long term neuropsychological sequelae associated with fractionated RT.

Author	RS dev	N° Pt	Me/Med FU mos.	Clinical Results			Perm. Sympt.
				No def. / Impr	Stable	Wors.	Compl.
Kim 2008	GK	6	57.3/55.5	-	-	-	-
Lekovic 2007	GK	1	96.0	-	-	-	0.0
Eder 2001	GK	1	-	-	1	-	0.0
Duke 1997	GK	1	17.0	Excellent	-	-	0.0
Present series	GK	8	92.6/71.8	2/8	2/8	4/8‡	0.0

RS dev = Radiosurgical device; N° Pt = number of treated patients; Me = Mean; Med = Median; mos. = months; No def./Impr = No pre-GK neurological deficit/Neurological improvement; Wors. = Neurological worsening; Perm. Sympt. Compl. = permanent symptomatic complications; GK = Gamma Knife.

‡: 3/4 due to tumor distant progression and 1/4 due to local and distant progression.

Table 8. Clinical data in previous and present series of CPP treated with GKRS.

Author	N° Pt	Ov. Surv. %	Act. Surv. %		Ov. Local TGC%	Act. Local PFS%	
			At 5y	At 10y		At 5y	At 10y
Kim 2008	6	66.7	-	-	36.4 (with some aggressive tumors)	-	-
Lekovic 2007	1	100.0	-	-	100.0	-	-
Eder 2001	1	100.0	-	-	100.0 (Ped. Pt.)	-	-
Duke 1997	1	100.0	-	-	100.0	-	-
Present series	8	75.0‡	90.0	80.0	87.5	90.0	90.0

N° Pt = number of treated patients; Ov. Surv. = overall survival; Act. Surv. = actuarial survival; Ov. Local TGC = overall local tumor growth control; Act. Local PFS = Actuarial local progression-free survival; Ped. Pt. = Pediatric patient.

‡: 2 deaths: 1 due to tumor distant progression and 1 due to local and distant progression.

Table 9. Radiosurgical outcome in previous and present series of CPP.

4.4 Central neurocytoma (CN)

CN was characterized by Hassoun (Hassoun et al., 1982) in the 1980's as a distinct histological entity with a typical immunohistochemical profile and ultrastructural features of neuronal differentiation. CN accounts for approximately 0.1% of all the primary CNS tumors and it is a typically disease of young adulthood, occurring in the second and third decades of life (Matsunaga et al., 2010; Tyler-Kabara et al., 2001). This unusual LGPNT usually arise from the neuronal cells of the septum pellucidum, fornix, or subependymal plate of the lateral and third ventricle, so these tumors are surrounded by cerebrospinal fluid and occur as a small tumor attached to normal structures. CN is defined as grade II according to the WHO classification. This neoplasm is generally considered a benign, slow-growing tumor. Histological study shows a pattern composed of uniform small round cells, usually with clear cytoplasm and round nuclei (Figure 7). Its features match those of oligodendroglioma or ependymoma, leading to frequent misdiagnosis when further investigations are not performed. Immunohistochemistry is very useful for the diagnosis of neurocytoma, which shows a dot-like positivity for synaptophysin, negativity for glial fibrillary acidic protein and constant expression of neuron-specific enolase (Martin et al., 2003). Typical neurocytomas are characterized by a MIB-1 labeling index ≤3% and the absence of histologic atypia (Rades & Schild, 2006). Standard initial treatment for CNs is a total resection whenever possible. The prognosis is usually favorable after gross total resection, generally leading to cure and long-term survival. Furthermore, tumor resection not only provides a histological diagnosis but also restores the intracranial cerebrospinal fluid circulation. But, tumors in more than half of patients with CN cannot be completely resected. Furthermore, recurrences, even after complete resection, and tumor progression after subtotal resection have been reported up to 33% of cases (Matsunaga et al., 2010, Kim et al., 2007, Yen et al., 2007, Martin et al., 2003, Cobery et al., 2001). Finally, malignant transformation is known to occur in a few cases, resulting in tumor progression, intracerebral hemorrhage, or craniospinal dissemination (Matsunaga et al., 2010). For treatment of residual or recurrent CNs, fractionated RT has been advocated because these tumors tend to have high radiosensitivity due to their high vascularity. The results showed effective local tumor control. However, because of the benign clinical course of CN, the young mean age of the affected patients and the well-known long-term adverse effects of conventional RT, such as cognitive dysfunction and secondary tumor formation, routine use of conventional RT for residual or recurrent CN has been critized by several authors (Kim et al., 2007, Yen et al., 2007, Martin et al., 2003). The advantage of a focused radiation is that a

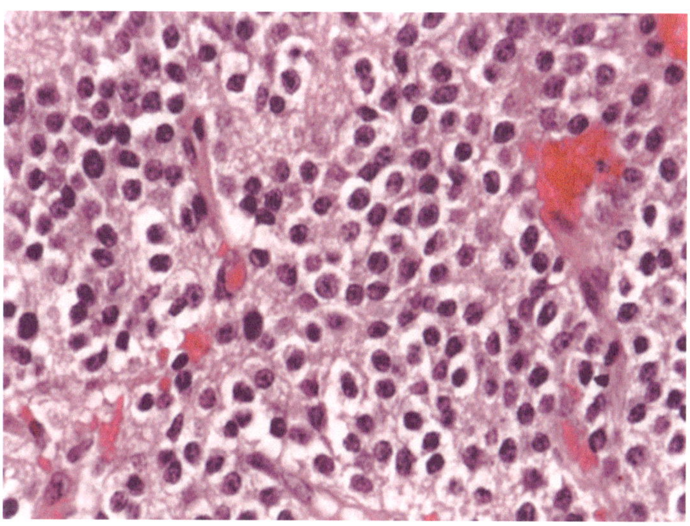

Fig. 7. CN: X100 H-E. Olicodendroglial like cells with round nuclei and clear haloes.

high dose with a steep fall off in radiation can be delivered precisely in one single treatment session. In addition, the residual or recurrent CNs are usually characterised by highly vascularized and well demarkated small volumes with generally intraventricular growth; therefore, they tend to be surrounded by CSF, and only a small part of the tumor has contact with the brain tissue. This makes them ideal targets for GKRS, as most of the dose surplus hits the CSF and the radiation burden to the neighbouring brain tissue can be kept at a minimum. In this way, the side effects of radiosurgery are minimised. All these advantages have led to the emergence of GKRS as an attractive alternative to conventional RT in the treatment of residual or recurrent CNs. The first CN patient treated with radiosurgery was described by Schild (Schild et al., 1997) in 1997. Since 1997, several studies of CNs treated with radiosurgery have demonstrated good response and high TGC. The mechanism of tumor response to GKRS is not yet clear. Several hypothesis have been formulated to explain the TV shrinkage: 1) cytotoxic effect; 2) accelerated programmed cell death; or 3) obliteration of nutritive vessels (Yen et al., 2007). The latter was reported by Kulkarni (Kulkarni et al., 2002) after they observed a decrease in contrast enhancement in the tumors after RT. The shrinkage of the residual neurocytoma began approximately 1 year after fractionated RT; this timing corresponds to the endothelial damage caused by irradiation which induces the proliferation of smooth muscle cells and the production of extracellular collagen by these cells, which leads to progressive stenosis and obliteration of the cAVM nidus. In addition, the contractile activity of these gamma ray-activated, spindle-shaped smooth muscle cells and the transformation of the resting cells into an activated form after irradiation may be relevant to the shrinking process and eventual occlusion of AVMs after radiosurgery. The activation of this obliteration mechanism is earlier in pediatric patients and young adults than in adults due to the greater number of nonresting cells found in young patients' vessels, as reported in an our previous study on cerebral arteriovenous malformations (Nicolato et al., 2005). To date, more than 50 patients treated with radiosurgery for CN has been described (Table 10). From the neurological point of view, the outcome was favourable in most cases. Only in one patient, a radiosurgery-related clinical worsening occurred: she was treated with a 6 MV LINAC system for a 8.09 cc left lateral ventricle CN. Radiation necrosis and brain edema were developed and ventriculo-peritoneal shunt was needed (Martin et al., 2003). The overall survival reported by the different authors varies between 67% and 100%, but none of the patients died due to the tumor progression. Rades (Rades & Schild, 2006) reviewed the data of all the CN patients reported since 1997. There were 21 cases treated with incomplete tumor resection followed by stereotactic radiosurgery, GK in 15 and Linac in 6 CNs. The median follow up period was 42 months. The 5-year actuarial survival and local PFS rates was 100% and 100%, respectively. The 4 patients of our series were observed for a median period of 180.6 months. The 10-year survival rate was 100%. Local tumor control was achieved in 75% of cases: in only one patient, tumor progression was documented at 9.3 months from GKRS. He was operated and he was alive and well at last follow-up. In conclusion, we suggest GKRS for residual CNs after incomplete resection or early detection of tumor recurrence with relatively small volume, which will reduce the long-term risk of radiation injury to the surrounding normal brain tissue compared with conventional RT. Because CN tends to show local recurrence leading to clinical malignant sequelae such as tumor progression, intracranial hemorrhage, or craniospinal dissemination and rarely malignant transformation, we strongly recommend GKRS for small residual or recurrent tumors rather than conservative follow up to obtain good tumor growth control.

Author	RS dev	N° Pt	Me/Med FU mos.	Clinical Results			Perm. Sympt. Compl.
				No def. /Impr	Stable	Wors.	
Matsunaga 2010	GK	7	63.6 Me	-	-	-	0.0
Kim 2007	GK	13	53.7/61.0	-	100.0	-	0.0
Yen 2007	GK	7	60.0 Me	100.0	-	-	0.0
Lekovic 2007	GK	1	54.0	-	1/1	-	0.0
Rades 2006 (reviews)	GK Linac	15 6	42 Med	-	-	-	-
Martin 2003	Linac	4	33.0/37.5	75.0	-	25.0	25.0
Javedan 2003	GK	1	25.0	1/1	-	-	0.0
Kim 2003	Linac	1	51.0	-	-	-	0.0
Hara 2003	GK	1	12.0	-	-	-	0.0
Tyler-Kabara 2001	GK	4	45.7/46.0	-	100.0	-	0.0
Anderson 2001	GK	4	16.5/13.0	100.0	-	-	0.0
Bertalanffy 2001	GK	3	32.0/24.0	67.0	33.0	-	0.0
Cobery 2001	GK	4	44.0/32.5	100.0	-	-	0.0
Pollock 2001	GK	1	34.0	1/1	-	-	0.0
Present series	GK	4	172.0/180.6	4/4	-	-	0.0

RS dev = Radiosurgical device; N° Pt = number of treated patients; Me = Mean; Med = Median; mos. = months; No def./Impr = No pre-GK neurological deficit/Neurological improvement; Wors. = Neurological worsening; Perm. Sympt. Compl. = permanent symptomatic complications; GK = Gamma Knife; Linac = Linear accelerator.

Table 10. Clinical data in previous and present series of CN treated with GKRS.

4.5 Pleomorphic xanthoastrocyroma (PXA)

PXA is a rare tumor accounting for less than 1% of all astrocytic neoplasms. At MRI, PXA does not show peculiar imaging features. This unusual LGPNT of the brain belongs to grade II according to WHO classification. Histopathological patterns includes cellular pleomorphism, focal eosinophilic protein droplets, and regions with an interstitial reticulin fiber network (Figure 8). Maximum surgical removal is considered the first treatment of choice. The efficacy of adjuvant radiotherapy has not yet been established, largely because of the relative rarity of this disease. Chemotherapy for PXA has been generally considered ineffective. The only described case of PXA treated with GKRS showed anaplastic features (Koga et al., 2009). Nevertheless, the authors chose to perform radiosurgery on 8 distinct intracranial tumor nodules in six different GKRS sessions during a 50 month follow up

Author	N° Pt	Ov. Surv. %	Act. Surv. %		Ov.Local TGC%	Act. Local PFS%	
			At 5y	At 10y		At 5y	At 10y
Matsunaga 2010	7	-	-	-	87.5	-	-
Kim 2007	13	-	-	-	84.6	-	-
Yen 2007	7	85.7	-	-	88.9	-	-
Lekovic 07	1	-	-	-	1/1	-	-
Rades 2006 (rews.)	156	100.0	100.0	-	95.2	100.0	-
Martin 2003	4	100.0	-	-	100.0	-	-
Javedan 2003	1	1/1	-	-	1/1	-	-
Kim 2003	1	1/1	-	-	1/1	-	-
Hara 2003	1	1/1	-	-	1/1	-	-
Tyler-Kabara 2001	4	100.0	-	-	100.0	-	-
Anderson 2001	4	100.0	-	-	100.0	-	-
Bertalanffy 2001	3	67.0	-	-	100.0	-	-
Cobery 2001	4	100.0	-	-	100.0	-	-
Pollock 2001	1	1/1	-	-	1/1	-	-
Present series	4	100.0	100.0	100.0	75.0	83.0	83.0

N° Pt = number of treated patients; Ov. Surv. = overall survival; Act. Surv. = actuarial survival; Ov. Local TGC = Overall local tumor growth control; Act. Local PFS = Actuarial local progression-free survival.

Table 11. Radiosurgical outcome in previous and present series of CN.

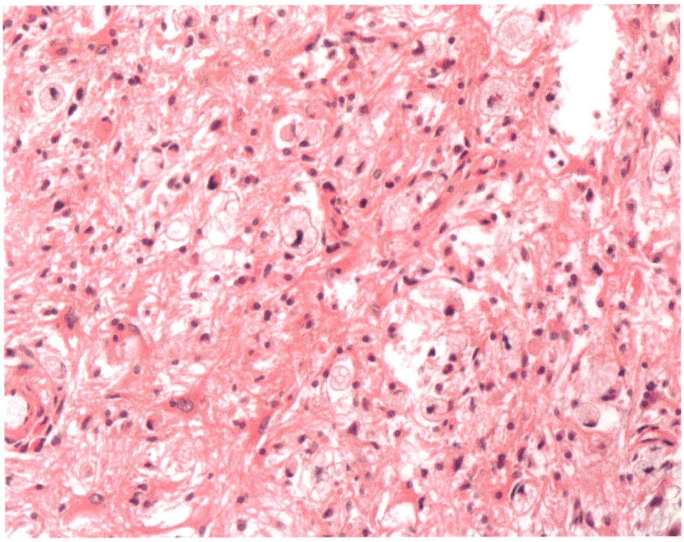

Fig. 8. PXA. X200 H-E. Presence of pleomorphic bizarre xanthomized cells in a fibrillary background.

Author	RS dev	N° Pt	Me/Med FU mos.	Clinical Results			Perm. Sympt. Compl.
				No def. /Impr	Stable	Wors.	
Koga 2009	GK	1	50.0	-	-	-	0.0
Present series	GK	3	45.6/43.7	1/3	1/3	1/3‡	0.0

RS dev = Radiosurgical device; N° Pt = number of treated patients; Me = Mean; Med = Median; mos. = months; No def./Impr = No pre-GK neurological deficit/Neurological improvement; Wors. = Neurological worsening; Perm. Sympt. Compl. = permanent symptomatic complications; GK = Gamma Knife.
‡: due to tumor distant progression.

Table 12. Clinical data in previous and present series of PXA treated with GKRS.

Author	N° Pt	Ov. Surv %	Act. Surv %		Ov. Local TGC%	Act. Local PFS%	
			At 5y	At 10y		At 5y	At 10y
Koga 2009	1	0.0	-	-	100.0	-	-
Present series	3	66.7‡	80.0	80.0	66.7	80.0	80.0

N° Pt = number of treated patients; Ov. Surv. = overall survival; Act. Surv. = actuarial survival; Ov. Local TGC = Overall local tumor growth control; Act. Local PFS = Actuarial local progression-free survival.
‡: dead due to tumor local and distant progression.

Table 13. Radiosurgical outcome in previous and present series of PXA.

period achieving a successful local control of all treated lesions without radiosurgery-related permanent side effects. The patient died 66 months after the disease onset; the cause of death was identified with a distant craniospinal axis tumor nodule dissemination. In this chapter, we report 3 patients affected with grade II PXA who underwent GKRS and followed up for a median period of 43.7 months. To our knowledge, this is the only reported "small" series of low-grade PXA treated with GKRS. One patient affected with a brain stem PXA died at 22.1 months from GKRS due to local and distant tumor progression. In the other 2 cases, a long term PFS was achieved and they are well and alive at last follow up performed at 43.7 months and 70.9 months from radiosurgical treatment.

4.6 Others (Miscellaneous)

This heterogeneous group of patients is represented by different histological types of extremely unusual LGPNT of the brain: gangliolgioma, mixed oligoastrocytoma, subependymoma, and papillary glioneuronal tumor. The results of our experience with GKRS is excellent: negative or stable neurologic conditions in all cases, no radiosurgery-related complications, 100% survival and local TGC rate. Obviously, other experiences with GKRS on such rare tumors are limited or even absent (Tables 14 and 15). In the few reported cases, the authors described encouraging responses to radiosurgery, as well. The results seems to be particularly encouraging when GKRS is employed. To our knowledge, there are no other patients affected with papillary glioneuronal tumor who underwent GKRS reported in the literature; therefore, the case of the present series represents the first papillary glioneuronal tumor treated with radiosurgery.

Histology	Author	RS dev	N° Pt	FU mos.	Clinical Results			Perm. Sympt. Compl.
					No def. /Impr	Stable	Wors.	
Ganglioglioma	Kim 1999	GK	1	14.0	-	-	-	0.0
	Schröttner 2002	GK	3	-	-	-	-	-
	Present series	GK	2	68.4	-	2/2	-	0.0
Subependymoma	Ecker 2004	GK	1	54.0	-	1/1	-	0.0
	Seol 2003	Lin	1	24	-	-	-	0.0
	Im 2003	GK Lin	2	22.5	-	-	-	0.0
	Roos 2000	Lin	1	16	1/1	-	-	0.0
	Present series	GK	1	31.2	1/1	-	-	0.0
Oligoastrocytoma	Sarkar 2002	GK	11 les	-	-	-	-	0.0
	Present series	GK	1	68.3	1	-	-	0.0
Papillary Gl. Tumour	Present series	GK	1	104.0	1/1	-	-	0.0

RS dev = Radiosurgical device; N° Pt = number of treated patients; mos. = months; No def./Impr = No pre-GK neurological deficit/Neurological improvement; Wors. = Neurological worsening; Perm. Sympt. Compl. = permanent symptomatic complications; GK = Gamma Knife; Lin = Linear accelerator; les = lesions; Papillary Gl. Tumour = Papillary Glioneuronal Tumour.

Table 14. Clinical data in previous and present series of rare unusual LGPNTs treated with GKRS.

Histology	Author	RS dev	N° Pt	Ov. Surv.	Ov. Local TGC%	Act. Local PFS% At 5y	Prognostic Factors
Ganglioglioma	Kim 1999	GK	1	-	1/1 solid compon.	-	-
	Schröttner 2002	GK	3				
	Present series	GK	2	2/2	2/2	-	None
Subependymoma	Ecker 2004	GK	1	1/1	1/1	-	-
	Seol 2003	Lin	1	1/1	0/1	-	-
	Im 2003	GKLin	2	2/2	0/2	-	-
	Roos 2000	Lin	1	1/1	1/1	-	-
	Present series	GK	1	1/1	1/1	-	None
Oligoastrocytoma	Sarkar 2002	GK	11 les	-	-	42.0	Younger age Smaller TVs
	Present series	GK	1	1/1	1	100.0	None
Papillary Gl. Tumour	Present series	GK	1	1/1	1/1	100.0	None

RS dev = Radiosurgical device; N° Pt = number of treated patients; Ov. Surv. = Overall survival; Ov. Local TGC = Overall local tumor growth control; Act. Local PFS = Actuarial local progression-free survival; GK = Gamma Knife; compon. = component; Lin = Linear accelerator; TVs = Tumor volumes.

Table 15. Radiosurgical outcome in previous and present series of rare unusual LGPNTs.

4.7 Future research/perspectives

The results described with the GKRS treatment in such unusual LGPNTs are very intersting. Nevertheless, the need for further future perspectives and researches emerge from all these studies. First of all, the application of multisession GKRS with the Extend system (Elekta instruments, AB) on larger TVs with the aim of increasing the local TGC without exposing the patients to higher risk of radiation toxicity on the surrounding normal brain tissue need to be studied. Second, it should be interesting to investigate if there is any potential correlation between biomarker expression (Ki67, MGMT, PCNA, p53, etc.) in such unusual LGPNTs and GKRS outcome. Finally, basing on the literature data and our experience results, it should be suitable that GKRS is included in the international guidelines for good clinical practice as part of the therapeutic armamentarium for the management of unusual LGPNTs, particularly as concerns pineocytoma and CN.

5. Conclusion

GKRS may be already considered an effective and safe treatment alternative in multimodality approach for selected cases with pineocytoma and CNs, thus eliminating the need for reoperation of residual or recurrent tumors and avoiding the potential long-term side effects of conventional RT in these young adult patients. In the unusual LGPNTs with a limited number of treated patients - CPP, PXA, and other rare tumors - radiosurgery seems to be a valid complementary treatment tool in these rarer tumors, also. Nevertheless, multidisciplinary studies on large series of patients and long follow-up period with statistical analysis are needed to convincingly demonstrate the efficacy and safety of GKRS on such primary low-grade brain tumors.

6. Acknowledgment

The authors thank Giovanni Nicolato, for his assistance in the preparation of this manuscript.

7. References

Anderson, R.C., Elder, J.B., Parsa, A.T., Issacson, S.R., Sisti, M.B. (2001). Radiosurgery for the treatment of recurrent central neurocytomas. *Neurosurgery,* Vol.48, pp 1231–1238.

Backlund, E.O., Rahn, T., Sarby, B. (1974). Treatment of pinealomas by stereotaxic radiation surgery. *Acta Radiol Ther Phys Biol,* Vol.13, pp 368–376.

Bertalanffy, A., Roessler, K., Dietrich, W., Aichholzer, M., Prayer, D., Ertl, A., Kitz, K. (2001). Gamma knife radiosurgery of recurrent central neurocytomas: a preliminary report. *J Neurol Neurosurg Psychiatry,* Vol.70, pp 489–493

Boethius, J., E Ulfarsson, T Rahn, B Lippitz. (2002). Gamma Knife radiosurgery for pilocytic astrocytomas. *J Neurosurg,* Vol.(Suppl 5)97, pp 677-680.

Breslaw, N. (1974). Covariance analysis of censored survival date. *Biometrics,* Vol.30, pp 89-99.

Bruce, J.N., Ogden, A.T. (2004). Surgical strategies for treating patients with pineal region tumors. *J Neuro-Oncol,* Vol.69, pp 221-236.

Chiechi, M.V., Smirniotopoulos, J.G., Mena, H. (1995). Pineal parenchymal tumors: CT and MR features. *J Comput Assist Tomogr,* Vol.19, pp 509–517.

Cobery, S.T., Noren, G., Friehs, G.M., Chougule, P., Zheng, Z., Epstein, M.H., Taylor, W. (2001). Gamma knife surgery for treatment of central neurocytomas. Report of four cases. *J Neurosurg,* Vol.94, pp 327–330.

Deshmukh, V.R., Smith, K.A., Rekate, H.L., Coons, S., Spetzler, R.F. (2004). Diagnosis and management of pineocytomas. *Neurosurgery,* Vol.55, pp 349–357.

Duke, B.J., Kindt, G.W., Breeze, R.E. (1997). Pineal region choroid plexus papilloma treated with stereotactic radiosurgery: a case study. *Comput Aided Surg,* Vol.2, pp 135–138.

Ecker, R.D., Pollock, B.E. (2004). Recurrent Subependymoma Treated with Radiosurgery. *Stereotact Funct Neurosurg,* Vol.82, pp 58–60.

Eder, H.G., Leber, K.A., Eustacchio, S., Pendl, G. (2001). The role of gamma knife radiosurgery in children. *Childs Nerv Syst,* Vol.17, pp 341–346.

Friedman, J.A., Lynch, J.J., Buckner, J.C., Scheithauer, B.W., Raffel, C. (2001). Managment of malignant pineal germ cell tumors with residual mature teratome. *Neurosurgery,* Vol.48, pp 518-523.

Grimoldi, N., Tomei, G., Stankov, B., Lucini, V., Masini, B., Caputo, V., Repetti, M.L., Lazzarini, G., Gaini, S.M. (1998). Neuroendocrine , himmunohistochemical, and ultrastructural study of pineal region tumors. *J Pineal Res,* Vol.25, pp 147-158.

Hadjipanayis, C.D., Kondziolka, D., Gardner, P., Niranjan, A., Dagam, S., Flickinger, J.C., Lunsford, L.D. (2002). Stereotactic radiosurgery for pilocytic astrocytomas when multimodal therapy is necessary. *J Neurosurg,* Vol.97, pp 56-64.

Hadjipanayis, C.G., Niranjan, A., Tyler-Kabara, E., Kondziolka, D., Flickinger, J.C., Lunsford, L.D. (2002). Stereotactic radiosurgery for well-circumscribed fibrillary grade II astrocytomas: an initial experience. *Stereotactic Funct Neurosurg,* Vol.79, pp 13-24.

Hara, M., Aoyagi, M., Yamamoto, M., Maehara, T., Takada, Y., Nojiri, T., Ohno, K. (2003). Rapid shrinkage of remnant central neurocytoma after gamma knife radiosurgery: a case report. *J Neurooncol,* Vol.62, pp 269–273.

Hasegawa, T., Kondziolka, D., Hadjipanayis, C.G., Flickinger, J.C., Lunsford, L.D. (2002). The role of radiosurgery for the treatment of pineal parenchymal tumors. *Neurosurgery,* Vol.51, pp 880-889.

Hassoun, J., Gambarelli, D., Grisoli, F., Pellet, W., Salamon, G., Pellissier, J.F., Toga, M. (1982). Central neurocytoma. An electron-microscopic study of two cases. *Acta Neuropathol,* Vol.56, pp 151–156.

Heppner, P.A., Sheehan, J.P., Steiner, L.E. (2005). Gamma knife surgery for low-grade gliomas. Neurosurgery, Vol.57, No.6, pp 1132-1139.

Im, S.-H., , Paek, S.H., Choi, Y.-L., Chi, J.G., Kim, D.G., Jung, H.W., Cho, B.-K. (2003). Clinicopathological study of seven cases of symptomatic supratentorial subependymoma. *Journal of Neuro-Oncology,* Vol.61, pp 57–67.

Javedan, S.P., Manwaring, K., Smith, K.A. (2003). Treatment of posterior third ventricular central neurocytoma with endoscopic biopsy, endoscopic third ventriculostomy and stereotactic radiosurgery. *Minim Invasive Neurosurg,* Vol.46, pp 165–168.

Kano, K., Kondziolka, D., Niranjan, A., Flickinger, J.C., Lunsford, L.D. (2009). Stereotactic radiosurgery for pilocytic astrocytomas part 1: outcome in adult patients. *J Neurooncol,* Vol.95, pp 211-218.

Kano, K., Niranjan, A., Kondziolka, D., Flickinger, J.C., Pollack, I., Jakacki, R., Lunsford, L.D. (2009) Stereotactic radiosurgery for pilocytic astrocytomas part 2: outcome in pediatric patients. *J Neurooncol,* Vol.95, pp 219-229.

Kano, H., Niranjan, A., Khan, A., Flickinger, J.C., Kondziolka, D., Lieberman, F., Lunsford, L.D. (2009). Does radiosurgery have a role in the management of oligodendrogliomas? *J Neurosurg,* Vol.110, pp 564–571.

Kano, H., Niranjan, A., Kondziolka, D., Flickinger, J.C., Kondziolka, D., Lunsford, L.D. (2009). Role of stereotactic radiosurgery in the managment of pineal parenchymal tumors, In: *Pineal Region Tumors. Diagnosis and treatment options,* T. Kobayashi & L.D. Lunsford, (Eds.), 44-58, ISSN 0079-6492, S. Karger AG, ISBN 978-3-8055-9077-8, Basel, Switzerland.

Kaplan, E.L.; Meier, P. (1958). Nonparametric estimation from incomplete observations. *J Am Stat Assoc*, Vol.53, pp 457-481.

Kida, Y., T Kobayashi, Y Mori. (2000). Gamma knife radiosurgery for low-grade astrocytomas: results of long term follow-up. J Neurosurg, Vol.(Suppl 3)93, pp 42-46.

Kim, M.S., Lee, S.I., Sim, J.H. (1999). Brain tumors with cysts treated with gamma knife radiosurgery: is microsurgery indicated ? *Stereotact Funct Neurosurg*, Vol. 72 (Suppl.), pp 38-44.

Kim, C.Y., Paek, S.H., Kim, D.G. (2003). Linear accelerator radiosurgery for central neurocytoma: a case report. *J Neurooncol*, Vol.61, pp 249–254.

Kim, C.Y., Paek, S.H., Jeong, S.S., Chung, H.T., Han, J.H., Park, C.K., Jung, H.W., Kim, D.G. (2007). Gamma Knife Radiosurgery for Central Neurocytoma. Primary and Secondary Treatment. *Cancer*, Vol.110, pp 2276–84.

Kim, I-Y., Niranjan, A., Kondziolka, D., Flickinger, J.C., Lunsford, L.D. (2008). Gamma knife radiosurgery for treatment resistant choroid plexus papillomas. *J Neurooncol*, Vol.90, pp 105–110.

Kobayashi, T., Kida, Y., Mori, Y. (2001). Stereotactic gamma radiosurgery for pineal and related tumors. *J Neurooncol*, Vol.54, pp 301–309.

Koga, T., Morita, A., Maruyama, K., Tanaka, M., Ino, J., Shibahara, J., Louis, D.N., Reifenberger, G., Itami, J., Hara, R., Saito, N., Todo, T. (2009). Long-term control of disseminated pleomorphic xanthoastrocytoma with anaplastic features by means of stereotactic irradiation. *Neuro-Oncology*, Vol.11, pp 446–451.

Krishnan, S., Brown, P.D., Scheithauer, B.W., Ebersold, M.J., Hammack, J.E., Buckner, J.C. (2004). Choroid plexus papillomas: a single institutional experience. *J Neurooncol*, Vol.68, pp 49–55.

Kulkarni, V., Rajshekhar, V., Haran, R.P., Chandi, S.M. (2002). Long-term outcome in patients with central neurocytoma following stereotactic biopsy and radiation therapy. *Br J Neurosurg*, Vol.16, pp 126–132.

Lekovic, G.P., Gonzales, L.F., Shetter, A.G., Porter, R.W., Smith, K.A., Brachman, D., Spetzler, R.F. (2007). Role of Gamma Knife surgery in the management of pineal region tumors. *Neurosurg Focus*, Vol.23, No.6, PP E12.

Louis, D.N., Ohgaki H., Wiestler, O.D., Cavenee, W.K., Burger, P.C., Jouvet, A., Scheithauer, B.W., Kleihues, P. (2007). The 2007 WHO Classifcation of Tumours of the Central Nervous System. Acta Neuropathol, Vol.114, pp 97–109.

Lunsford, L.D., Flickinger, J., Lindner, G., Maitz, A. (1989). Stereotactic radiosurgery of the brain using the first United States 201 cobalt-60 source gamma knife. Neurosurgery, Vol.24, pp 151–159.

Martin, J.M., Katati, M., Lopez, E., Bullejos, J.A., Arregui, G., Busquier, H., Minguez, A., Olivares, G:; Hernandez, V., Arjona, V. (2003). Linear accelerator radiosurgery in treatment of central neurocytomas. *Acta Neurochir (Wien)*, Vol.145, pp 749–754.

Matsunaga, S., Shuto, T., Suenaga, J., Inomori, S., Fujino H. (2010). Gamma Knife Radiosurgery for Central Neurocytomas. *Neurol Med Chir (Tokio)*, Vol.50, pp 107-113.

Mori, Y., Kobayashi, T., Hasegawa, T., Yoshida, K., Kida, Y. (2009). Stereotactic radiosurgery for pineal and related tumors, In: *Pineal Region Tumors. Diagnosis and treatment options,* T. Kobayashi & L.D. Lunsford, (Eds.), 107-118, ISSN 0079-6492, S. Karger AG, ISBN 978-3-8055-9077-8, Basel, Switzerland.

Nicolato, A., Gerosa, M., Ferraresi, P., Piovan, E., Pasoli, A., Perini, S., Mazza, C. (1997). Stereotactic radiosurgery for the treatment of arteriovenous malformations in childhood. *J Neurosurg Sci,* Vol.41, pp 359-371.

Nicolato, A., F Lupidi, MF Sandri, R Foroni, P Zampieri, C Mazza, A Pasqualin , A Beltramello, M Gerosa (2006). Gamma knife radiosurgery for cerebral arteriovenous malformations in children/adolescents and adults. Part II: differences in obliteration rates, treatment-obliteration intervals, and prognostic factors. *Int J Radiat Oncol Biol Phys,* Vol.64, pp 914-921.

Pollock, B.E., Stafford, S.L. (2001). Stereotactic radiosurgery for recurrent central neurocytoma: case report. *Neurosurgery,* Vol.48, pp 441-443.

Rades, D., Schild, S.E. (2006). Value of postoperative stereotactic radiosurgery and conventional radiotherapy for incompletely resected typical neurocytomas. *Cancer,* Vol.106, pp 1140-1143.

Reyns, N., M Hayashi, O Chinot, L Manera, J-C Peragut, S Blond, J Regis. The role of Gamma Knife radiosurgery in the treatment of pineal parenchymal tumours. *Acta Neurochir (Wien)* 2006;148:5-11.

Roos, D.E., Brophy, B.P., Zavgorodni, S.F., Francis, J.W. (2000). Radiosurgery at the Royal Adelaide Hospital: The first 4 1/2 years' clinical experience. *Australas Radiol,* Vol.44:, pp 85-192.

Sarkar, A., Pollock, B.E., Brown, P.D., Gorman, D.A. (2002). Evaluation of gamma knife radiosurgery in the treatment of oligodendrogliomas and mixed oligodendroastrocytomas. *J Neurosurg,* Vol.97(5 Suppl), pp 653-656.

Schild, S.E., Scheithauer, B.W., Haddock, M.G., Schiff, D., Burger, P.C., Wong, W.W., Lyons, M.K. (1997). Central neurocytomas. *Cancer,* Vol.79, 790-795.

Schild, S.E., Scheithauer, B.W., Haddock, M.G., Wong, W.W., Lyons, M.K., Marks, L.B., Norman, M.G., Burger, P.C. (1996). Histologically confirmed pineal tumors and other germ cell tumors of the brain. *Cancer,* Vol.78, pp 2564-2571.

Schröttner, O., Unger, F., Eder, H.G., Feichtinger, M., Pendl, G. (2002). Gamma-Knife radiosurgery of mesiotemporal tumour epilepsy observations and long-term results. *Acta Neurochir Suppl.,* Vol.84, pp 49-55.

Seol, H.J., Hwang, S.-K., Choi, Y.L., Chi, J.G., Jung, H.W. (2003). A case of recurrent subependymoma with subependymal seeding: case report. *Journal of Neuro-Oncology,* Vol.62 pp 315-320.

Simonova, G., J Novotny, R Lisckac. (2005). Low-grade gliomas treated by fractionated gamma knife surgery. *J Neurosurg,* Vol.(Suppl)102, pp 19-24.

Subach, B.R., Lunsford, L.D., Kondziolka, D. (1998). Stereotactic radiosurgery in the treatment of pineal region tumors. *Prog Neurol Surg,* Vol.14, pp 175-194.

Talacchi, A., De Micheli, E., Lombardo, C., Turazzi, S., Bricolo, A. (1999). Choroid plexus papilloma of the cerebellopontine angle: a twelve patient series. *Surg Neurol,* Vol.51, pp 621-629.

Tyler-Kabara, E., Kondziolka, D., Flickinger, J.C., Lunsford, L.D. (2001). Stereotactic radiosurgery for residual neurocytoma. Report of four cases. *J Neurosurg,* Vol.95, pp 879-882.

Yen, C.P., Sheehan, J., Patterson, G., Steiner, L. (2007). Gamma Knife surgery for neurocytoma. *J Neurosurg*, Vol.107, pp 7–12.

Part 2

Functional and Vascular Disorders

6

Clinical, Anatomo-Radiological and Dosimetric Features Influencing Pain Outcome After Gamma Knife Treatment of Trigeminal Neuralgia

José Lorenzoni[1,2], Adrián Zárate[1], Raúl de Ramón[2], Leonardo Badínez[2,3], Francisco Bova[2] and Claudio Lühr[2]
[1]*Department of Neurosurgery, Pontificia Universidad Católica de Chile, Santiago*
[2]*Centro Gamma Knife de Santiago, Santiago*
[3]*Department of Radiation Oncology, Fundación Arturo López Pérez, Santiago*
Chile

1. Introduction

Gamma Knife radiosurgery has become nowadays a well validated and accepted option for the treatment of trigeminal neuralgia and numerous publications support its role in the management of this disease. The results achieved with this technique in terms of pain outcome are quite similar to other ablative treatments such as radiofrequency thermo-coagulation, balloon micro-compression or glycerol gangliolysis, nevertheless, complications seem to be less frequent (López 2004a).

In contrast to the mentioned treatments, radiosurgery does not mitigate pain immediately, existing a "latency period" for pain relief of about 2 to 6 weeks. Initially, favorable results (Barrow Neurological institute I -IIIb) are obtained in more than 80% of the cases, then, because of recurrences over time, at 3 to 5 years after the treatment, the percentage of patient which maintains this outcome is near 50%. (Kondziolka, 2010; Longhi, 2007; lópez, 2004a; 2004b; Pollock, 2002; Regís, 2009; Sheehan, 2005; Verheul, 2010).

From the evidence based medicine point of view, either for radiosurgery as well as for all other medical and surgical treatment options for trigeminal neuralgia, there is lacking of comparative randomized prospective trials and the majority of publications correspond to observational data, categorized in Class III studies, then, in general the level of evidence is poor (Cruccu, 2008; López, 2004b; Zakrzewska, 2007).

The aim of the present chapter consists in a systematic review of the literature searching and categorizing information about the prognostic factors involved in pain improvement after Gamma knife radiosurgery for trigeminal neuralgia.

A search in Pub med was done crossing the key words: Gamma Knife, and Trigeminal Neuralgia. Secondarily, other key words were introduced: Radiosurgery, Multiple sclerosis, Atypical, Secondary, postherpethic, anatomy, Neurovascular compression, contact or conflict, Nerve Atrophy, Target, root entry zone, Proximal, Retrogasserian and Distal. For the purposes of this study 67 Manuscripts published between 1997 and 2011 were selected.

Because of the relative low level of existing evidence, more than to state definitive conclusions about the influence on pain outcome of the different variables studied, each variable was arranged in one of 5 powered categories according to the number of publications and the agreement of their findings.

1. **Consistent agreement:** there are clear coincidental conclusions among the publications, without controversial findings. In this category is highly possible that the conclusion is right.
2. **Reasonable agreement:** there are more coincidental conclusions among the publications, but with some controversial findings. In this category is quite possible that the conclusion is right.
3. **Some agreement with a trend:** there are less coincidental conclusions among the publications, more controversial findings but a trend is observed. In this category the conclusion could be right but more information is recommended.
4. **Scarce information with a trend:** A trend is observed, but because the small quantity of data more information is recommended for definitive conclusions.
5. **Scarce information with no clear trend or controversial findings:** In these cases more information is absolutely needed for having any conclusion.

Two plots for each variable were built showing the influence on pain control. The first plot represents the number of publications (papers) supporting the prognostic value of the variable and the second plot shows the number of patients enrolled in such studies: better (variable is a positive prognostic factor), unaffected (variable is not a prognostic factor) and worse (variable is a negative prognostic factor).

The variables studied were categorized in 3 types:

1. Clinical
2. Anatomo-radiological
3. Dosimetric.

2.1 Clinical variables

2.1.1 Age: Pan (Pan, 2010) communicated that younger patients obtained better result in terms of pain outcome. Han (Han, 2009), Sheehan (Sheehan, 2005), Regis (Regís, 2006) and Towk (Tawk, 2005) conversely described worse results in younger patients. In spite of these controversial results, the majority of authors have not found significant influence of the patient age in pain control (Aubuchon, 2010; Azar, 2009; Brisman, 2004; Dellaretti, 2008; Hayashi, 2009; Kondziolka, 2010; Little, 2008; Longhi, 2007; Massager, 2007a; Park, 2011; Petit, 2003; Riesenburger, 2010; Rogers, 2000; Young, 1998). **It seems that age is not a prognostic factor with "reasonable agreement".**

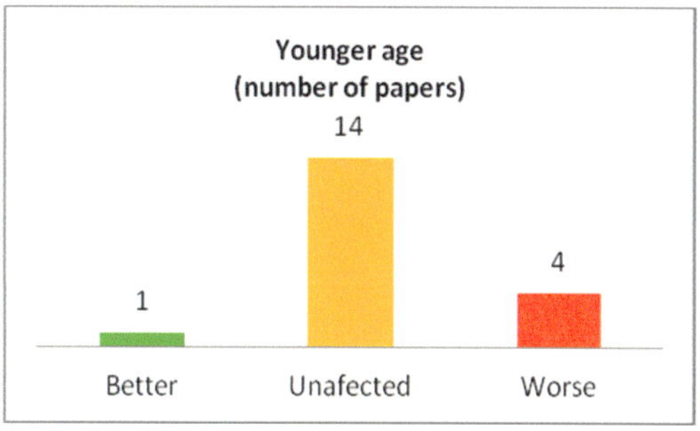

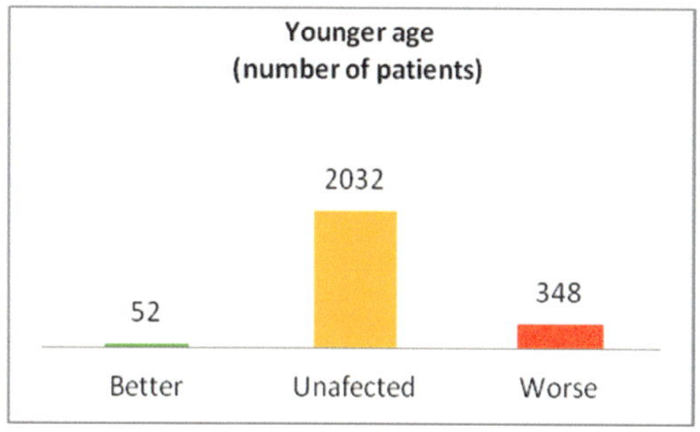

2.1.2 Gender: In spite of female gender seems to be slightly more frequent in the series (Brisman , 2004; Kondziolka, 2010; Longhi , 2007; Pollock, 2002;), concerning pain outcome it has been systematically communicated that this variable has not prognostic significance (Aubuchon, 2010; Azar, 2009; Brisman , 2004; Dellaretti, 2008; ; Hayashi, 2009; Kimball, 2010; Longhi, 2007; Massager 2007a Park, 2011; Riesenburger, 2010; ; Rogers, 2000; Sheehan, 2005; Tawk, 2005; Young, 1998): **There was found "Consistent agreement" indicating that gender is not a prognostic variable for pain control.**

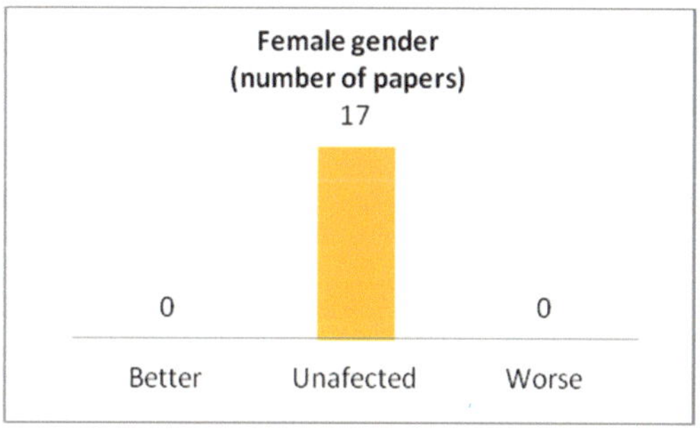

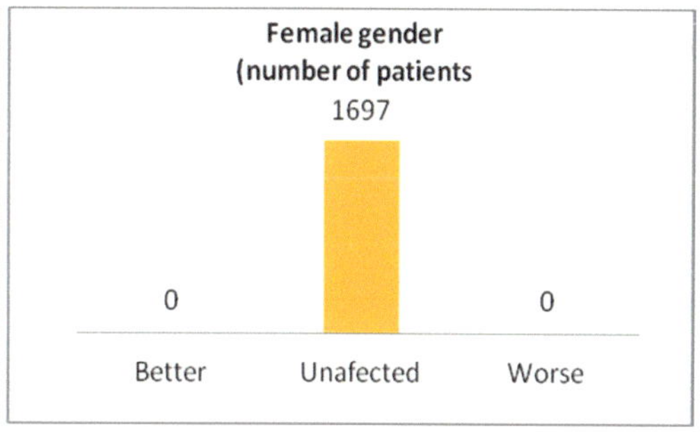

2.1.3 Side: Right side seems to be slightly more frequent (Aubuchon, 2010; Cheuk, 2004; Dhople, 2009; Huang, 2008; Kimball, 2010; Kondziolka, 2010; Pan, 2010; Park, 2011; Pollock, 2001 ; Regís, 2006; Shaya, 2004; Tawk, 2005), Most authors coincide that the side of the neuralgia has not a prognostic factor (Brisman, 2004; Hayashi, 2009; Kimball, 2010; Little, 2008; Massager , 2007a; ; Park, 2011; Riesenburger, 2010; Tawk, 2005). Sheehan (Sheehan, 2005) on the other hand, found better results in patients with right side neuralgia. **It seems that the side of the trigeminal neuralgia has not influence on pain outcome with "reasonable agreement" of findings.**

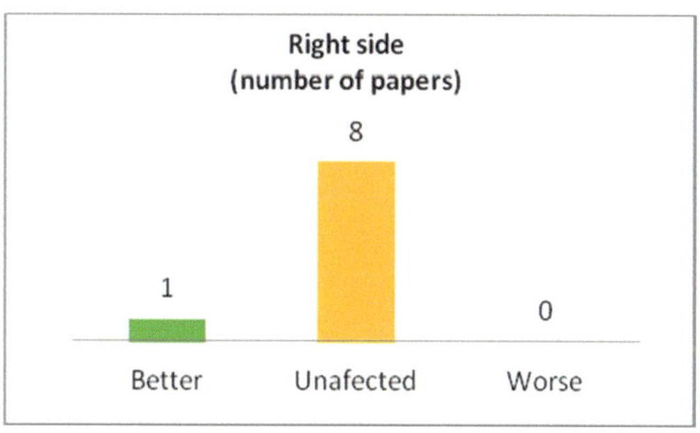

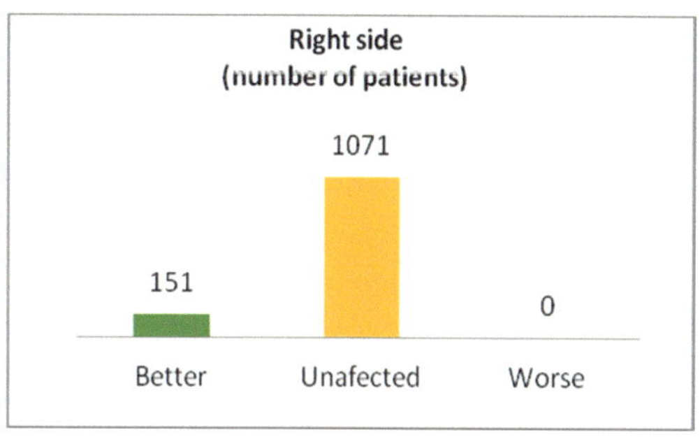

2.1.4 Pain distribution: All revised papers conclude that pain distribution does not affect the clinical outcome of trigeminal neuralgia after Gamma Knife treatment (Abuchon, 2010; Hayashi, 2009; Jawahar, 2005; Little, 2008; Massager, 2007a; Sheehan, 2005). **For this variable a "Consistent agreement" was observed.**

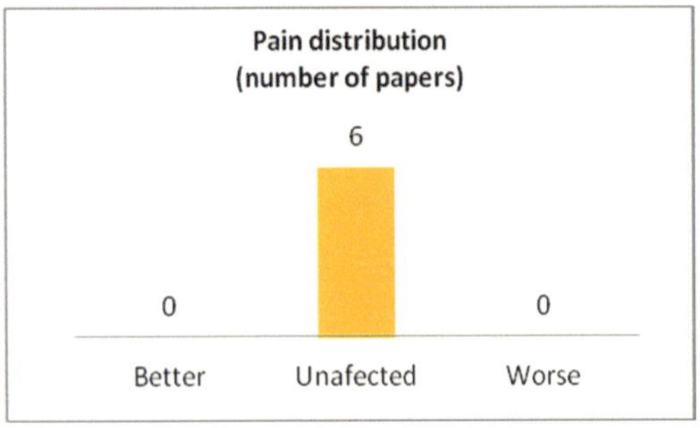

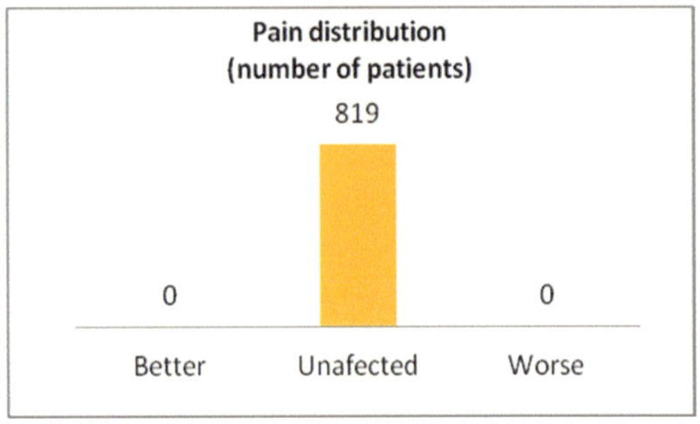

2.1.5 Single branch involvement: Kano, **(Kano, 2010)**, found a significant favorable pain outcome in patients with a single branch compromise, nevertheless other two publications mentioned no influence on pain outcome of a single branch compromise (Massager, 2007a; Tawk, 2005). No publication was found mentioning worse results when a unique branch is affected. **"Scarce information with a trend" suggests that single branch involved could be a positive prognostic variable.**

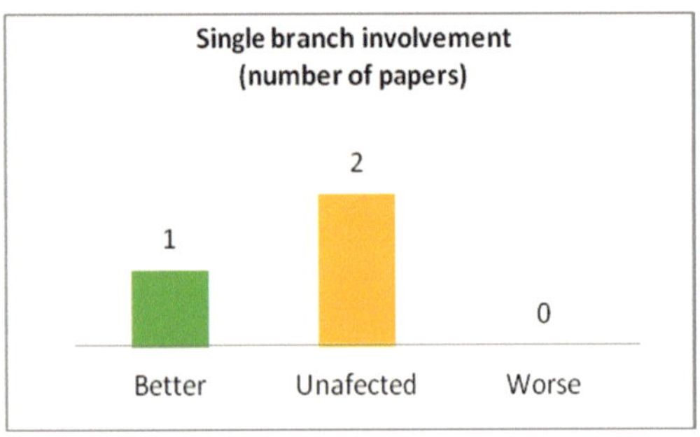

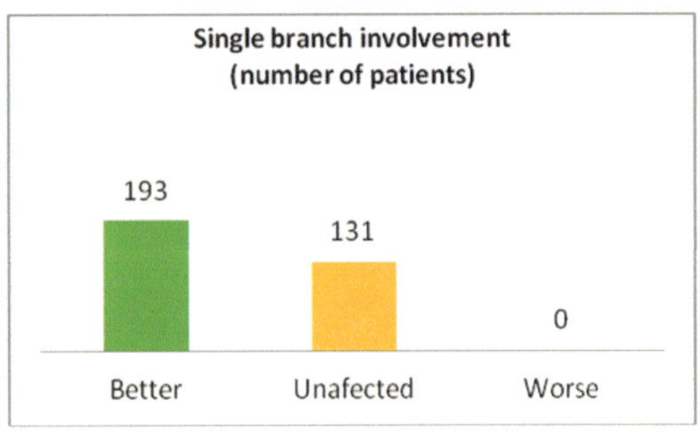

2.1.6 Atypical neuralgia: More reports found worse pain outcome in patients with atypical neuralgia (Brisman, 2004; Dhople, 2007; Kano,2010; Longhi, 2007; Maesawa, 2001; Rogers, 2000; Varheul, 2010; Young, 1998). Other authors did not found influence of atypical neuralgia on pain improvement (Aubuchon, 2010; Petit, 2003; Pollock, 2002; Regís, 2009; Sheehan, 2005). No publications informing better results in patients with atypical facial pain were found. **"Some agreement with a trend" indicates that atypical facial pain could responds worse to Gamma Knife treatment.**

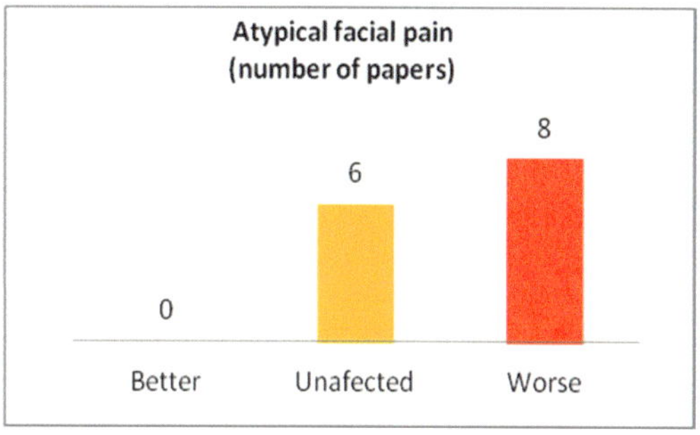

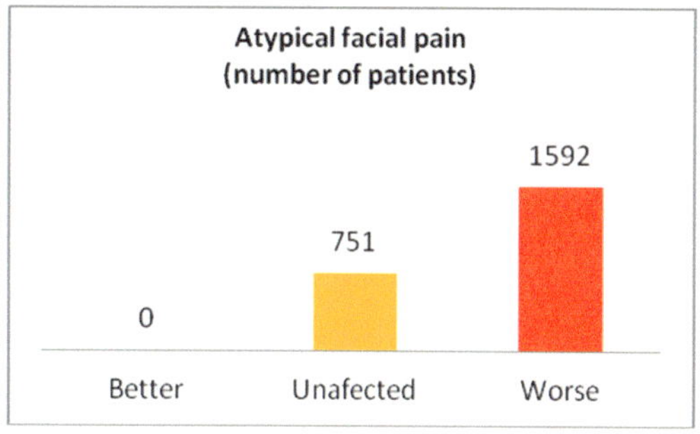

2.1.7 Secondary neuralgia: Young (Young, 1997) reported 88% of pain relief in 9 patient treated targeting the tumor, Regis (Regis 2001), obtained pain cessation in 79.5% of 46 patients targeting the tumor, in 3 cases the target was the nerve and in 4 the target was the tumor with the nerve together. Pollock (Pollock, 2000) treated 23 patients (16 meningiomas and 8 malignant tumors). After treatment 50% of patients were initially pain free and 46% experience significant pain improvement. Chang (Chang, 1999) in a series of 27 patients (mainly meningiomas and schwannomas) targeting the tumor found 40% of pain improvement and a slower response. If the analysis is done in those series that compare classic trigeminal neuralgia and secondary neuralgia (Chang, 2000), worse results in patients with secondary trigeminal neuralgia were found. Verheul (Verheul, 2010) on the other hand, did not found differences in clinical results between secondary and classic trigeminal pain. **"Scarce information with a trend" could suggest that secondary trigeminal neuralgia could be a negative prognostic variable.**

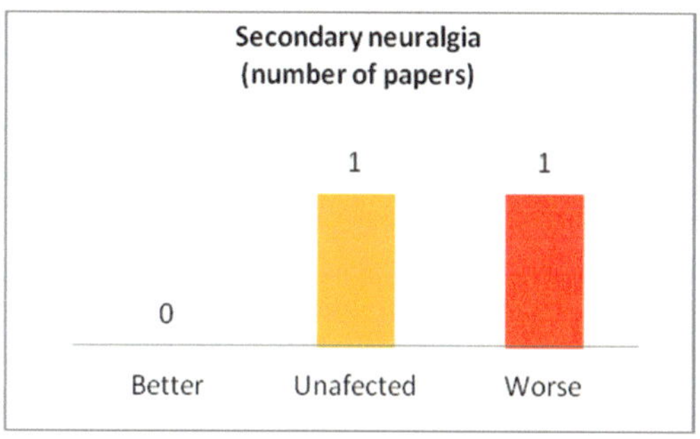

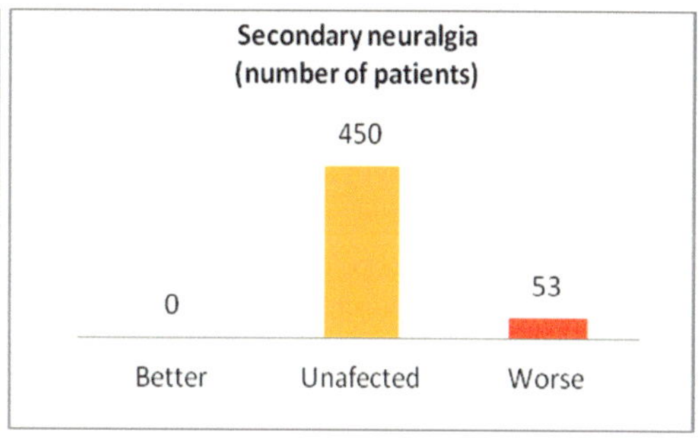

2.1.8 Association with Multiple sclerosis: When specific publications for multiple sclerosis were analized, some authors (Huang, 2002; Rogers, 2002; Zorro, 2009) communicated quite similar results of Gamma Knife radiosurgery in patients harboring trigeminal neuralgia secondary to multiple sclerosis. If the analysis is done in those series that compare classic trigeminal neuralgia and neuralgia associated to multiple sclerosis, some authors reported worse results in cases of multiple sclerosis (Brisman 2000a; Cheng, 2005; Morbidini-gaffney, 2006; Verheul, 2010; Young, 1998). Other manuscripts did not report significant differences in pain control between classic trigeminal neuralgia and neuralgia secondary to multiple sclerosis (Cheuk, 2004; Petit, 2003; Regís, 2009; Riesenburger, 2010; ; Rogers, 2000). No communication exists informing better results when multiple sclerosis is present. **With "Some agreement with a trend" It seems that trigeminal neuralgia secondary to multiple sclerosis could respond worse to Gamma Knife treatment.**

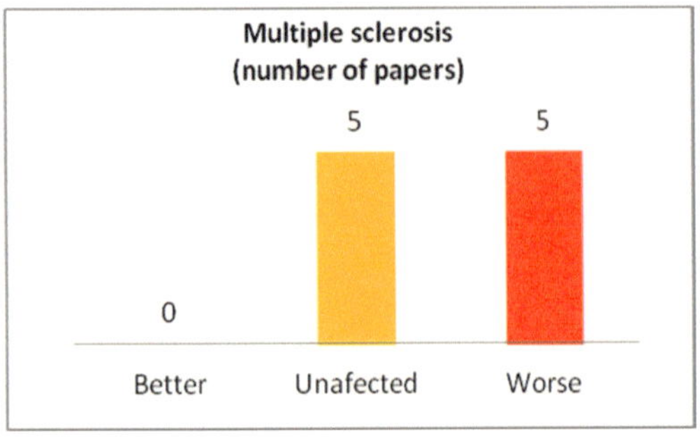

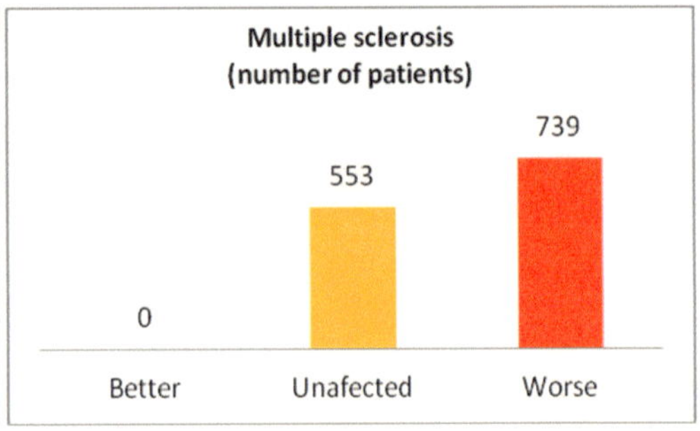

2.1.9 Postherpetic neuralgia: There was found only one study concerning Gamma Knife treatment for post herpetic neuralgia. Urgosík (Urgosík, 2000) It comprised 16 patients and the favorable pain response was 44%, results quite inferior to those communicated in the literature for classic trigeminal neuralgia. **"Scarce information with a trend" suggests that post herpetic trigeminal neuralgia could not respond well to Gamma Knife treatment.**

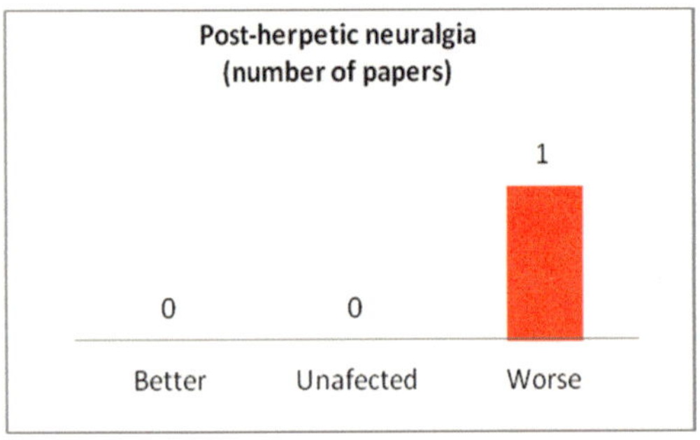

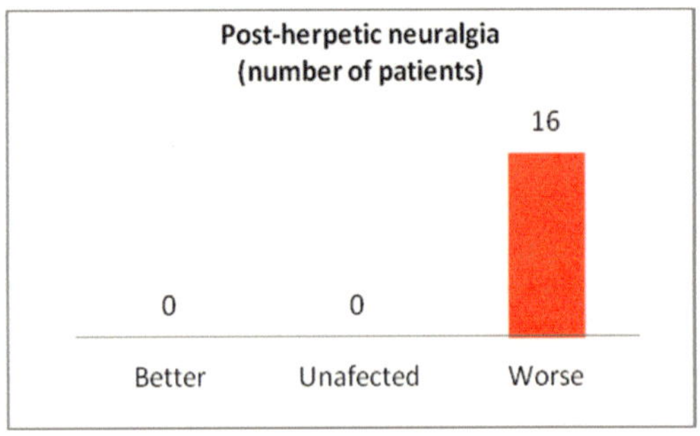

2.1.10 Previous treatments: The majority of studies found worse pain outcome in patients with the antecedent of previous treatments of the trigeminal neuralgia. (Brisman, 2000a; Dellanretti, 2008; Dhople, 2009; Kondziolka, 2010; Little, 2008; Longhi, 2007; Pan, 2010; Petit, 2003; Pollock, 2002; Regís, 2009; Tawk, 2005; Verheul, 2010; Young 1997), lesses number of articles found no influence of this variable (Dhople, 2009 ; Fountas, 2007; Hayashi, 2009; Massager, 2007a; Park, 2011; Reisenburger, 2010; Sheehan, 2005). Only one study showed better pain outcome in those patients previously treated (Rogers, 2000). **It seems that the antecedent of previous surgical treatments is a negative prognostic factor with "reasonable agreement".**

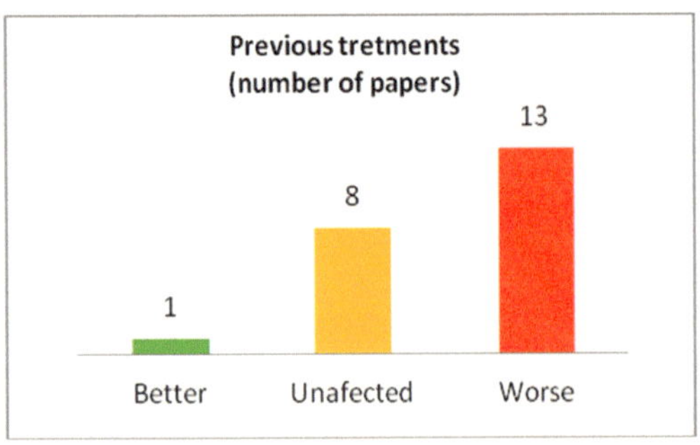

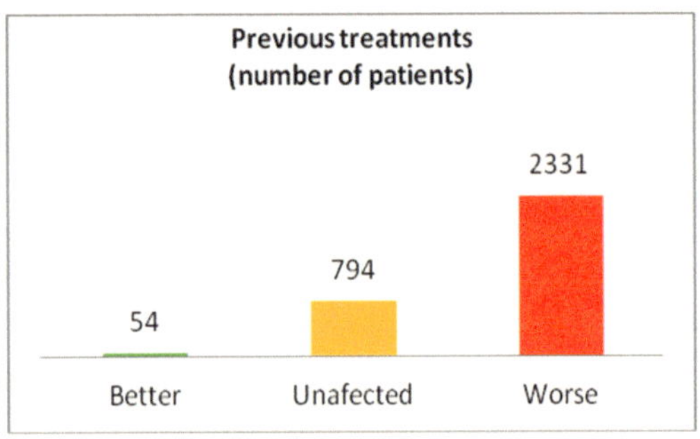

2.1.11 Longer duration of symtoms: Kondziolka (Kondziolk, 2010) found better results in patients with less than 3 years of disease. Pan (Pan, 2010) communicate better outcome in patients with less of 24 months of evolution and Petit (Petit, 2003) reported better pain control when the time of disease was less than 50 months. Other manuscripts did not confirm influence of this variable (Brisman, 2004; Dellaretti, 2008; Hayashi, 2009; Kano, 2010; Kimball, 2010; Little, 2008; Pollock, 2002; Reisenburger, 2010; Sheehan, 2005; Tawk, 2005; Young, 1998). No communication exist informing better results when the illness was present for a longer time. **A longer time of evolution of the trigeminal neuralgia could be a variable associated to a worse prognosis wit "Some agreement with a trend".**

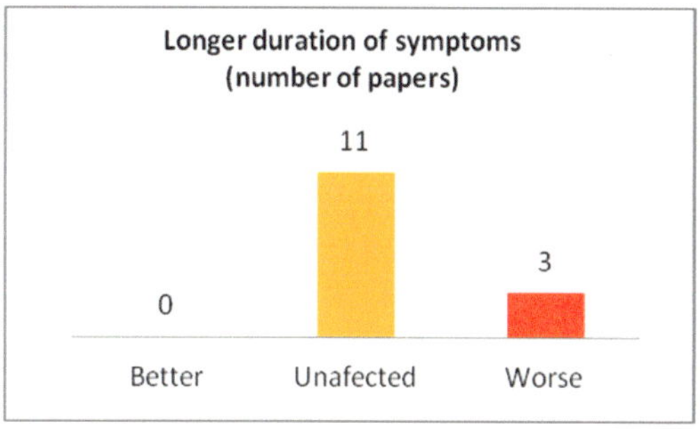

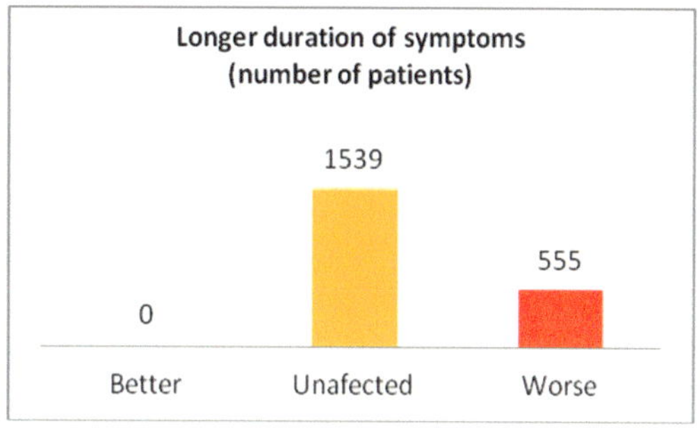

2.1.12 Pre-treatment sensory deficit: Kondziolka (Kondziolka, 2010) found better pain control in patients without previous sensory deficit; nevertheless this variable could be associated with other variable (no previous treatments). Pollock (Pollock 2002) and Sheehan (Sheehan, 2005) did not find this association. No communication was found informing better results in cases with pre-treatment sensory deficit. **"Scarce information with a trend" suggests that pre-treatment sensory deficit could be associated to a worse pain control.**

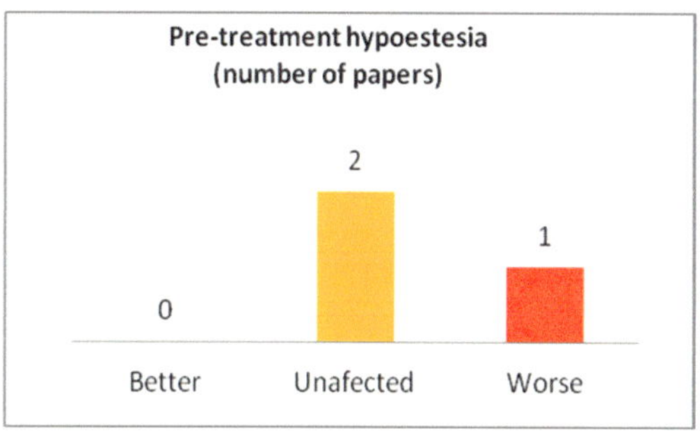

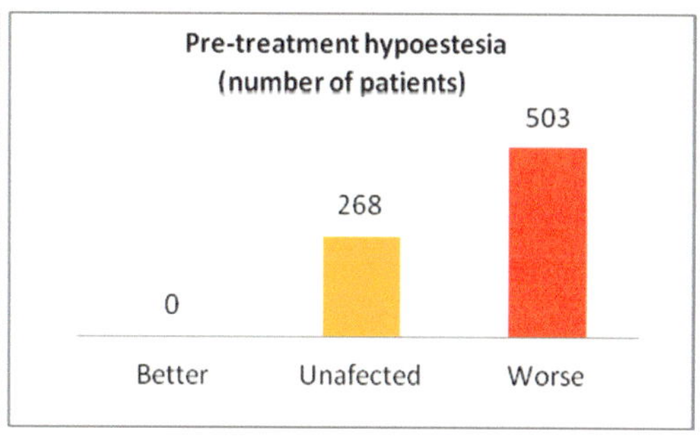

2.1.13 Post-treatment sensory deficit: Clear predominance was found concerning the association between post-treatment sensory deficit and better pain outcome (Aubuchon, 2010; Dellaretti, 2008; Huang, 2008; Kimball, 2010; Kondziolka, 2010; Massager 2007a; Matsuda, 2010; Pollock, 2002; Rogers, 2000; Tawk, 2005). Four authors reported no influence of this variable (Cheuk, 2004; Petit 2003; Reisenburger, 2010; Sheehan, 2005). No publications informing worse pain control in patients with post operative sensitive deficit was got. **Post Gamma knife sensory dysfunction is associated with better pain outcome with "reasonable agreement of findings".**

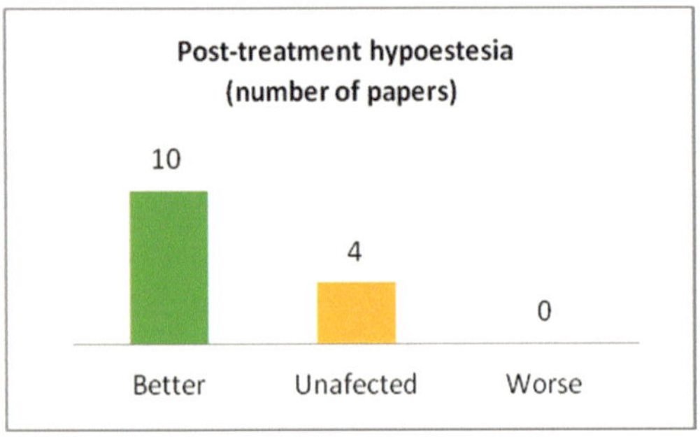

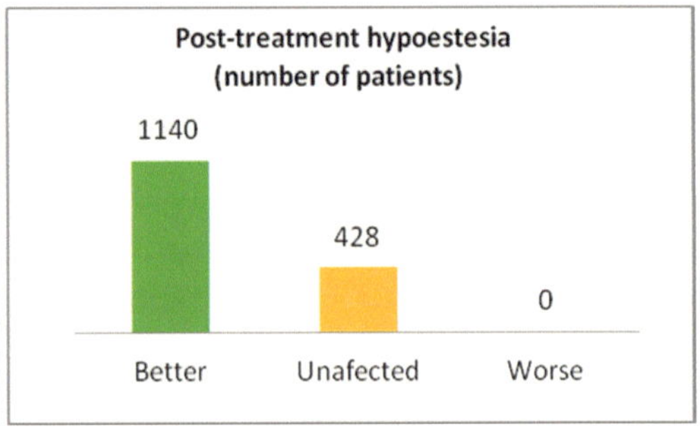

2.1.14 Repeated gamma Knife treatment: With regard a second treatment by Gamma Knife, two studies report no difference in term of pain control compared with the results obtained after a first Gamma Knife treatment (Huang, 2010; Verheul, 2010). Pollock (Pollock, 2005) found even better pain outcome after the second treatment. All these three studies report significant more trigeminal dysfunction after the second treatment. **"Scarce information with a trend" suggests that pain control after a second Gamma Knife treatment could be similar or better compared with the first treatment; nevertheless, it is associated to higher nerve toxicity.**

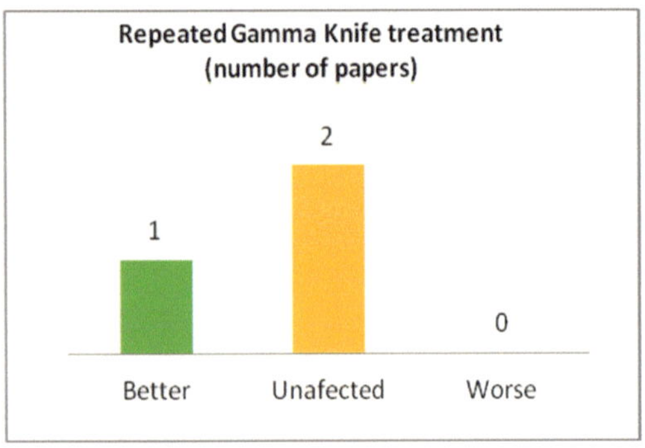

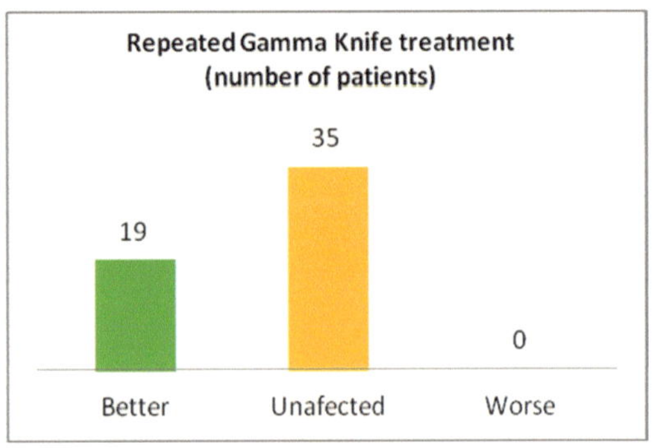

2.2 Anatomo-radiological variables

2.2.1 Neurovascular compression on magnetic resonance: Erbay (Erbay, 2006), Pan (Pan, 2010) and Brisman (Brisman ,2002a) report better pain control in those patients with neurovascular compression visualized on magnetic resonance. Other authors (Cheuk, 2004; Lorenzoni, 2008; Park, 2011; Shaya, 2004; Sheehan, 2010) did not find significant influence of this variable. No paper informing better outcome in patients without neurovascular compression in the magnetic resonance was found. Based in this, **"Some agreement with a trend" suggests that a neurovascular compression visualized on MR could be a neutral or good prognostic factor but not a negative factor.**

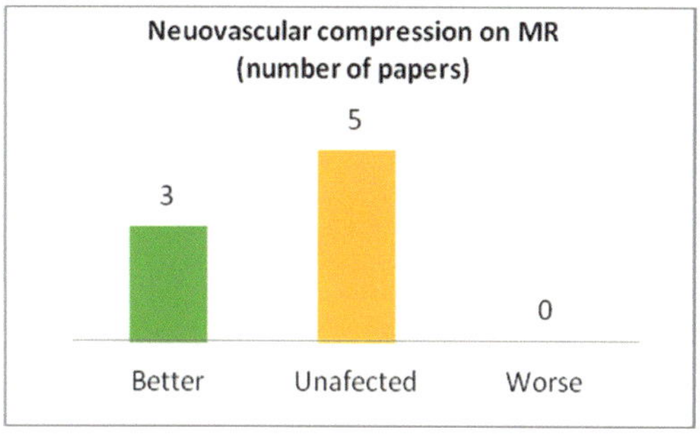

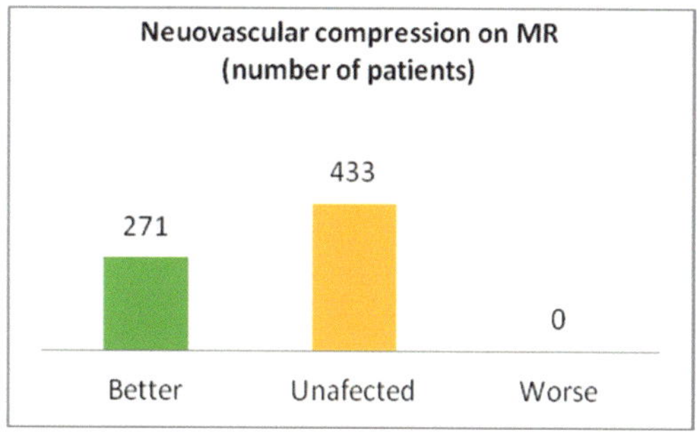

2.2.2 Nerve deformation or dislocation by the vessel: Lorenzoni et al (Lorenzoni 2008) found no influence of this factor on pain outcome. In spite of these findings, **"Scarce information with a trend" exists and this fact needs to be validated with further studies.**

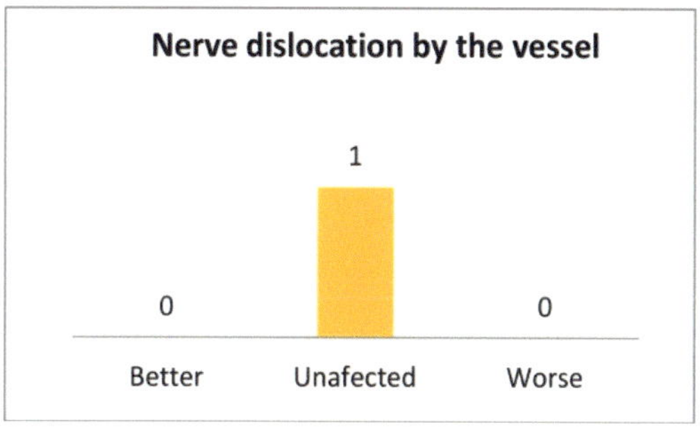

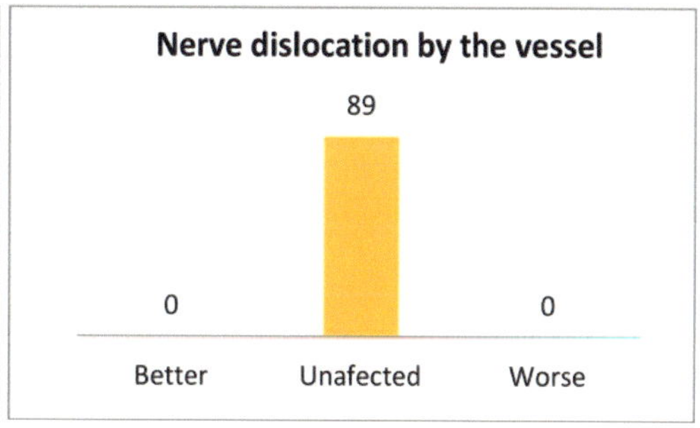

2.2.3 Large vessel involved in the neurovascular compression: Lorenzoni and co-workers (Lorenzoni, 2008) informed that a neurovascular compression by a large vessel such as a dolicoectatic basilar artery or a tortuous vertebral artery is a negative factor for pain mitigation. In spite of these findings, **"Scarce information with a trend" exists and these findings need to be validated with further studies.**

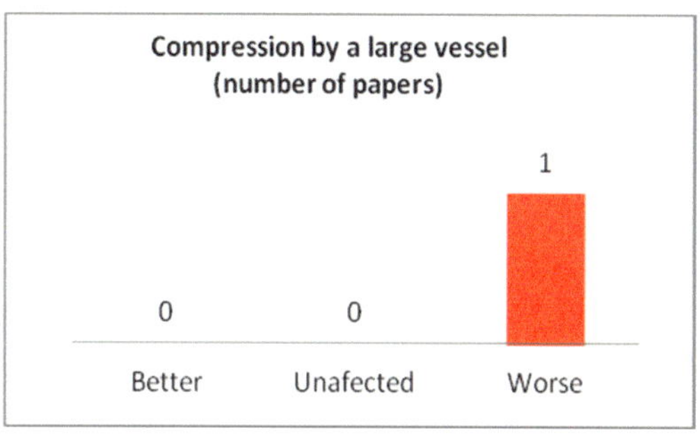

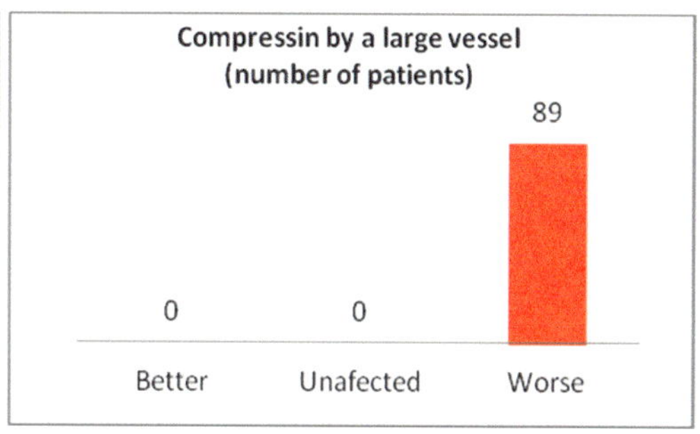

2.2.4 Proximal neurovascular compression: Lorenzoni et al (Lorenzoni, 2008; Lorenzoni, 2009) communicated that neurovascular compression can be located at any place along the trajectory of the trigeminal nerve. Proximal neurovascular compressions (less than 3 mm to the nerve emergency in the brainstem), was associated to a worse pain control (Lorenzoni 2008). **"Scarce information with a trend" exists and this fact needs further confirmation.**

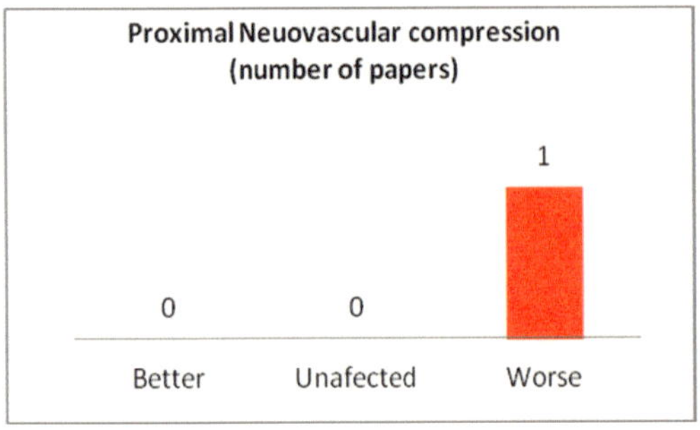

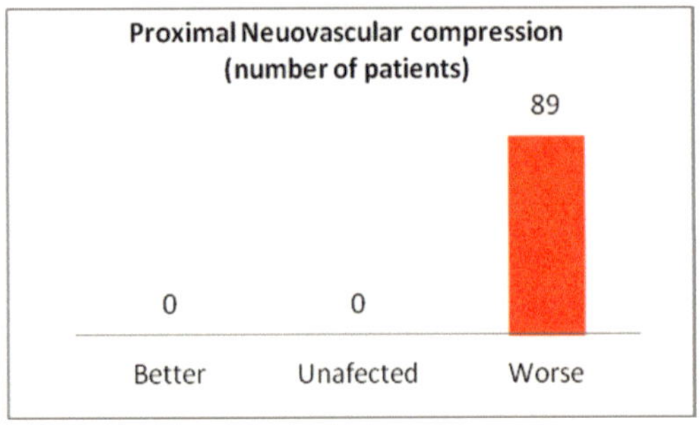

2.2.5 Nerve atrophy: Two articles (Hayashi, 2009; Lorenzoni, 2008) found no influence of this variable on pain response. **"Scarce information with a trend" suggests that nerve atrophy could not be a predictive factor; nevertheless, because of the little information available, more studies are desirable for a definitive conclusion.**

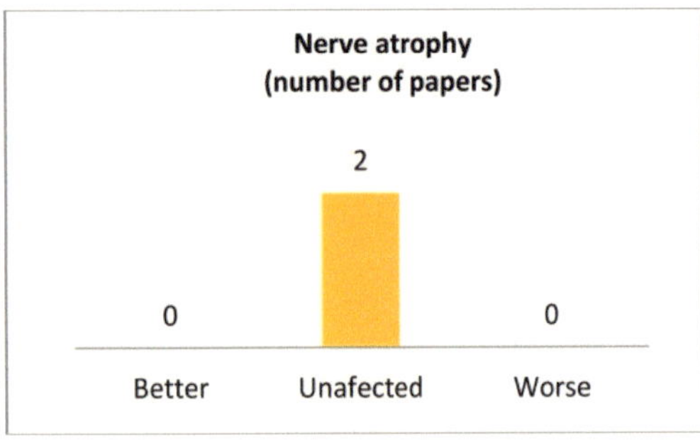

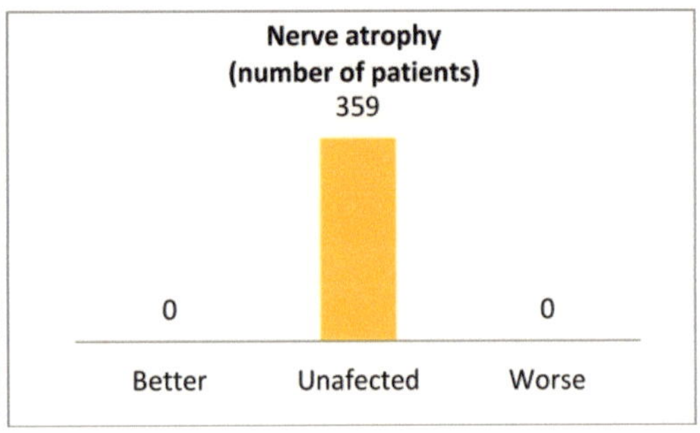

2.2.6 Nerve enhancement after treatment: In many cases, but not always, contrast enhancement of the trigeminal nerve is visualized on magnetic resonance some weeks or months after the Gamma Knife treatment. Fountas (Fountas, 2007), reports this phenomenon in 79% of the treated patients. This finding confirms the zone that received the irradiation. Alberico (Alberico, 2001) studied 15 patients and in 10 there was nerve enhancement. This finding was not related with pain response. Massager (Massager 2004) in a series of 47 patients did not find a prognostic value of this variable. Based on these two articles, it was considered that there is **"Scarce information with a trend" suggests that nerve contrast enhancement after treatment is not related to pain results.**

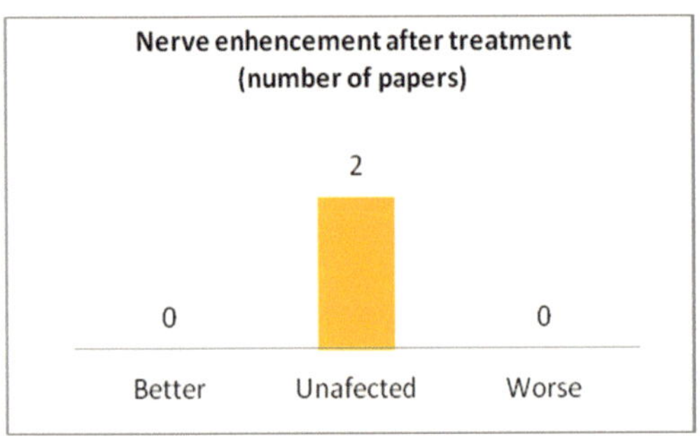

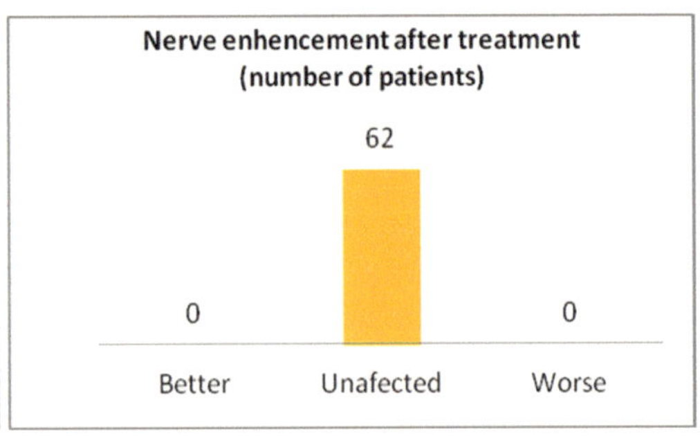

2.2.7 Brainstem enhancement after treatment: Sheehan (Sheehan, 2005) reported that brainstem contrast enhancement after treatment did not correlate with results of the Gamma Knife treatment. **"Scarce information with a trend" suggests that brainstem contrast enhancement after treatment is not related to pain control.**

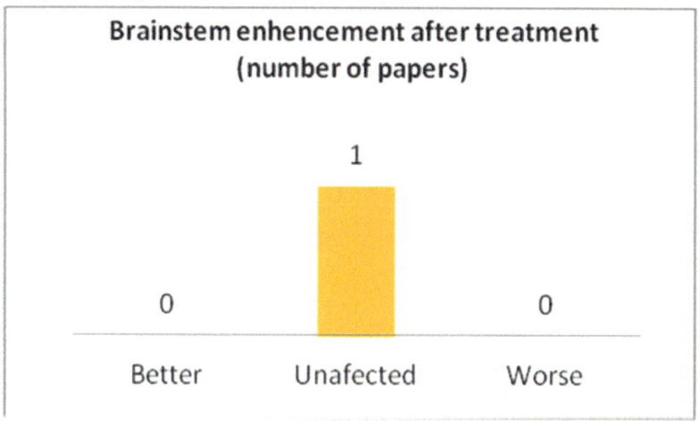

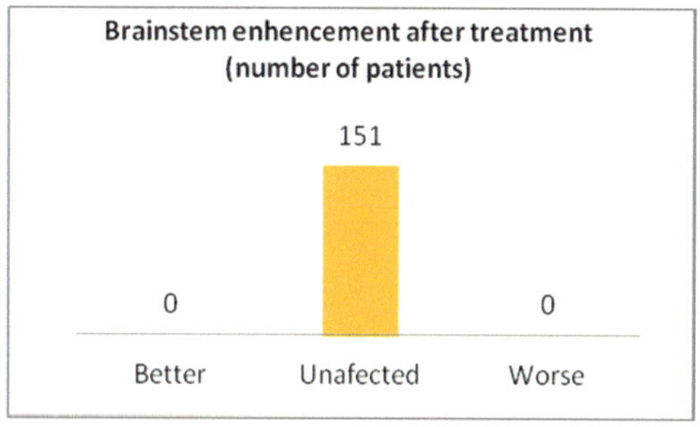

2.3 Dosimetric variables

2.3.1 Maximal dose administered to the nerve: For the analysis of the maximal dose delivered (in the range of 70 to 90 Gray), Many authors (Alpert, 2005; Kim, 2010; Longhi, 2007; Massager, 2007b; Morbidini-Gaffnay, 2006; Regis, 2009; Park, 2011; Shaya, 2004), communicate that using a maximal prescribed dose in the range of 80 to 90 Gray the patients response is better compared with treatment with a lower dose. On the other hand, other authors communicated that maximal dose of irradiation is not a prognostic factor (Aubuchon, 2010; Azar, 2009; Brisman, 2004; Dellaretti, 2008; Hayashi, 2009; Kondziolka, 2010; Little, 2008; Longhi, 2007; Park, 2011; Petit, 2003; Riesenburger, 2010; Rogers, 2000; Young, 1998;). Conversely, no study has shown better results using a lower dose. Concerning this fact, **"Some agreement with a trend" suggests that the use of a higher dose of irradiation (in the range of 80 to 90 Gray) achieve better results.**

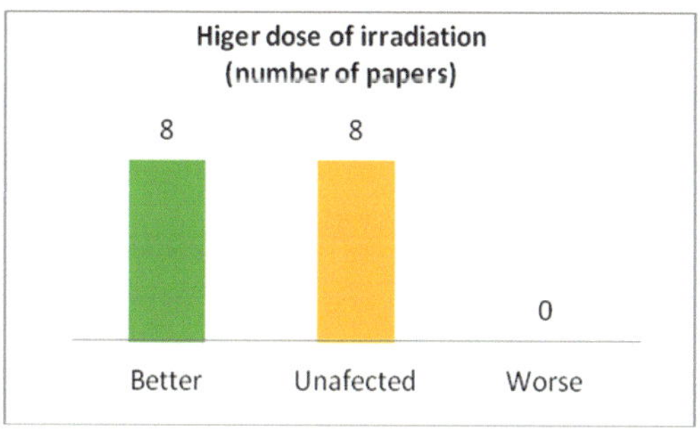

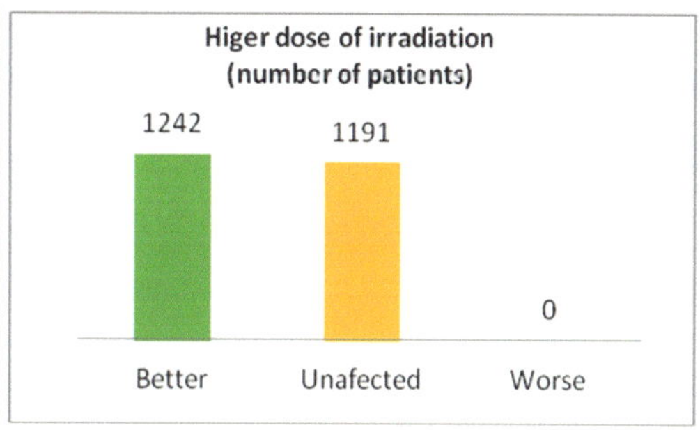

2.3.2 Proximal nerve targeting: Two zones in the trigeminal nerve has been described as targets for radiosurgical treatment of trigeminal neuralgia, a proximal target located at the root entry zone and a distal one located at the retrogaserian portion of the nerve. It seems that clinical results are quite similar using either the proximal target (Brisman 2004; Cheuk, 2004; Dhople, 2007; Han, 2009; Huang, 2008; Kim, 2010; Kondziolka, 2010; Little, 2008; Longhi, 2007; 2005 Matsuda, 2010; Nicol, 2000; Pan, 2010; Park, 2011; Pollock, 2002; Rogers, 2000 Tawk; Verheul, 2010; Young, 1998) as well as the distal one (Dellaretti, 2008; Hayashi 2009; Massager, 2007a; Regis, 2009). Matsuda (Matsuda 2008) in a series of 100 patients reports better pain control and lesser morbidity in patients treated with a proximal compared with those treated with a distal target. Conversely, Park (Park 2010) in a series of 39 patients found that a distal target was associated to more rapid response, better pain control and lower nerve morbidity. With the data available in the literature there are not clear differences in terms of clinical results between the two targets, then, considering any of these two targets as prognostic variable **"scarce information with no clear trend or controversial findings" exist.**

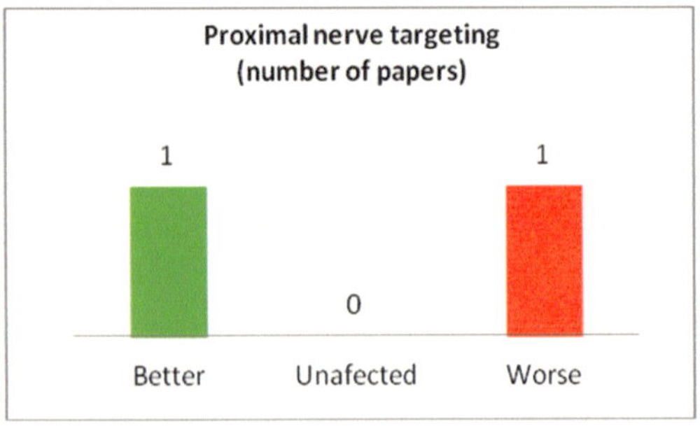

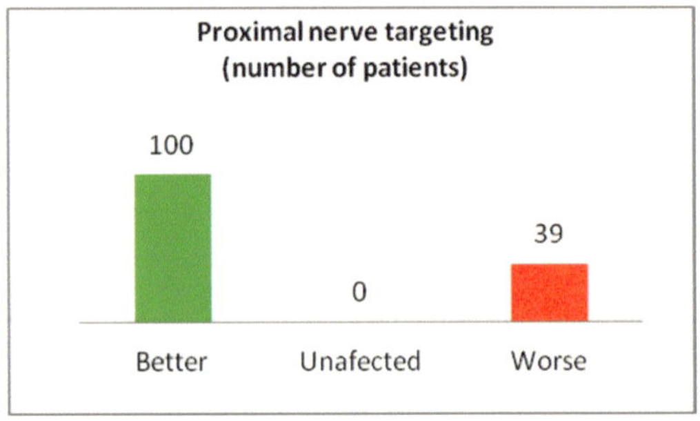

2.3.3 Shorter distance from the isocenter to the brainstem: Regís (Regís, 2009) and massager (Massager 2007a) using distal retrogaserian targeting report better pain control when the distance between the isocenter and the brainstem is less. Sheehan (Sheehan, 2005) and Aubuchon (Aubuchon, 2010) found no influence. No article showing worse outcome when a smaller distance from the isocenter to the brainstem was identified. This variable could be linked with the next variable analyzed (higher dose of irradiation received by the brainstem) **"Scarce information with a trend" suggests that a shorter distance from the isocenter to the brainstem is a good prognostic variable.**

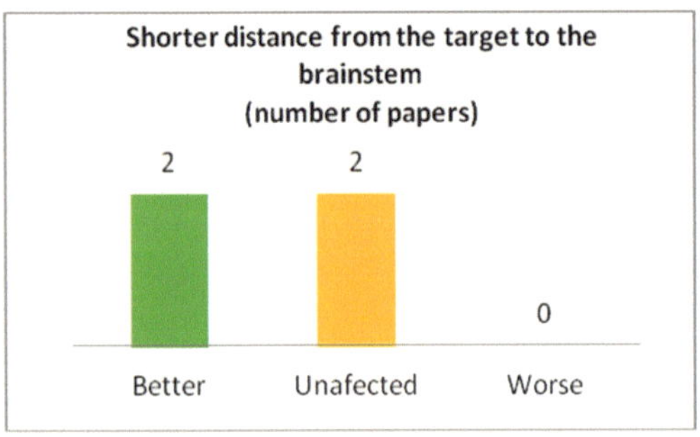

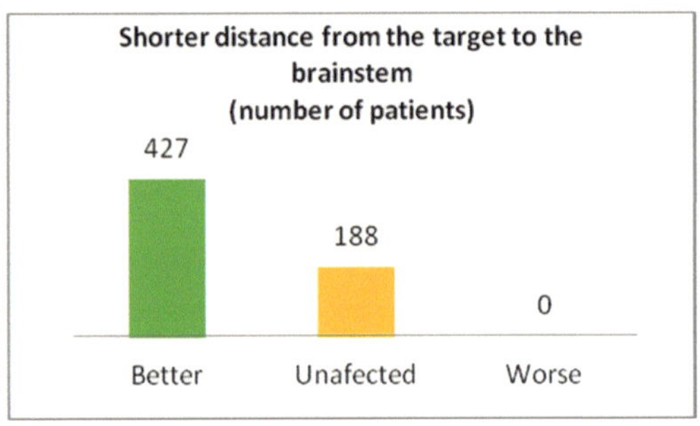

2.3.4 Higher dose received by the brainstem: A higer dose of irradiation received by the brainstem was associated to better results in 3 papers (Brisman, 2000b; Massager, 2007a; Regís 2009). Cheuk (Cheuk, 2004) in a series of 112 patients did not find this correlation. No manuscript showing worse results when a lower dose is received by the brainstem was recognized. As it was previously mentioned, this variable could be linked to the precedent variable (Shorter distance from the isocenter to the brainstem). **There is "reasonable agreement" suggesting better results when the brainstem receives a higher dose of irradiation.**

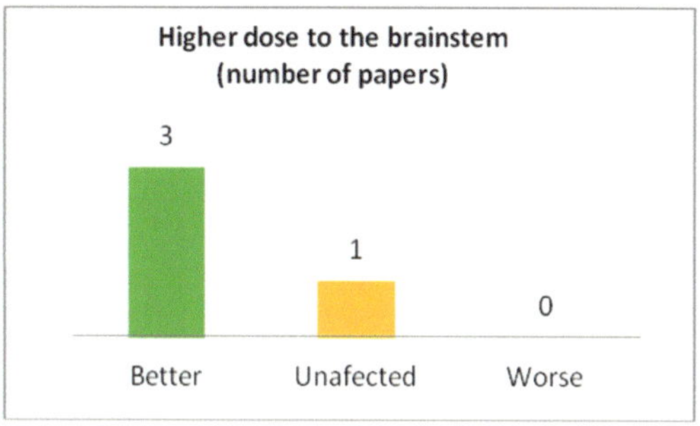

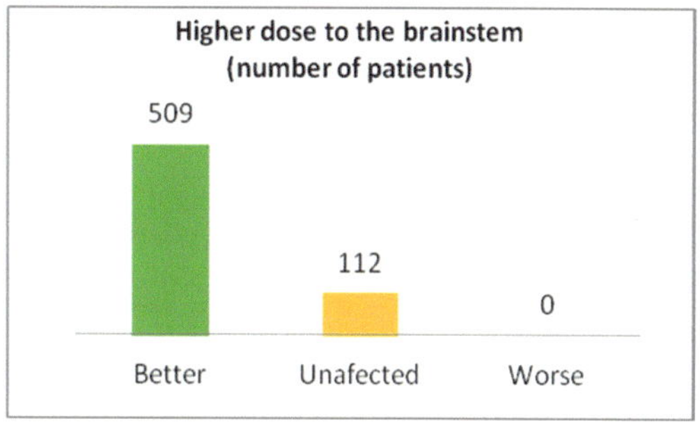

2.3.5 Higher volume of nerve irradiated (multiple isocenters or plugging): This topic is related to the concept of "integral dose", in other words, the quantity of energy received by the nerve in a determined volume. A higher integral dose can be augmented either using of two isocenters or using of plugs. Morbidini-Gaffney (Morbidini-Gaffney, 2006) and Alpert (Alpert, 2005) found better pain control using two isocenters, Conversely Flickinger (Flickinger 2001) in a randomized prospective study found no differences using one or two isocenters and Fountas (Fountas, 2007) reports no differences using one, 2 or 3 isocenters. Nevertheless, nerve dysfunction was more important in the group of patients treated with multiple isocenters. With regard the length of nerve irradiated Sheehan (Sheehan, 2005) and Delarenti (Dellaretti, 2008) reported that this variable did not correlate with pain control. Massager (Massager, 2006; Massager, 2007b), found a larger volume of nerve irradiated and a higher integral dose received by the trigeminal nerve when plugs are used. In these cases better pain outcome but higher nerve toxicity was achieved. The author recommends avoiding the use of plugs in patients treated with a maximal dose of 90 Gray. **"Some agreement with a trend" suggests that a larger irradiated volume of the nerve could correlate with better pain control but associated with more nerve dysfunction.**

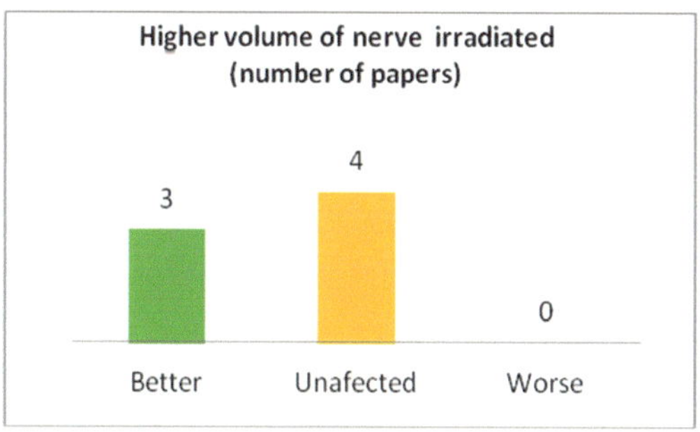

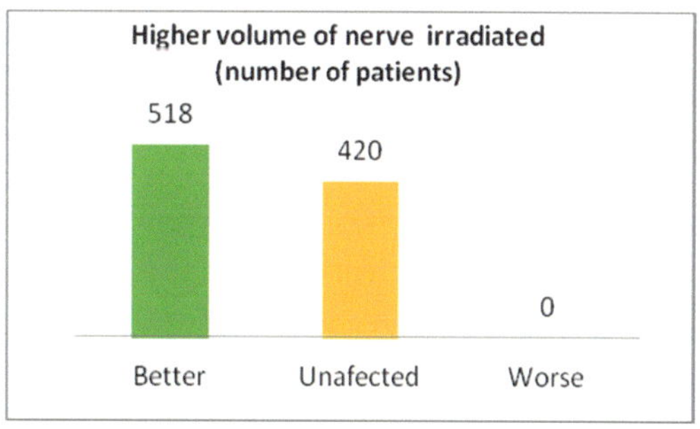

2.3.6 Dose received by the nerve at the level of neurovascular compression: Lorenzoni (Lorenzoni, 2008) found no correlation between the dose of irradiation received by the nerve at the level of the neurovascular compression visualized on magnetic resonance imaging, Sheehan (Sheehan, 2010) by the contrary communicate that pain relief correlated with a higher dose to the point of contact between the impinging vessel and the nerve. With regard to this variable **"scarce information with no clear trend or controversial findings" exist.**

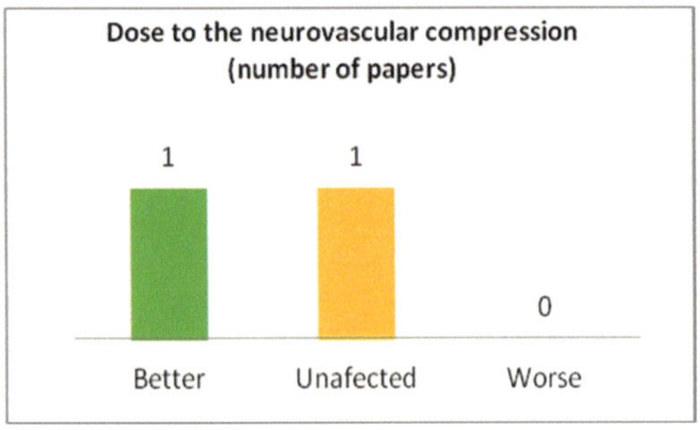

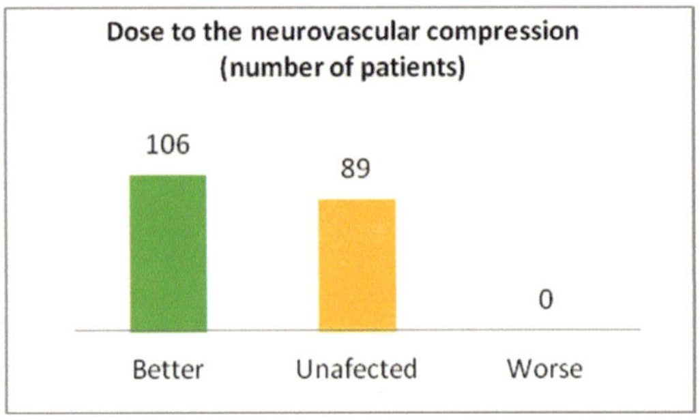

2.3.7 Dose rate: Along the time the cobalt sources decay and the irradiation of the Gamma unit is progressively less, then, for to obtain the same physical dose of irradiation a longer time of treatment is needed. A concern may exist because a longer time of irradiation can allow more tissue reparation with a theoretically less biologic effect. Despite this theory, Arai (Arai, 2010) and Massager (Massager, 2007a) concluded that Gamma Knife dose rate do not affect outcomes (pain control or morbidity). Concerning this variable there is **"Scarce information with a trend".**

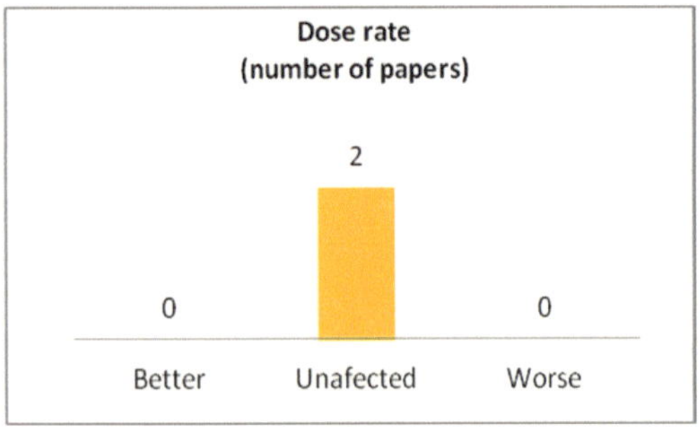

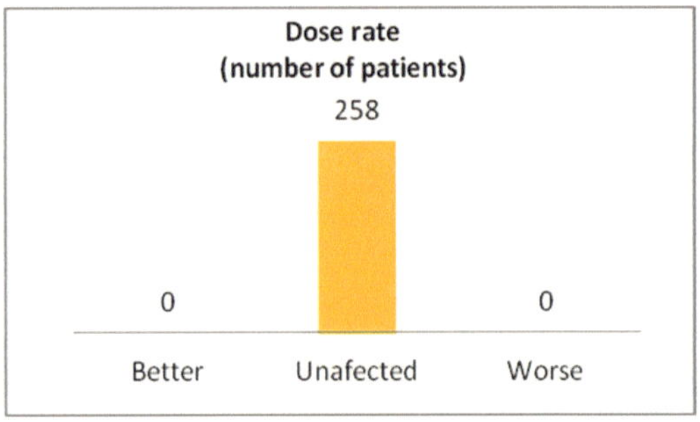

3. Conclusions

3.1 There is consistent agreement for the following variables

1. Gender is not a prognostic factor
2. Pain distribution is not a prognostic factor

3.2 There is reasonable agreement for the following variables

1. Age is not a prognostic factor
2. Side is not a prognostic factor
3. Previous treatments is a negative prognostic factor
4. Post-treatment hypoesthesia is a positive prognostic factor

3.3 There is some agreement with a trend for the following variables

1. Atypical facial pain is a negative prognostic factor
2. Multiple sclerosis is a negative prognostic factor
3. A longer duration of the symptoms is a negative prognostic factor

4. A neurovascular compression visualized on MR is a positive prognostic factor
5. A higher dose of irradiation is a positive prognostic factor
6. A higher volume of nerve irradiated is a positive prognostic factor

3.4 There is scarce information with some trend for the following variables

1. A single branch involved is a positive prognostic factor
2. Secondary trigeminal neuralgia is a negative prognostic factor
3. Post-herpetic neuralgia is a negative prognostic factor
4. Pre-treatment hypoesthesia is a negative prognostic factor
5. Repeated Gamma knife treatment is not prognostic for pain control but associated ith more nerve dysfunction
6. Nerve deformation or dislocation by the vessel is not a prognostic factor
7. Compression by a large vessel (basilar or vertebral artery) is a negative prognostic factor
8. Proximal neurovascular compression is a negative prognostic factor
9. Nerve atrophy has not prognostic value
10. Nerve enhancement after treatment is not a prognostic factor
11. Brainstem enhancement after treatment is not a prognostic factor
12. Shorter distance between the target and the brainstem is a positive prognostic variable
13. Dose rate is not a prognostic factor

3.5 There is scarce information with no clear trend or controversial findings for the following variables

1. Proximal or distal targeting
2. Dose of irradiation received by the nerve at the neurovascular compression

When many papers are analyzed it is frequent to find some differences or even controversial findings in the results and conclusions, then, an overview of a constellation of manuscript could be necessary to have a more solid idea about the multiple variables concerned with Gamma Knife treatment of Trigeminal Neuralgia. A paper is a brick in the knowledge wall and it could be better to look the whole wall instead of focusing the attention in just one brick.

4. References

Alberico R., fenstermaker R., Lobel J (2001) Focal enhancement of cranial nerve V after radiosurgery with the Leksell Gamma Knife: Experience in 15 patients with medically refractory trigeminal neuralgia AJNR 22: 1944-8.

Alpert, T.E., Chung, C.T., Mitchell, L.T., Hodge, C.J., Montgomery, C.T., Bogart, J.A., Kim, D.Y., Bassano, D.A., Hahn, S.S. (2005) Gamma knife surgery for trigeminal neuralgia: improved initial response with two isocenters and increasing dose. J Neurosurg 102 Suppl, 185-188.

Arai, Y., Kano, H., Lunsford, L.D., Novotny, J., Jr., Niranjan, A., Flickinger, J.C., Kondziolka, D. (2010) Does the Gamma Knife dose rate affect outcomes in radiosurgery for trigeminal neuralgia? J Neurosurg 113 Suppl, 168-171.

Aubuchon, A.C., Chan, M.D., Lovato, J.F., Balamucki, C.J., Ellis, T.L., Tatter, S.B., McMullen, K.P., Munley, M.T., Deguzman, A.F., Ekstrand, K.E., Bourland, J.D., Shaw, E.G. (2010) Repeat Gamma Knife Radiosurgery for Trigeminal Neuralgia. Int J Radiat Oncol Biol Phys.

Azar, M., Yahyavi, S.T., Bitaraf, M.A., Gazik, F.K., Allahverdi, M., Shahbazi, S., Alikhani, M. (2009) Gamma knife radiosurgery in patients with trigeminal neuralgia: quality of life, outcomes, and complications. Clin Neurol Neurosurg 111, 174-178.

Brisman, R. (2000) Gamma knife radiosurgery for primary management for trigeminal neuralgia. J Neurosurg 93 Suppl 3, 159-161.

Brisman, R., Mooij, R. (2000) Gamma knife radiosurgery for trigeminal neuralgia: dose-volume histograms of the brainstem and trigeminal nerve. J Neurosurg 93 Suppl 3, 155-158.

Brisman, R., Khandji, A.G., Mooij, R.B. (2002) Trigeminal Nerve-Blood Vessel Relationship as Revealed by High-resolution Magnetic Resonance Imaging and Its Effect on Pain Relief after Gamma Knife Radiosurgery for Trigeminal Neuralgia.

Brisman, R. (2004) Gamma knife surgery with a dose of 75 to 76.8 Gray for trigeminal neuralgia. J Neurosurg 100, 848-854.

Neurosurgery 50, 1261-1266, discussion 1266-1267.

Chang, J.W., Kim, S.H., Huh, R., Park, Y.G., Chung, S.S. (1999) The effects of stereotactic radiosurgery on secondary facial pain. Stereotact Funct Neurosurg 72 Suppl 1, 29-37.

Chang, J.W., Chang, J.H., Park, Y.G., Chung, S.S. (2000) Gamma knife radiosurgery for idiopathic and secondary trigeminal neuralgia. J Neurosurg 93 Suppl 3, 147-151.

Cheng, J.S., Sanchez-Mejia, R.O., Limbo, M., Ward, M.M., Barbaro, N.M. (2005) Management of medically refractory trigeminal neuralgia in patients with multiple sclerosis. Neurosurg Focus 18, e13.

Cheuk, A.V., Chin, L.S., Petit, J.H., Herman, J.M., Fang, H.B., Regine, W.F. (2004) Gamma knife surgery for trigeminal neuralgia: outcome, imaging, and brainstem correlates. Int J Radiat Oncol Biol Phys 60, 537-541.

Cruccu, G., Gronseth, G., Alksne, J., Argoff, C., Brainin, M., Burchiel, K., Nurmikko, T., Zakrzewska, J.M. (2008) AAN-EFNS guidelines on trigeminal neuralgia management. Eur J Neurol 15, 1013-1028.

Dellaretti, M., Reyns, N., Touzet, G., Sarrazin, T., Dubois, F., Lartigau, E., Blond, S. (2008) Clinical outcomes after Gamma Knife surgery for idiopathic trigeminal neuralgia: review of 76 consecutive cases. J Neurosurg 109 Suppl, 173-178.

Dhople, A., Kwok, Y., Chin, L., Shepard, D., Slawson, R., Amin, P., Regine, W. (2007) Efficacy and quality of life outcomes in patients with atypical trigeminal neuralgia treated with gamma-knife radiosurgery. Int J Radiat Oncol Biol Phys 69, 397-403.

Dhople, A.A., Adams, J.R., Maggio, W.W., Naqvi, S.A., Regine, W.F., Kwok, Y. (2009) Long-term outcomes of Gamma Knife radiosurgery for classic trigeminal neuralgia: implications of treatment and critical review of the literature. Clinical article. J Neurosurg 111, 351-358.

Erbay, S.H., Bhadelia, R.A., Riesenburger, R., Gupta, P., O'Callaghan, M., Yun, E., Oljeski, S. (2006) Association between neurovascular contact on MRI and response to gamma knife radiosurgery in trigeminal neuralgia. Neuroradiology 48, 26-30.

Flickinger, J.C., Pollock, B.E., Kondziolka, D., Phuong, L.K., Foote, R.L., Stafford, S.L., Lunsford, L.D. (2001) Does increased nerve length within the treatment volume improve trigeminal neuralgia radiosurgery? A prospective double-blind, randomized study. Int J Radiat Oncol Biol Phys 51, 449-454.

Fountas, K.N., Smith, J.R., Lee, G.P., Jenkins, P.D., Cantrell, R.R., Sheils, W.C. (2007) Gamma Knife stereotactic radiosurgical treatment of idiopathic trigeminal neuralgia: long-term outcome and complications. Neurosurg Focus 23, E8.

Han, J.H., Kim, D.G., Chung, H.T., Paek, S.H., Kim, Y.H., Kim, C.Y., Kim, J.W., Jeong, S.S. (2009) Long-term outcome of gamma knife radiosurgery for treatment of typical trigeminal neuralgia. Int J Radiat Oncol Biol Phys 75, 822-827.

Hayashi, M. (2009) Trigeminal neuralgia. Prog Neurol Surg 22, 182-190.

Huang, E., Teh, B.S., Zeck, O., Woo, S.Y., Lu, H.H., Chiu, J.K., Butler, E.B., Gormley, W.B., Carpenter, L.S. (2002) Gamma knife radiosurgery for treatment of trigeminal neuralgia in multiple sclerosis patients. Stereotact Funct Neurosurg 79, 44-50.

Huang, C.F., Tu, H.T., Liu, W.S., Chiou, S.Y., Lin, L.Y. (2008) Gamma Knife surgery used as primary and repeated treatment for idiopathic trigeminal neuralgia. J Neurosurg 109 Suppl, 179-184.

Huang, C.F., Chiou, S.Y., Wu, M.F., Tu, H.T., Liu, W.S. (2010) Gamma Knife surgery for recurrent or residual trigeminal neuralgia after a failed initial procedure. J Neurosurg 113 Suppl, 172-177.

Jawahar, A., Wadhwa, R., Berk, C., Caldito, G., DeLaune, A., Ampil, F., Willis, B., Smith, D., Nanda, A. (2005) Assessment of pain control, quality of life, and predictors of success after gamma knife surgery for the treatment of trigeminal neuralgia. Neurosurg Focus 18, E8.

Kano, H., Kondziolka, D., Yang, H.C., Zorro, O., Lobato-Polo, J., Flannery, T.J., Flickinger, J.C., Lunsford, L.D. (2010) Outcome predictors after gamma knife radiosurgery for recurrent trigeminal neuralgia. Neurosurgery 67, 1637-1644; discussion 1644-1635.

Kim, Y.H., Kim, D.G., Kim, J.W., Han, J.H., Chung, H.T., Paek, S.H. (2010) Is it effective to raise the irradiation dose from 80 to 85 Gy in gamma knife radiosurgery for trigeminal neuralgia? Stereotact Funct Neurosurg 88, 169-176.

Kimball, B.Y., Sorenson, J.M., Cunningham, D. (2010) Repeat Gamma Knife surgery for trigeminal neuralgia: long-term results. J Neurosurg 113 Suppl, 178-183.

Kondziolka, D., Zorro, O., Lobato-Polo, J., Kano, H., Flannery, T.J., Flickinger, J.C., Lunsford, L.D. (2010) Gamma Knife stereotactic radiosurgery for idiopathic trigeminal neuralgia. J Neurosurg 112, 758-765.

Little, A.S., Shetter, A.G., Shetter, M.E., Bay, C., Rogers, C.L. (2008) Long-term pain response and quality of life in patients with typical trigeminal neuralgia treated with gamma knife stereotactic radiosurgery. Neurosurgery 63, 915-923; discussion 923-914.

Longhi, M., Rizzo, P., Nicolato, A., Foroni, R., Reggio, M., Gerosa, M. (2007) Gamma knife radiosurgery for trigeminal neuralgia: results and potentially predictive parameters--part I: Idiopathic trigeminal neuralgia. Neurosurgery 61, 1254-1260; discussion 1260-1251.

Lopez, B.C., Hamlyn, P.J., Zakrzewska, J.M. (2004) Systematic review of ablative neurosurgical techniques for the treatment of trigeminal neuralgia. Neurosurgery 54, 973-982; discussion 982-973.

Lopez, B.C., Hamlyn, P.J., Zakrzewska, J.M. (2004) Stereotactic radiosurgery for primary trigeminal neuralgia: state of the evidence and recommendations for future reports. J Neurol Neurosurg Psychiatry 75, 1019-1024.

Lorenzoni, J.G., Massager, N., David, P., Devriendt, D., Desmedt, F., Brotchi, J., Levivier, M. (2008) Neurovascular compression anatomy and pain outcome in patients with classic trigeminal neuralgia treated by radiosurgery. Neurosurgery 62, 368-375; discussion 375-366.

Lorenzoni, J., David, P, Levivier M.. (2011) Patterns of neurovascular compression in patients with classic trigeminal neuralgia: A high-resolution MRI-based study. Eur J Radiol.(In press)

Maesawa, S., Salame, C., Flickinger, J.C., Pirris, S., Kondziolka, D., Lunsford, L.D. (2001) Clinical outcomes after stereotactic radiosurgery for idiopathic trigeminal neuralgia. J Neurosurg 94, 14-20.

Massager, N., Lorenzoni, J., Devriendt, D., Desmedt, F., Brotchi, J., Levivier, M. (2004) Gamma knife surgery for idiopathic trigeminal neuralgia performed using a far-anterior cisternal target and a high dose of radiation. J Neurosurg 100, 597-605.

Massager, N., Lorenzoni, J., Devriendt, D., Levivier, M. (2007) Radiosurgery for trigeminal neuralgia. Prog Neurol Surg 20, 235-243.

Massager, N., Murata, N., Tamura, M., Devriendt, D., Levivier, M., Regis, J. (2007) Influence of nerve radiation dose in the incidence of trigeminal dysfunction after trigeminal neuralgia radiosurgery. Neurosurgery 60, 681-687; discussion 687-688.

Massager, N., Nissim, O., Murata, N., Devriendt, D., Desmedt, F., Vanderlinden, B., Regis, J., Levivier, M. (2006) Effect of beam channel plugging on the outcome of gamma knife radiosurgery for trigeminal neuralgia. Int J Radiat Oncol Biol Phys 65, 1200-1205.

Matsuda, S., Serizawa, T., Nagano, O., Ono, J. (2008) Comparison of the results of 2 targeting methods in Gamma Knife surgery for trigeminal neuralgia. J Neurosurg 109 Suppl, 185-189.

Matsuda, S., Nagano, O., Serizawa, T., Higuchi, Y., Ono, J. (2010) Trigeminal nerve dysfunction after Gamma Knife surgery for trigeminal neuralgia: a detailed analysis. J Neurosurg 113 Suppl, 184-190.

Morbidini-Gaffney, S., Chung, C.T., Alpert, T.E., Newman, N., Hahn, S.S., Shah, H., Mitchell, L., Bassano, D., Darbar, A., Bajwa, S.A., Hodge, C. (2006) Doses greater than 85 Gy and two isocenters in Gamma Knife surgery for trigeminal neuralgia: updated results. J Neurosurg 105 Suppl, 107-111.

Nicol, B., Regine, W.F., Courtney, C., Meigooni, A., Sanders, M., Young, B. (2000) Gamma knife radiosurgery using 90 Gy for trigeminal neuralgia. J Neurosurg 93 Suppl 3, 152-154.

Pan, H.C., Sheehan, J., Huang, C.F., Sheu, M.L., Yang, D.Y., Chiu, W.T. (2010) Quality-of-life outcomes after Gamma Knife surgery for trigeminal neuralgia. J Neurosurg 113 Suppl, 191-198.

Park, S.H., Hwang, S.K., Kang, D.H., Park, J., Hwang, J.H., Sung, J.K. (2010) The retrogasserian zone versus dorsal root entry zone: comparison of two targeting techniques of gamma knife radiosurgery for trigeminal neuralgia. Acta Neurochir (Wien) 152, 1165-1170.

Park, Y.S., Kim, J.P., Chang, W.S., Kim, H.Y., Park, Y.G., Chang, J.W. (2011) Gamma knife radiosurgery for idiopathic trigeminal neuralgia as primary vs. secondary treatment option. Clin Neurol Neurosurg 113, 447-452.

Petit JH, Herman JM, Nagda S, diBiase SJ, Chin LS (2003) Radiosurgical treatment of trigeminal neuralgia: evaluating quality of life and treatment outcomes. Int J Radiat Oncol Biol Phys 56, 1147-53.

Pollock, B.E., Iuliano, B.A., Foote, R.L., Gorman, D.A. (2000) Stereotactic radiosurgery for tumor-related trigeminal pain. Neurosurgery 46, 576-582; discussion 582-573.

Pollock, B.E., Phuong, L.K., Foote, R.L., Stafford, S.L., Gorman, D.A. (2001) High-dose trigeminal neuralgia radiosurgery associated with increased risk of trigeminal nerve dysfunction. Neurosurgery 49, 58-62; discussion 62-54.

Pollock B.E., Phuong L.K., Gorman D.A., Foote R.L., Stafford S.L. (2002) Stereotactic radiosurgery for idiopathic trigeminal neuralgia. J. Neurosurg 97, 347-53.

Pollock BE, Foote RL, Link MJ, Stafford SL, Brown PD, Schomberh PJ (2005) Repeat radiosurgery for idiopathic trigeminal neuralgia. Int J Radiat Oncol Biol Phys 61, 192-5.

Regis, J., Metellus, P., Dufour, H., Roche, P.H., Muracciole, X., Pellet, W., Grisoli, F., Peragut, J.C. (2001) Long-term outcome after gamma knife surgery for secondary trigeminal neuralgia. J Neurosurg 95, 199-205.

Regis, J., Metellus, P., Hayashi, M., Roussel, P., Donnet, A., Bille-Turc, F. (2006) Prospective controlled trial of gamma knife surgery for essential trigeminal neuralgia. J Neurosurg 104, 913-924.

Regis, J., Arkha, Y., Yomo, S., Murata, N., Roussel, P., Donnet, A., Peragut, J.C. (2009) [Radiosurgery in trigeminal neuralgia: long-term results and influence of operative nuances]. Neurochirurgie 55, 213-222.

Riesenburger, R.I., Hwang, S.W., Schirmer, C.M., Zerris, V., Wu, J.K., Mahn, K., Klimo, P., Jr., Mignano, J., Thompson, C.J., Yao, K.C. (2010) Outcomes following single-treatment Gamma Knife surgery for trigeminal neuralgia with a minimum 3-year follow-up. J Neurosurg 112, 766-771.

Rogers, C.L., Shetter, A.G., Fiedler, J.A., Smith, K.A., Han, P.P., Speiser, B.L. (2000) Gamma knife radiosurgery for trigeminal neuralgia: the initial experience of The Barrow Neurological Institute. Int J Radiat Oncol Biol Phys 47, 1013-1019.

Rogers, C.L., Shetter, A.G., Ponce, F.A., Fiedler, J.A., Smith, K.A., Speiser, B.L. (2002) Gamma knife radiosurgery for trigeminal neuralgia associated with multiple sclerosis. J Neurosurg 97, 529-532.

Shaya, M., Jawahar, A., Caldito, G., Sin, A., Willis, B.K., Nanda, A. (2004) Gamma knife radiosurgery for trigeminal neuralgia: a study of predictors of success, efficacy, safety, and outcome at LSUHSC. Surg Neurol 61, 529-534; discussion 534-525.

Sheehan, J., Pan, H.C., Stroila, M., Steiner, L. (2005) Gamma knife surgery for trigeminal neuralgia: outcomes and prognostic factors. J Neurosurg 102, 434-441.

Sheehan, J.P., Ray, D.K., Monteith, S., Yen, C.P., Lesnick, J., Kersh, R., Schlesinger, D. (2010) Gamma Knife radiosurgery for trigeminal neuralgia: the impact of magnetic resonance imaging-detected vascular impingement of the affected nerve. J Neurosurg 113, 53-58.

Tawk, R.G., Duffy-Fronckowiak, M., Scott, B.E., Alberico, R.A., Diaz, A.Z., Podgorsak, M.B., Plunkett, R.J., Fenstermaker, R.A. (2005) Stereotactic gamma knife surgery for trigeminal neuralgia: detailed analysis of treatment response. J Neurosurg 102, 442-449.

Urgosik, D., Vymazal, J., Vladyka, V., Liscak, R. (2000) Treatment of postherpetic trigeminal neuralgia with the gamma knife. J Neurosurg 93 Suppl 3, 165-168.

Verheul, J.B., Hanssens, P.E., Lie, S.T., Leenstra, S., Piersma, H., Beute, G.N. (2010) Gamma Knife surgery for trigeminal neuralgia: a review of 450 consecutive cases. J Neurosurg 113 Suppl, 160-167.

Young, R.F., Vermeulen, S.S., Grimm, P., Blasko, J., Posewitz, A. (1997) Gamma Knife radiosurgery for treatment of trigeminal neuralgia: idiopathic and tumor related. Neurology 48, 608-614.

Young, R.F., Vermulen, S., Posewitz, A. (1998) Gamma knife radiosurgery for the treatment of trigeminal neuralgia. Stereotact Funct Neurosurg 70 Suppl 1, 192-199.

Zakrzewska, J.M., Linskey, M.E. (2009) Trigeminal neuralgia. Clin Evid (Online) 2007.

Zorro, O., Lobato-Polo, J., Kano, H., Flickinger, J.C., Lunsford, L.D., Kondziolka, D. (2009) Gamma knife radiosurgery for multiple sclerosis-related trigeminal neuralgia. Neurology 73, 1149-1154.

7

Advanced Gamma Knife Treatment Planning of Epilepsy

Andrew Hwang and Lijun Ma
University of California San Francisco, California, USA

1. Introduction

1.1 Background

Epilepsy is not a single disease, but a broad group of conditions characterized by recurrent seizures resulting from the abnormal firing of cerebral neurons (1). Both medical and surgical treatments have been available for over a century, but there has been recent interest in radiosurgery as an alternative to open surgery for patients with medically intractable epilepsy.

Mesial temporal lobe epilepsy (MTLE) specifically consists of atrophy and gliosis within the limbic system and is the most frequent cause of medically intractable epilepsy in adults (2). Currently, the standard treatment for epilepsy is the use of anticonvulsants. Medically intractable cases may be treated with temporal lobectomy, consisting of removal of parts of the superior temporal gyrus, temporal portion of the amygdala, and the hippocampus.

Other causes of epilepsy include hypothalamic hamartomas (HH) and vascular malformations. Hypothalamic hamartomas are benign lesions composed of varying amounts of glia, neurons, and myelinated fibers. These tumors are often associated with gelastic seizures, precocious puberty, and behavioral problems (3) and often do not respond well to anticonvulsant therapy. As a result, surgical resection and stereotactic radiofrequency thermocoagulation have been used to treat HH (4). Epilepsy is also a symptom of cerebral vascular malformations. In particular, patients with cavernous malformations (CM) frequently present with drug-resistant epilepsy (5).

Given the toxicity of open surgery and poor quality of life for patients with medically intractable epilepsy, stereotactic radiosurgery (SRS) with the Gamma Knife has been proposed as a viable alternative to open surgery for treating these patients. Preliminary data have shown that Gamma Knife radiosurgery is highly promising in terms of safety and efficacy for the treatment of MTLE (6-8). Potential advantages of Gamma Knife radiosurgery include lower morbidity and lower cost with equal effectiveness. One potential disadvantage of radiosurgery is the latency of response, which may be up to two years (9). Although much of the data are promising, the results of Vojtěch et al suggest that more study is needed (10). Based on these data, an international clinical trial is currently being conducted for determining the role of radiosurgery for managing MTLE.

1.2 Radiosurgery for MTLE

Because radiosurgery for MTLE is still an experimental procedure, a multi-center Phase III clinical trial known as the ROSE trial (Radiosurgery or Open Surgery for Epilepsy) was initiated in 2009 to investigate the use of Gamma Knife radiosurgery as an alternative to open surgery for the treatment of medically intractable mesial temporal lobe epilepsy (11, 12). The primary objective of this study is to demonstrate the equivalence of radiosurgery with temporal lobectomy in terms of freedom from seizures. Other endpoints include quality of life, neuropsychological outcomes, and cost-effectiveness.

Due to the location of the target volume and proximity of critical structures, Gamma Knife radiosurgery for mesial temporal lobe epilepsy (MTLE) is technically challenging. In this chapter we will discuss the methods used for planning Gamma Knife radiosurgery treatments for epilepsy, the equipment used for delivering these treatments, and challenges specific to the treatment of MTLE and other causes of epilepsy.

Similar to the traditional surgical approach to treatment of MTLE with temporal lobectomy, the proposed radiosurgical treatment target is comprised of the amygdala, anterior 2 cm of the hippocampus, and the parahippocampal gyrus. Images of a representative target volume are shown in FIG. 1. The current target prescription dose is 24 Gy, which is based on the results of an earlier study in which lower doses were shown to result in reduced efficacy (13). The total irradiated volume is maintained to be less than 7.5 mL in order to minimize late radiation sequelae such as festering radiation necrosis.

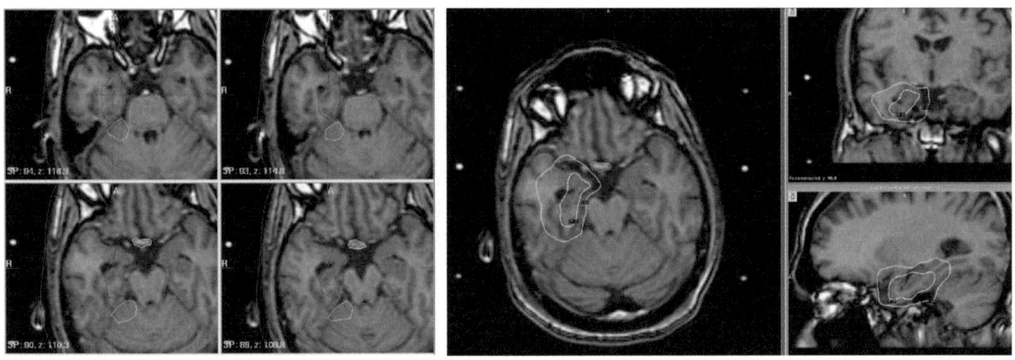

Fig. 1. (left) MR image showing target volume (red), brainstem (pink), and optical chiasm (blue). The target volume consists of the amygdala, anterior hippocampus, and parahippocampal gyrus. (right) A typical dose distribution is shown with the prescription (24 Gy) isodose line shown in yellow and the 8 Gy isodose line in green.

1.3 Radiosurgery for hypothalamic harmatomas and cavernous malformations

Studies have demonstrated that the use of stereotactic radiosurgery for treatment of epilepsy associated with hypothalamic hamartomas is safe and effective (14-22). In 2000, Régis *et al* reported the results of a multi-center study that involved ten patients treated at seven sites with Gamma Knife SRS (15). The median follow-up was 28 months and the results demonstrated a clear relationship between dose and efficacy and the authors recommended a margin dose of 18 Gy or more. Selch *et al* described the use of linac based SRS for the treatment of HH (18). A good summary of the various treatment options for HH including SRS has been published by Régis *et al* (20). This report also includes the results of a prospective study of Gamma Knife SRS for hypothalamic hamartomas. At the time of publication, the authors had sufficient (3 years) follow-up to report results for 27 patients and found that a very good result was obtained in 60% of the patients.

Data have also been published regarding the use of radiosurgery for treatment of epilepsy associated with cavernous malformations (23-28). In 1999, Bartolomei *et al* reported the results of a retrospective study to evaluate the feasibility of using radiosurgery to treat epilepsy associated with cavernous malformations (23, 29). Data from forty nine patients were included in this study, with over 70% either seizure-free or with a significant reduction

Study	Year	No. of Patients	Findings
Hypothalamic Hamartomas			
Régis *et al* (15)	2000	10	40% patients were seizure free.
Unger *et al* (16)	2002	4	No patients seizure free
Barajas *et al* (17)	2005	3	No patients seizure free
Selch *et al* (18)	2005	3	67% seizure free
Matthieu *et al* (19)	2006	4	75% of patients showed improvement
Régis *et al* (20)	2006	27	Very good result in 60% of patients.
Abla *et al* (21)	2010	10	40% were seizure free after SRS.
Mathieu *et al* (22)	2010	9	4/6 patients with smaller tumors seizure free. 0/3 with larger tumors seizure free.
Cavernous Malformations			
Bartolomei *et al* (23)	1999	49	53% of patients seizure free.
Kim *et al* (24)	2005	12	75% of patients seizure free
Liscák *et al* (25)	2005	44	45% improved after radiosurgery
Liu *et al* (26)	2005	28	53% reported good seizure control
Shih and Pan (27)	2005	16	25% remained seizure free.
Hsu *et al* (28)	2007	14	64% seizure free. Linac based radiosurgery.
Mesial Temporal Lobe Epilepsy			
Régis *et al* (7)	1999	7	83% of patients were seizure free.
Régis *et al* (6)	2004	20	65% were seizure free.
Vojtech *et al* (10)	2009	14	18, 20, or 25 Gy. No seizure control achieved.
Quigg *et al* (8)	2011	26	Patients received 20 or 24 Gy. No neuropsychological changes from baseline at 24 months.

Table 1. Published Studies for Radiosurgical Treatment of Epilepsy Due to Various Causes.

in the number of seizures. Shih and Pan reported on 46 patients treated with surgery or radiosurgery for supratentorial cavernous malformations (27). Of this group, 24 of 46 patients presented with seizures. The results suggested that patients undergoing craniotomy had better bleeding and seizure control than those receiving Gamma Knife radiosurgery.

A brief summary of the literature regarding radiosurgical treatment of epilepsy due to various causes can be found in TABLE 1. We also refer the reader to the literature reviews on this topic by Quigg and Barbaro (2) and Romanelli *et al* (30).

2. Methods and techniques

2.1 Mesial temporal lobe epilepsy

The dosimetric criteria for the ROSE trial included: 1) prescription dose of 24 Gy to the 50% isodose line (*i.e.,* maximum dose of 48 Gy), 2) total volume receiving 24 Gy (V-24 Gy) within the range of 5.5-7.5 cm^3, 3) maximum brainstem dose of 10 Gy, and 4) maximum dose of 8 Gy to the optical apparatus.

2.2 Hypothalamic hamartomas

Planning for hypothalamic hamartomas is challenging due to the proximity of the brainstem and the optical apparatus (FIG. 2). However, compared to MTLE, planning for HH is less challenging due to lower doses and smaller target volumes for hypothalamic hamartomas. In our institution, target doses range from 15-18 Gy. Target volumes have ranged from 0.3 to 2.1 cm^3, with a mean volume of 0.81 cm^3 (N=4).

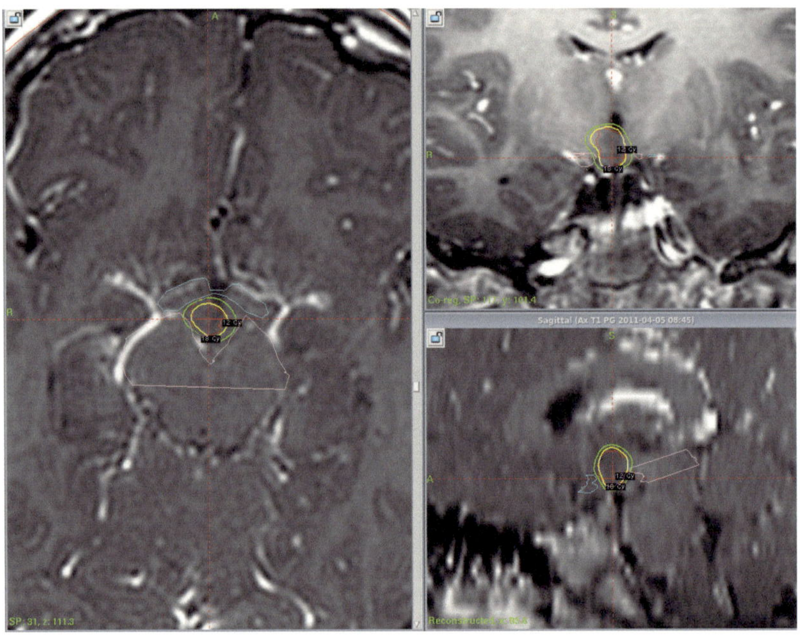

Fig. 2. Radiosurgery treatment for hypothalamic hamartoma. Note the proximity of the brainstem and the optical chiasm to the target volume. The prescription isodose line is shown in yellow and the 12 Gy isodose line in green.

2.3 Benchmarking treatment planning practices

Due to the critical location of these lesions, special radiosurgical treatment planning techniques are applied to minimize the dose to the surrounding normal brain and functional structures. In order to achieve optimal dose fall-off outside of the target, it is preferable to use small collimators (i.e., 4-mm diameter) for treating such lesions. Selective blocking of individual beamlets is a must for enhancing the dose gradient toward a nearby critical structure. However, selective blocking and planning techniques are known to vary significantly among different Gamma Knife models and individual users. To benchmark such differences, a pre-clinical trial quality assurance procedure was developed. The results of such a study are summarized in the following section.

3. Comparison among present gamma knife models for treating MTLE

There are multiple models of the Leksell Gamma Knife currently in use. The newest is the Perfexion model introduced in 2006 (5-7). The Perfexion uses 192 Cobalt-60 sources (versus 201 Cobalt-60 sources of prior Gamma Knife models) focused on a single point, the isocenter. The sources are arranged and divided conically into 8 sectors each containing 24 sources. The sources can be collimated to form circular beams with a 4-mm, 8-mm, or 16-mm diameter respectively or blocked entirely, with each sector being independently controlled, which is fundamentally different from previous models.

By contrast, the previous model Gamma Knife (Model 4C) uses 201 Cobalt-60 sources. The sources are collimated to form circular beams with 4 mm, 8 mm, 14 mm, or 18 mm diameters. The collimator size is selected by switching helmets. All beams have the same diameter, but individual beams can be blocked by "plugging" the helmets. However, switching helmets and changing plugging patterns can be time consuming, so in reality only a limited number of plugging patterns are used. Despite these differences, the mechanical accuracy of all Gamma Knife models has been consistently maintained to be better than 0.4 mm. As a result, Gamma Knife has so far been the only radiosurgical modality reported for managing intractable mesial temporal lobe epilepsy.

As part of the physics review process for the ROSE trial, each center was required to submit a treatment plan based on a sample data set for the purpose of quality assurance. Image data for this sample patient were transferred to participating institutions. The target volume was then delineated and a treatment plan was created to satisfy the previously described dosimetric constraints. The plans were then transferred to the review center for a centralized review by the trial director. Plans that did not satisfy the dosimetric constraints were revised and resubmitted. Plans were submitted for the Gamma Knife Perfexion and C/4C models, depending on the device used at the individual centers. These data were analyzed to look for potential differences between the Perfexion and C/4C models.

A total of 13 plans from 8 institutions satisfied the dosimetric constraints and were included in the data analysis. This included seven plans for the Model 4/4C and six plans for the Perfexion. Details of the individual plans are shown in TABLE 2.

Parameters studied included beam-on time, number of shots, volume receiving 24 Gy (V-24Gy), minimum dose to the delineated target, and the gradient index. Beam-on time was

Plan	Institution	Machine	V-24Gy (cm^3)	Minimum dose (Gy)	Beam-on Time (min)	No. of Shots	Gradient Index
1	1	4C	5.6	6.7	128	17	3.16
2	2	4C	5.7	7.2	209	37	2.90
3	2	4C	5.6	6.0	209	26	2.95
4	3	4C	5.5	6.9	228	20	3.47
5	4	4C	6.2	3.2	180	22	2.86
6	4	4C	5.5	3.8	138	17	3.09
7	5	4C	6.2	9.9	51	4	2.71
All 4C		**4C**	**5.8±0.3**	**6.2±2.2**	**163±62**	**20.4±10.0**	**3.0±0.2**
8	2	Pfxn	6.7	7.1	197	23	3.02
9	6	Pfxn	7.5	5.2	158	17	2.93
10	7	Pfxn	5.6	6.4	120	17	3.02
11	2	Pfxn	5.5	7.0	246	26	2.96
12	8	Pfxn	7.5	7.2	123	19	2.87
13	8	Pfxn	7.4	8.7	88	12	2.95
All Pfxn		**Pfxn**	**6.7±0.9**	**6.9±1.1**	**155±58**	**19.0±4.9**	**3.0±0.1**

Table 2. Summary of Treatment Planning Results of a Single MLTE Case by 8 Individual Institutions.

calculated assuming a dose rate of 3.0 Gy/minute. The gradient index was defined as the volume receiving the prescription dose (24 Gy) divided by the volume receiving half the prescription dose (12 Gy).(31) The Wilcoxon rank-sum test was employed to check for statistical significance.

The average 24-Gy volume was larger for Perfexion plans as compared with Model 4/4C plans, suggesting more aggressive targeting of the treatment area while satisfying normal tissue constraints due to the added flexibility of the Perfexion. Plans created for the Perfexion tended to have a higher minimum dose to the target volume (FIG. 3), which is consistent with the above result. In addition, the results showed that the plans for the Perfexion tended to have shorter beam-on times (155±58 vs. 163±62) and used fewer shots (19±5 vs. 20±10). However the differences were not statistically significant due to the small sample size (FIG. 4). In particular, Plan 7 (for the 4C) used only four shots and had an extremely short beam-on time. After excluding Plan 7, the beam-on time and number of shots for the Model 4C increase to 182±41 minutes and 23±8 shots, respectively. The mean gradient index was 3.0 for both the Perfexion and the Model 4C.

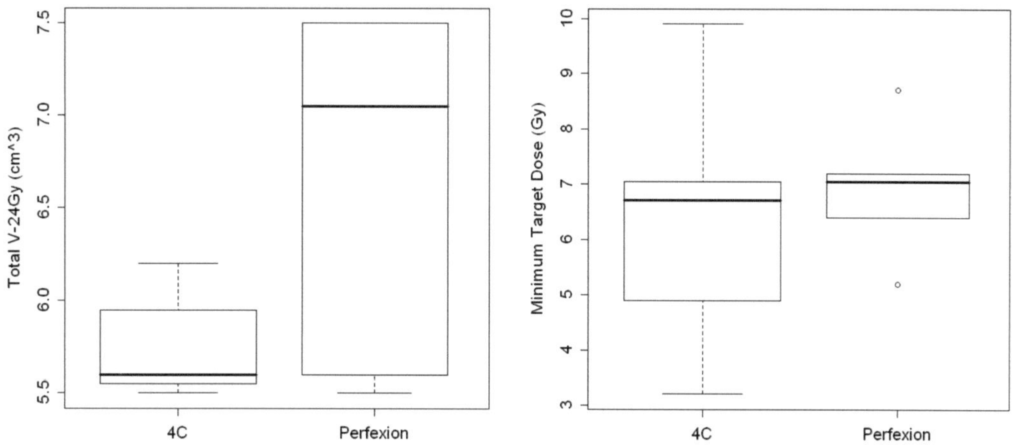

Fig. 3. Boxplots showing the total volume receiving the prescription dose and the minimum dose received by the target. Differences were not statistically significant, although the results suggest that plans generated for the Perfexion provide better target coverage.

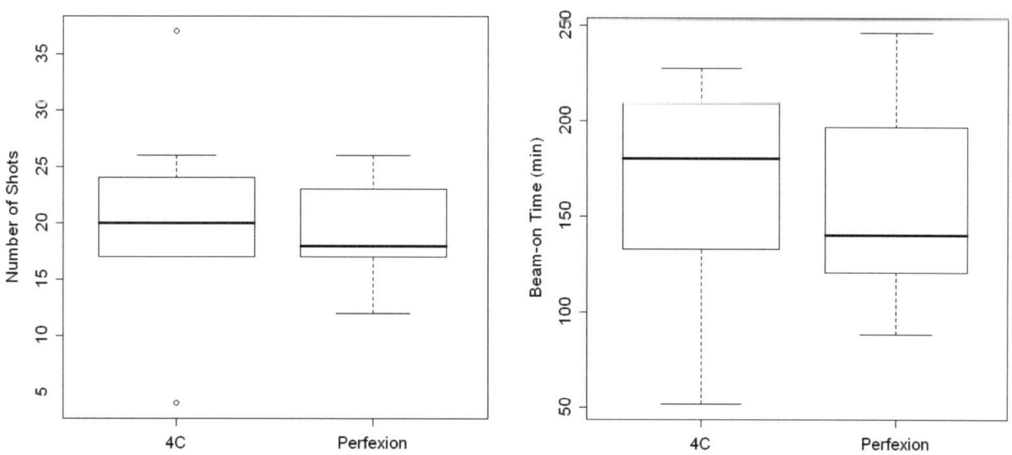

Fig. 4. Comparison of the number of shots and beam-on time of treatment plans for the Gamma Knife Perfexion and Model 4C. Due to high variability in the results, differences are not statistically significant. However, the mean number of shots and mean beam-on time are lower for the Perfexion.

4. Summary

Gamma Knife radiosurgery is being actively investigated as an alternative to open surgery for the treatment of MTLE and other forms of medically intractable epilepsy. Despite notable efficiency and practice differences between the various Gamma Knife models, consistent treatment planning practices and dosimetric parameters are demonstrated for a multi-institutional international trial setting. The final clinical results of such a trial for treating MTLE are forthcoming.

5. References

[1] Engle JJ, Pedley TA. Introduction: What is Epilepsy? In: Engle JJP, Timothy A, ed. Epilepsy: A comprehensive textbook. Philadelphia: Lippincott-Raven Publishers; 1997:1-7.

[2] Quigg M, Barbaro NM. Stereotactic Radiosurgery for Treatment of Epilepsy. *Arch Neurol* 2008; 65:177-83.

[3] Kuzniecky R, Guthrie B, Mountz J, *et al.* Intrinsic epileptogenesis of hypothalamic hamartomas in gelastic epilepsy. *Annals of Neurology* 1997; 42:60-7.

[4] Harvey AS, Freeman JL. Newer operative and stereotactic techniques and their application to hypothalamic hamartoma. In: Wylie EG, Ajay, Lachhwani DK, eds. The treatment of epilepsy:principles and practice 4th ed. Philadelphia: Lippincott Williams & Wilkins; 2006:1169-74.

[5] Casazza M, Broggi G, Franzini A, *et al.* Supratentorial Cavernous Angiomas and Epileptic Seizures: Preoperative Course and Postoperative Outcome. *Neurosurgery* 1996; 39:26-34.

[6] Régis J, Rey M, Bartolomei F, *et al.* Gamma Knife Surgery in Mesial Temporal Lobe Epilepsy: A Prospective Multicenter Study. *Epilepsia* 2004; 45:504-15.

[7] Régis J, Bartolomei F, Rey M, *et al.* Gamma Knife Surgery for Mesial Temporal Lobe Epilepsy. *Epilepsia* 1999; 40:1551-6.

[8] Quigg M, Broshek DK, Barbaro NM, *et al.* Neuropsychological outcomes after Gamma Knife radiosurgery for mesial temporal lobe epilepsy: A prospective multicenter study. *Epilepsia* 2011; 52:909-16.

[9] Régis J, Bartolomei F, Rey M, *et al.* Gamma knife surgery for mesial temporal lobe epilepsy. *Journal of Neurosurgery* 2000; 93:141-6.

[10] Vojtěch Z, Vladyka V, Kalina M, *et al.* The use of radiosurgery for the treatment of mesial temporal lobe epilepsy and long-term results. *Epilepsia* 2009; 50:2061-71.

[11] Barbaro NM, Quigg M. Epilepsy - radiosurgery for epilepsy. *Rev Neurol Dis* 2009; 6:39.

[12] Barbaro NM, Quigg M, Broshek DK, *et al.* A multicenter, prospective pilot study of gamma knife radiosurgery for mesial temporal lobe epilepsy: seizure response, adverse events, and verbal memory. *Ann Neurol* 2009; 65:167-75.

[13] Bartolomei F, Hayashi M, Tamura M, *et al.* Long-term efficacy of gamma knife radiosurgery in mesial temporal lobe epilepsy. *Neurology* 2008; 70:1658-63.

[14] Arita K, Kurisu K, Iida K, *et al.* Subsidence of seizure induced by stereotactic radiation in a patient with a hypothalamic hamartoma. *Journal of Neurosurgery* 1998; 89:645-8.

[15] Régis J, Bartolomei F, de Toffol B, *et al.* Gamma Knife Surgery for Epilepsy Related to Hypothalamic Hamartomas. *Neurosurgery* 2000; 47:1343-52.

[16] Unger F, Schröttner O, Feichtinger M, *et al.* Stereotactic radiosurgery for hypothalamic hamartomas. *Acta Neurochir Suppl* 2002; 84:57-63.

[17] Barajas MA, G. Ramírez-Guzmán M, Rodríguez-Vázquez C, *et al.* Gamma knife surgery for hypothalamic hamartomas accompanied by medically intractable epilepsy and precocious puberty: experience in Mexico. *Special Supplements* 2005; 102:53-5.

[18] Selch MT, Gorgulho A, Mattozo C, *et al.* Linear Accelerator Stereotactic Radiosurgery for the Treatment of Gelastic Seizures due to Hypothalamic Hamartoma. *Minim Invasive Neurosurg* 2005; 48:310,4.

[19] Mathieu D, Kondziolka D, Niranjan A, *et al.* Gamma Knife Radiosurgery for Refractory Epilepsy Caused by Hypothalamic Hamartomas. *Stereotactic and Functional Neurosurgery* 2006; 84:82-7.

[20] Régis J, Scavarda D, Tamura M, *et al.* Epilepsy related to hypothalamic hamartomas: surgical management with special reference to gamma knife surgery. *Child's Nervous System* 2006; 22:881-95-95.

[21] Abla AA, Shetter AG, Chang SW, *et al.* Gamma Knife surgery for hypothalamic hamartomas and epilepsy: patient selection and outcomes. *Special Supplements* 2010; 113:207-14.

[22] Mathieu D, Deacon C, Pinard C-A, *et al.* Gamma Knife surgery for hypothalamic hamartomas causing refractory epilepsy: preliminary results from a prospective observational study. *Special Supplements* 2010; 113:215-21.

[23] Bartolomei F, Régis J, Kida Y, *et al.* Gamma Knife radiosurgery for epilepsy associated with cavernous hemangionmas: a retrospective study of 49 cases. *Stereotactic and Functional Neurosurgery* 1998; 72:22-8.

[24] Kim MS, Pyo SY, Jeong YG, *et al.* Gamma knife surgery for intracranial cavernous hemangioma. *Special Supplements* 2005; 102:102-6.

[25] Liscák R, Vladyka V, Simonová G, *et al.* Gamma knife surgery of brain cavernous hemangiomas. *Special Supplements* 2005; 102:207-13.

[26] Liu K-D, Chung W-Y, Wu H-M, *et al.* Gamma knife surgery for cavernous hemangiomas: an analysis of 125 patients. *Special Supplements* 2005; 102:81-6.

[27] Shih Y-H, Pan DH-C. Management of supratentorial cavernous malformations: craniotomy versus gammaknife radiosurgery. *Clinical Neurology and Neurosurgery* 2005; 107:108-12.

[28] Hsu PW, Chang CN, Tseng CK, *et al.* Treatment of Epileptogenic Cavernomas: Surgery versus Radiosurgery. *Cerebrovascular Diseases* 2007; 24:116-20.

[29] Régis J, Bartolomei F, Kida Y, *et al.* Radiosurgery for Epilepsy Associated with Cavernous Malformation: Retrospective Study in 49 Patients. *Neurosurgery* 2000; 47:1091-7.

[30] Romanelli P, Muacevic A, Striano S. Radiosurgery for hypothalamic hamartomas. *Neurosurgical Focus* 2008; 24:E9.

[31] Paddick I, Lippitz B. A simple dose gradient measurement tool to complement the conformity index. *J Neurosurg* 2006; 105 Suppl:194-201.

8

Hemorrhage from Arteriovenous Malformation Following Gamma Knife Radiosurgery: Pathophysiology of Rupture Early in the Latency Period

Juanita M. Celix, James G. Douglas and Robert Goodkin
University of Washington
USA

1. Introduction

Arteriovenous malformations (AVM) are uncommon congenital abnormalities with a prevalence of 10-18 per 100, 000 adults (Al-Shahi et al. 2002; Berman et al. 2000) and an incidence of 1. 3 per 100, 000 person-years. (Stapf et al. 2003) Arteriovenous malformations typically present with hemorrhage, seizure, or focal neurological deficit. Intracranial hemorrhage is the most common clinical presentation of an AVM, resulting in significant morbidity and mortality. The natural risk of primary hemorrhage in untreated AVMs is 2% to 4% per year. (Barrow and Reisner 1993; Brown et al. 1988; Crawford et al. 1986; Davis and Symon 1985; Forster, Steiner, and Hakanson 1972; Fults and Kelly 1984; Graf, Perret, and Torner 1983; Mast et al. 1997; Ondra et al. 1990; Pollock et al. 1996) The primary goal of AVM treatment is elimination of the risk of hemorrhage by removal of the bleeding potential of the abnormal vasculature. Currently, the therapeutic options for AVM treatment include microsurgical resection, stereotactic radiosurgery (SRS), and endovascular embolization, alone or in combination. Small AVMs or those that are surgically inaccessible in deep brain or eloquent cortex are typically amenable to stereotactic radiosurgery.

Complete obliteration of the vascular malformation and concomitant elimination of the risk of hemorrhage are the goals of radiosurgical treatment for AVM. There is generally a latency period of 2 to 3 years to achieve the vessel obliteration that results from radiation-induced changes to the abnormal vasculature, and 80%-95% of patients will achieve angiographic obliteration by 5 years. (Colombo et al. 1994; Friedman, Bova, and Mendenhall 1995; Karlsson, Lindquist, and Steiner 1997; Lindqvist et al. 2000) During the interval from treatment to AVM obliteration, a risk of rupture persists, but there is debate as to the direction and magnitude of the influence of radiosurgery on the risk of AVM hemorrhage during the latency period. Conflicting reports in the literature provide evidence for a decreased risk of hemorrhage, (Karlsson, Lax, and Soderman 2001; Karlsson, Lindquist, and Steiner 1996; Kjellberg et al. 1983; Levy et al. 1989; Maruyama et al. 2005; Maruyama et al. 2007; Yen et al. 2007) an unchanged risk of hemorrhage, (Friedman et al. 1996; Kjellberg 1986; Lunsford et al. 1991; Maesawa et al. 2000; Nataf et al.

2004; Pollock et al. 1996; Steiner et al. 1992) and an increased risk of hemorrhage. (Colombo et al. 1994; Fabrikant et al. 1992; Steinberg et al. 1990) There is also evidence that a risk of hemorrhage persists even after radiographic obliteration of the AVM. (Izawa et al. 2005; Lindqvist et al. 2000; Matsumoto et al. 2006; Shin et al. 2005; Yamamoto et al. 1992; Prat et al. 2009)

Hemorrhage in the early period following SRS is a rare occurrence, with few reports in the literature (Table 1). In the 30-day period following SRS, most reported cases of post-radiosurgery hemorrhage within 72 hours of radiosurgery occurred in patients with irradiated tumors. (Franco-Vidal et al. 2007; Izawa et al. 2006; Park et al. 2000; Suzuki et al. 2003; Uchino et al. 2003) There is only one report of AVM hemorrhage within 72 hours following SRS. (Nataf et al. 2004) Within 4 to 30 days following SRS there are a few more documented cases of post-radiosurgery AVM hemorrhage. (Chang et al. 2004; Colombo et al. 1994; Pollock et al. 1994; Shimizu et al. 2001; Shin et al. 2004; Yen et al. 2007; Zabel-du Bois et al. 2007; Celix et al. 2009) With two exceptions, the cases reported in the literature of AVM hemorrhage in the early period following radiosurgery are presented in the context of retrospective observational cohort studies and the clinical and radiographical details of the cases are not described. One published case report of rupture of a pial AVM 29 days following SRS was associated with pretreatment partial thrombosis of a distal draining vein varix. (Shimizu et al. 2001) The authors of this chapter recently published a case of AVM hemorrhage occurring 9 days after gamma knife radiosurgery, with radiographic documentation of venous thrombus formation immediately preceding intracranial hemorrhage. (Celix et al. 2009) We posit that the pathophysiology of AVM rupture in the early period following SRS differs from rupture occurring months after radiosurgery.

There is a substantial literature on AVM hemorrhage and the associated factors that increase hemorrhage risk both prior to treatment and following radiosurgery. Clinical and morphological risk factors for AVM rupture during the latency period have been proposed, but little is known about the mechanism of and risk factors for hemorrhage in the early period following radiosurgery. The histological effects of radiation on abnormal AVM vessels, the resultant alterations in cerebral hemodynamics, and the timing of vascular changes in relation to the timing of AVM rupture post-radiosurgery have not been extensively studied, but the available literature evidence supports the association among tissue irradiation, acute inflammatory response, and vessel thrombosis in the pathophysiology of early hemorrhage following AVM radiosurgery.

2. Risk factors for AVM hemorrhage – Untreated AVMs

Based on observational studies, there are several characteristics that are hypothesized to predispose to hemorrhage in untreated AVMs. Patient age (Crawford et al. 1986; Graf, Perret, and Torner 1983; Karlsson et al. 1997; Mast et al. 1997) and pregnancy status (Dias and Sekhar 1990; Forster, Kunkler, and Hartland 1993; Horton et al. 1990; Robinson, Hall, and Sedzimir 1974) are proposed factors with insufficient evidence to support their association with an increased risk of AVM hemorrhage. Arteriovenous malformation size (Crawford et al. 1986; Graf, Perret, and Torner 1983; Guidetti and Delitala 1980; Itoyama et al. 1989; Kader et al. 1994; Karlsson et al. 1997; Langer et al. 1998; Parkinson and Bachers 1980; Spetzler et al. 1992; Waltimo 1973) and AVM location (Crawford et al. 1986; Duong et al.

Author	Dx	Treatment Modality	Study Type	Prescription Dose (Gy) Range, Mean	Maximum Dose (Gy) Range, Mean	Isodose Line (%) Range, Mean	Age (yrs), Sex	Time Course	Outcome
Celix 2009	AVM	GK	CR	18	36	50	57, M	9 Day	Died
Zabel-du Bois 2007	AVM	LINAC	Cohort	15 - 22, 18 (Median)	(18.8 - 27.5)†	80	NR, NR	6 Day	NR
Yen 2007	AVM	GK	Cohort	15 - 31, 22.5	22 - 90, 41.3	30 - 91, 50 (Median)	NR, NR	30 Day	NR
Franco-Vidal 2007	VS	GK	CR	13	(26)†	50	20, M	24 Hr	Hearing Loss
Izawa 2006	Met	GK	CR	20	(40)†	50	46, F	15 Min	Died
Chang 2004	AVM	NR	Cohort	12 - 20, 19.3	15 - 25, 24.1	80	NR, NR	30 Day	NR
Nataf 2004	AVM	LINAC	Cohort	19 - 28, 23	(27 - 56)	50 - 70, 70 (Median)	NR, NR	< 24 Hr	NR
Shin 2004	AVM	GK	Cohort	17 - 28, 20 (Median)	25 - 60, 40 (Median)	NR	NR, NR	< 30 Day	NR
Suzuki 2003	Met	LINAC	Cohort	20 - 25	NR	NR	NR, NR	1 Day	NR
							NR, NR	14 Day	NR
							NR, NR	14 Day	NR
							NR, NR	30 Day	NR
							NR, NR	30 Day	NR
Uchino 2003	Met	NR	CR	20	25 - 30	(67 - 80)†	44, F	2 Hr	Transient Aphasia
Shimizu 2001	AVM	GK	CR	20	40	50	50, M	29 Day	ND
Park 2000	Met	GK	CR	10	(20)†	50	69, M	3 Day	Died
Pollock 1994	AVM	GK	Cohort	15 - 25, 21	22.2 - 50, 36	≥50‡	35, F	30 Day	ND
							NR, NR	30 Day	ND
Colombo 1994	AVM	LINAC	Cohort	(13 – 36)†	18.7 - 40, 28.2	70 - 90	NR, NR	6 Day	NR

Dx=diagnosis; AVM=arteriovenous malformation; VS=vestibular schwannoma; Met=metastasis; GK=gamma knife; LINAC=linear accelerator; CR=case report; Cohort=retrospective observational cohort; Gy=gray; NR=not reported; ND=no deficit.
† Values in parenthesis were calculated from available data.
‡ 98% of patients were treated at ≥50% isodose line.

Table 1. Cases of hemorrhage within 30 days following stereotactic radiosurgery.

1998; Langer et al. 1998; Marks et al. 1990; Stefani et al. 2002; Turjman et al. 1995; Willinsky et al. 1988) are proposed risk factors that may have a confounded association with an increased risk of hemorrhage. Arteriovenous malformation size and location may be associated with hemorrhagic presentation and may not truly represent characteristics that increase the risk of AVM hemorrhage. Arteriovenous malformation size and location may also be associated with other AVM characteristics, such as feeding artery pressure and venous drainage pattern, respectively, that could independently predispose to AVM rupture. (Duong et al. 1998; Spetzler et al. 1992; Stefani et al. 2002)

Several studies provide evidence of independent risk factors for AVM hemorrhage. Deep venous drainage, (Kader et al. 1994; Langer et al. 1998; Duong et al. 1998; Marks et al. 1990; Mast et al. 1997) AVM size, (Kader et al. 1994; Langer et al. 1998) diffuse AVM morphology, (Pollock et al. 1996) feeding artery pressure, (Duong et al. 1998) intranidal aneurysms, (Marks et al. 1990) deep, periventricular or intraventricular AVM location, (Marks et al. 1990; Zipfel et al. 2004; Stefani et al. 2002) a single draining vein, (Pollock et al. 1996; Stefani et al. 2002) and venous ectasias (Stefani et al. 2002) have been shown to be independent risk factors. Studies also suggest other risk factors for AVM hemorrhage. Multiple aneurysms, (Turjman et al. 1995) perforating feeding vessels, (Turjman et al. 1995) and venous outflow compromise (Miyasaka et al. 1992; Vinuela et al. 1985) have been proposed to influence the risk of AVM hemorrhage.

There is additional evidence that a history of prior AVM hemorrhage predisposes to an increased risk of subsequent hemorrhage. (Crawford et al. 1986; Forster, Steiner, and Hakanson 1972; Fults and Kelly 1984; Graf, Perret, and Torner 1983; Halim et al. 2004; Itoyama et al. 1989; Kjellberg 1986; Mast et al. 1997; Pollock et al. 1996; da Costa et al. 2009) Studies have reported annual hemorrhage rates of 6% to 33% in the first year after a primary hemorrhage. (Forster, Steiner, and Hakanson 1972; Fults and Kelly 1984; Graf, Perret, and Torner 1983; Itoyama et al. 1989; Mast et al. 1997; da Costa et al. 2009) There is disagreement as to whether this risk remains elevated for the long term or only a short period following the initial hemorrhage, and some argue against the hypothesis that prior AVM hemorrhage increases the natural risk of subsequent hemorrhage. (Ondra et al. 1990; Stefani et al. 2002)

3. Risk factors for AVM hemorrhage – Radiosurgically treated AVMs

Since the first use of radiosurgery for AVM was reported in 1972, observational cohort studies have provided us with valuable information on rates of AVM rupture and risk factors associated with AVM hemorrhage during the latency period (Table 2). In one of the largest follow-up studies, the risk of AVM rupture during the latency period was reported to be 4. 8% per year during the first 2 years and 5. 0% per year for 3 to 5 years following SRS. (Pollock et al. 1996) Other studies report the risk to be 1. 2% to 6. 5% per year prior to obliteration. (Friedman et al. 1996; Friedman and Bova 1992; Karlsson, Lax, and Soderman 2001; Karlsson, Lindquist, and Steiner 1996; Maruyama et al. 2007; Miyawaki et al. 1999; Nataf et al. 2004; Nicolato et al. 2006; Pollock et al. 1994; Shin et al. 2004; Steiner et al. 1992)

The data from observational cohort studies have been used to propose risk factors associated with AVM hemorrhage after SRS. These studies have demonstrated that several of the risk factors for hemorrhage after SRS may be different from those associated with hemorrhage prior to treatment. The risk of AVM hemorrhage during the latency period is

Table 2. (Continued)

Author, (Yr)	Tx	Number Patients	Study Period	Prescription Dose (Gy) Range, Mean	Maximum Dose (Gy) Range, Mean	Isodose Line (%) Range, Mean	Follow-up Period (Months) Range, Mean	Latency Hemorrhage Number, (%)	Latency Hemorrhage Cumulative Incidence	Latency Period Annualized Hemorrhage Rate	Latency Hemorrhage Risk Factors****
Zabel-du Bois (2007)	LINAC	50	1996-2002	15-22, 18 (Median)	(18.75-27.5)	80	8.5-180, 37 (Median)	6 (12)	ND	ND	Obliteration status, AVM size, AVM volume, AVM score (RBAS), Dose†
Yen (2007)	GK	159	1970-2004	15-31, 22.5	22-90, 41.3	30-91, 50 (Median)	5-185, 59.4	1 (0.63)	ND	ND	ND
Moreno-Jimenez (2007)	LINAC	40	Jan 2003-Dec 2003	10.5-20, 15.4	13-22, 18.5	63-95, 84	23-34, 29	1 (2.5)	ND	ND	ND
Maruyama (2007)	GK	182	1990-2004	21	40.9	NR	NR	11 (6.0)	ND	2.0%	None†
Nicolato (2006)	GK	362**	Feb 1993-Dec 2004	16.8-43.3, 28.6	20-62.5, 40.5 (Median)	22-90, 54.2 (Median)	1.1-130.7, 30.6 (Median)	8 (2.7)	ND	1.2%	ND
Maruyama (2005)	GK	500	July 1990-June 2003	21	40.9	50	93.6 (Median)	23 (5.0)	ND	ND	ND
Zabel (2005)	LINAC	110	1998-2001	14-22, 18 (Median)	(17.5-27.5)	80	7.8-86, 30 (Median)	9 (8.2)	3.7% 1yr 3.0% 2yr 3.5% 3yr	ND	AVM size, Obliteration status†
Nataf (2004)	LINAC	756	Jan 1984-Dec 1999	19-28, 23	NR	50-70, 70 (Median)	0-178, 26	51 (6.7)	ND	3.1%	AVM size, SM grade, Reference isodose, Minimum dose, Intranidal/ paranidal aneurysm, Complete AVM coverage†
Shin (2004)	GK	400	June 1990-Nov 1999	17-28, 20 (Median)	25-60, 40 (Median)	NR	1-135, 63	21 (5.3)	4.6% 3yr 10.2% 5 yr 14.6% 10yr	1.9%	Age, AVM location, BA feeders, Cerebellar symptoms[A]
Zipfel (2004)	LINAC	268	NR	NR	NR	NR	NR	26 (9.7)	ND	ND	None†
Friedman (2003)	LINAC	269	Feb 1989-Feb 1999	NR	NR	NR	NR	28 (10)	ND	ND	None†
Inoue (2002)	GK	115	1991-1995	17-25, 20.1	NR	NR	NR	8 (7)	ND	ND	AVM flow rate[B]
Karlsson (2001)	GK	1593	1970-1995	NR	NR	NR	NR	56 (3.5)	ND	1.8%	Mimimum dose, Average dose, Age, AVM volume‡

Author, (Yr)	Tx	Number Patients	Study Period	Prescription Dose (Gy) Range, Mean	Maximum Dose (Gy) Range, Mean	Isodose Line (%) Range, Mean	Follow-up Period (Months) Range, Mean	Latency Hemorrhage Number, (%)	Latency Hemorrhage Cumulative Incidence	Latency Period Annualized Hemorrhage Rate	Latency Hemorrhage Risk Factors****
Miyawaki (1999)	LINAC	73	Mar 1988-Sept 1991	NR	17.5-46.5, 25 (Median)	23-90, 66 (Median)	NR	12 (16)	12%-16% 5yr 33%-55% 7yr	3.9%-5.5%	AVM size, venous drainage pattern, prior hemorrhage[C]
Pollock (1996)	GK	315	Aug 1987-Jan 1992	12-32, 20 (Median)	22-50, 35.7 (Median)	≥50***	47	21 (6.7)	ND	4.8%£ 5.0%ß	Unsecured proximal aneurysm[D]
Friedman (1996)	LINAC	201	May 1988-Feb 1995	15	NR	NR	NR	12 (6.0)	ND	4.8%€ 5.6%¥ 4.4%Æ	AVM volume, SM grade, Dose, Isodose line ≤70Gy[A]
Karlsson (1996)	GK	1604	Apr 1970-June 1992	NR	NR	NR	NR	49 (3.1)	ND	2.1%£	Minimum dose, Average dose, Age, AVM volume‡
Yamamoto (1995)	GK	121	Jan 1990-Dec 1993	16-22, 18	22-44, 35	50-70	12-60	7 (5.8)	ND	ND	None§
Pollock (1994)	GK	65	Aug 1987-Aug 1991	15-25, 21	22.2-50, 36	≥50***	24-60, 35	5 (7.7)	ND	3.7%	ND
Colombo (1994)	LINAC	180	Nov 1984-Apr 1992	NR	18.7-40, 28.2	70-90	1-88, 43.1	15 (8.3)	9.3% 1yr 13.3% 2yr	ND	Ratio maximum dose/peripheral dose[A]
Seifert (1994)	PB	68	Oct 1980-May 1990	NR	NR	NR	30-144	5 (7.9)	ND	ND	ND
Steiner (1992)	GK	247	Apr 1970-Dec 1983	NR	NR	NR	NR	9 (3.6)	3.4% 35mos 7.2% 2yr 11.2% 5yr	1.9%-6.5%	ND
Friedman (1992)	LINAC	80	May 1988-Aug 1991	10-25, 16.5	NR	70-90, 80	3-42, 19	2 (2.5)	ND	1.6%	ND
Lunsford (1991)	GK	227	Aug 1987-Aug 1990	12-27, 21.2	22-50, 36.5	40-90	3-36, 14	10 (4.4)	ND	ND	ND
Steinberg (1990)	PB	86	July 1983-Jan 1984	NR	NR	NR	24-72, 38	10 (12)	ND	ND	ND

AVM=arteriovenous malformation; Tx=treatment modality; LINAC=linear accelerator; GK=gamma knife; PB=proton beam; Gy-gray; NR=not reported; ND=not determined; RBAS=radiosurgery based AVM score; SM=Spetzler-Martin; BA=basilar artery.

**Separate analysis of patients age ≥21 years.

***98% of patients were treated at >=50% isodose line.

**** By univariate or multivariate analysis; † $p<0.05$; ‡ $p<0.01$; §=level of significance not reported.

A=$p<0.05$, level of significance not reported; *B*=$p=0.005$, level of significance not reported; *C*=$p<0.003$, level of significance not reported; *D*=$p<0.001$, level of significance not reported.
£=per year during years 1-2; ß=per year during years 3-5; €=per year 1st year; ¥=per year 2nd year; Æ=per year during years 1-5.

Table 2. AVM hemorrhage during the latency period following stereotactic radiosurgery.

hypothesized to be related to patient age, (Karlsson, Lax, and Soderman 2001; Karlsson, Lindquist, and Steiner 1996; Shin et al. 2004) AVM size/volume, (Friedman et al. 1996; Karlsson, Lax, and Soderman 2001; Karlsson, Lindquist, and Steiner 1996; Miyawaki et al. 1999; Nataf et al. 2004; Zabel et al. 2005; Zabel-du Bois et al. 2007) and radiation dose. (Colombo et al. 1994; Friedman et al. 1996; Karlsson, Lax, and Soderman 2001; Karlsson, Lindquist, and Steiner 1996; Nataf et al. 2004; Zabel-du Bois et al. 2007) The presence of intranidal, paranidal, or unsecured proximal aneurysms, (Nataf et al. 2004; Pollock et al. 1996) AVM flow rate, (Inoue and Ohye 2002) and the extent of AVM coverage (Nataf et al. 2004) are also reported to be associated with the risk of post-radiosurgery AVM hemorrhage.

The use of observational cohort studies, whether prospective or retrospective, natural history or descriptive, to determine truly independent risk factors for AVM hemorrhage is inadequate for several reasons. Arteriovenous malformations are uncommon, thus the conclusions suggested by many observational studies are limited by small sample size. Selection bias cannot be avoided in studies of AVM natural history and risk factors for hemorrhage due to physician referral practices, surgeon treatment preferences and standards of care, and fatal hemorrhages excluding those patients from analysis. In addition, the clinical, morphological, and physiological characteristics of AVMs that are surgically resected differ from those that are treated with radiosurgery and those that are followed without treatment. The confounded association of risk factors for AVM hemorrhage can be addressed by statistical methods to control for confounding, but, even in well-designed observational studies, residual confounding will likely persist after statistical adjustment. Given the limitations of the retrospective observational cohort study design, it is unlikely that we will be able to estimate the true risk of AVM hemorrhage for a particular population. From these studies, though, the identification of factors that may be associated with AVM hemorrhage during the latency period has enhanced our understanding of the disease and influenced the evolution of radiosurgical treatment for AVM.

With so few literature reports of AVM hemorrhage in the early period following SRS, little is known of the risk factors for or mechanisms of AVM hemorrhage during the early period. To begin to understand the potential differences between AVM hemorrhage in the early period following SRS and AVM hemorrhage that occurs months to years following radiosurgery, it is important to understand the histological and ultrastructural effects of radiation in the central nervous system and the hemodynamic alterations that can occur in different pathophysiological settings. There is an acute inflammatory response following tissue irradiation, resulting in structural and functional vascular changes that can lead to vessel thrombosis and AVM rupture.

4. Histopathological effect of radiation and vessel obliteration

The tissue effects of radiation have been documented and studied since the discovery of ionizing x-rays. Both the desired outcomes and the undesired complications of any radiation therapy are the result of the same pathophysiological processes in the irradiated tissue. The mechanisms of vascular obliteration after stereotactic radiosurgery are not completely understood, (O'Connor and Mayberg 2000) but several histological and ultrastructural studies have helped to elucidate the physiological basis. (Adams 1991; Chang et al. 1997; Schneider, Eberhard, and Steiner 1997; Szeifert et al. 1997; Szeifert, Major, and Kemeny 2005; Tu et al. 2006; Yamamoto et al. 1992) Focused irradiation causes damage to endothelial cells and induces the subsequent proliferation of smooth muscle cells, fibroblasts, and myofibroblasts in the subendothelial layer. The elaboration of collagenous extracellular matrix in the intimal layer follows, leading to progressive hyalinization and thickening of the intimal layer, stenosis of the irradiated vessels, and complete vessel occlusion and nidal obliteration.

The histological response of normal vessels to irradiation follows a predictable pattern, but the timing and extent of the response of both normal cerebral vessels to conventional irradiation and the abnormal vasculature of cerebral AVMs to radiosurgery is highly variable. (Fajardo and Berthrong 1988; Schneider, Eberhard, and Steiner 1997; Tu et al. 2006) A decrease in blood flow through AVMs, which is consistent with decreased luminal diameter due to intimal thickening, has been demonstrated on magnetic resonance (MR) imaging and angiography within a few months following radiosurgery. (Lunsford et al. 1991; Yamamoto et al. 1992) Arteriovenous malformations treated with radiosurgery may completely radiographically obliterate as early as a few months or more than 8 years after SRS, (Lunsford et al. 1991; Yen et al. 2007) and persistence of subtotal obliteration is documented during follow-up periods as great as 14 years after radiosurgery. (Yen et al. 2007) The vaso-occlusive effects of SRS, as demonstrated on MR imaging or angiography, progress slowly and heterogeneously, generally reaching a maximum at 1 to 3 years post-radiosurgery. Many studies have found that approximately 75% of AVMs are completely obliterated at 2 to 3 years post-radiosurgery. (Coffey, Nichols, and Shaw 1995; Guo et al. 1993; Lunsford et al. 1991; Shin et al. 2004; Yamamoto et al. 1993; Yamamoto et al. 1992) Observational studies utilizing MR imaging and angiography have documented the time course of the hemodynamic manifestations of vessel obliteration, (Quisling et al. 1991; Yamamoto et al. 1993) and the sequence of histological changes appears to correlate with the reduction in AVM size on imaging. (Schneider, Eberhard, and Steiner 1997) The true range of time to histological AVM obliteration, though, is unknown. There is evidence that radiographic obliteration does not correspond with histological obliteration. (Yamamoto et al. 1992) The difficulty in obtaining tissue during the early period following SRS results in a lack of histopathological studies of early AVM changes and a paucity of data concerning the time course of histological AVM obliteration.

Early radiation-induced obliteration of the venous system and resultant venous outflow impairment may increase the risk of early AVM hemorrhage following SRS, but there is a lack of literature evidence to support this hypothesis. There are no published ultrastructural or histopathological studies of AVMs in the early period following radiosurgery. Additionally, neither the histological effect of radiation on the venous drainage system of AVMs nor the variable radiosensitivity of the draining vessel walls compared to the nidus vessel walls has been explored. A case report of the histological findings at autopsy in a woman with an AVM treated with radiosurgery and confirmed by angiography to be obliterated at 2 years, who died of causes unrelated to the AVM, showed that obliteration occurs in nidal arteries before nidus-associated veins. (Yamamoto et al. 1995) Some studies have demonstrated an increased resistance of veins to radiation-induced changes compared to capillaries and arteries. (Fajardo 1982) A study of SRS for treatment of venous angioma showed a lower proportion of complete or partial obliteration compared to radiosurgically treated AVMs receiving similar doses. (Lindquist et al. 1993) These observations suggest that the abnormal veins associated with vascular malformations may be less radiosensitive than arteries. The decreased radiosensitivity of veins and slower venous obliteration provide evidence against the role of radiation-induced vessel changes in AVM hemorrhage in the immediate post-radiosurgery setting. Based on the current knowledge of cellular responses to tissue irradiation, the time course of progressive intimal thickening and vessel occlusion, even if abnormally accelerated, cannot explain AVM hemorrhage in the early period following SRS.

5. Hemodynamic alterations and AVM hemorrhage

Venous thrombosis is a proposed mechanism for intracranial hemorrhage and there are reports in the literature of hemorrhage from venous malformations associated with thrombosis of the draining vein. (Field and Russell 1995; Merten et al. 1998; Yamamoto et al. 1989) In these reports, thrombus formation preceding hemorrhage is the hypothesized mechanism based upon the presence of thrombosis and hemorrhage on the same imaging study, but none of the reports provide pre-hemorrhage imaging studies demonstrating the temporal relationship of thrombosis and hemorrhage. Venous outflow obstruction due to venous thrombus formation is a mechanism for AVM hemorrhage following SRS. Physiologically, venous outflow impairment is believed to cause venous hypertension in a retrograde manner leading to elevated intranidal pressure and rupture of abnormal AVM vessels. (Garcia Monaco et al. 1990; Vinuela et al. 1985) Intraoperative measurements of pre-stenotic draining vein pressure in patients with segmental venous stenosis and a history of AVM hemorrhage have demonstrated venous hypertension. (Miyasaka et al. 1994) Several studies have identified characteristics of AVM venous drainage that may play a role in the pathophysiology of AVM rupture. Venous stenosis or occlusion impairing venous drainage, (Miyasaka et al. 1994; Miyasaka et al. 1992; Vinuela et al. 1985) the number of draining veins, (Albert 1982; Albert et al. 1990; Miyasaka et al. 1992; Pollock et al. 1996; Stefani et al. 2002) the location of draining veins as deep, superficial, or mixed, (Duong et al. 1998; Kader et al. 1994; Langer et al. 1998; Marks et al. 1990; Mast et al. 1997; Miyasaka et al. 1992; Turjman et al. 1995) and the presence of venous aneurysms or varices are the venous drainage characteristics reported to influence AVM hemorrhage. (Albert et al. 1990; Stefani et al. 2002)

In the setting of AVMs, the risk of rupture due to venous stenosis or occlusion and the resultant venous drainage impairment is debated. (Marks et al. 1990; Miyasaka et al. 1994; Miyasaka et al. 1992; Turjman et al. 1995; Vinuela et al. 1985; Willinsky et al. 1988; Young et al. 1994) While impaired venous drainage is viewed by some as an essential determinant of the hemodynamics of the AVM nidus, (Wilson and Hieshima 1993) limited work has been done to investigate the influence of altered hemodynamics due to venous outflow impairment on the risk of AVM hemorrhage. Biomathematical models based on electrical network analysis have been developed and used to theoretically investigate the hemodynamics within an AVM nidus. (Hademenos and Massoud 1996, 1996; Hademenos, Massoud, and Vinuela 1996; Hecht, Horton, and Kerber 1991; Lo 1993, 1993; Lo et al. 1991; Nagasawa et al. 1996; Ornstein et al. 1994) One study examined the development of hyperperfusion during the AVM obliteration process and found that as AVM flow decreased during obliteration, feeding vessel pressure increased, draining vessel pressure decreased, and perfusion pressure in brain tissue surrounding the AVM increased. (Nagasawa et al. 1996) In another study of the theoretical risk of AVM rupture due to venous outflow obstruction, the investigators found that stenosis or occlusion of a high-flow draining vein was predictive of AVM rupture. (Hademenos and Massoud 1996)

Clinically, acute alteration in cerebral hemodynamics following surgical resection of an AVM is a known cause of postoperative hemorrhage. The risk of AVM hemorrhage due to acute alterations in hemodynamics is most commonly encountered in the setting of postoperative residual AVM. There is evidence suggesting that residual AVM is associated with early postoperative hemorrhage due to the persistence of high flow through a nidus with surgically impaired venous outflow. Hemodynamic changes following AVM resection are also theorized to play a causal role in neurological deterioration with or without hemorrhage or edema. Normal perfusion pressure breakthrough and occlusive hyperemia are two proposed hypotheses for neurological deterioration due to hemodynamic alterations following AVM resection. (al-Rodhan et al. 1993; Spetzler et al. 1978)

Occlusive hyperemia is a proposed hemodynamic mechanism for neurological decline following surgical removal of AVMs. (al-Rodhan et al. 1993) Based on angiographic findings in a group of patients who experienced neurological deterioration within 3 hours to 11 days following complete AVM resection, al-Rhodan and colleagues found that obstruction of the primary venous drainage or other venous structures accompanied by passive hyperemia was believed to be the cause of acute postoperative edema and/or hemorrhage in certain patients. Occlusive hyperemia in the setting of venous thrombosis has been proposed as a mechanism for neurological deterioration following radiosurgery for AVM. (Pollock 2000) Pollock provides radiographic evidence of acute draining vein thrombosis after radiosurgery in two patients with acute neurological deficits and hypothesizes that hemodynamic alterations occur in tissue surrounding the AVM after radiosurgery and lead to venous outflow impairment and perinidal edema that is manifest in neurological deficits. Pollock and colleagues propose that these changes are not due to radiation injury. Chapman and colleagues (Chapman, Ogilvy, and Loeffler 2004) provide further evidence supporting the hypothesis that venous occlusion and hyperemia may be one mechanism responsible for complications following radiosurgery. In their case report, they provide radiographic evidence of venous outflow impairment in two patients with acute neurological deficits developing months to years following SRS, and in one case offer the results of histological examination that failed to show radionecrosis.

Occlusive hyperemia in the postoperative setting can result in intracranial hemorrhage. Similarly, spontaneous venous thrombosis and venous hypertension may play a role in AVM hemorrhage following SRS. It is the opinion of some in the field that venous outflow restriction and resultant venous overload is a critical determinant of nidal and perinidal hemodynamics and often precedes AVM rupture. (Wilson and Hieshima 1993) Acute venous thrombus formation preceding intracranial hemorrhage is a physiologically sound mechanism for AVM hemorrhage, with radiographic support based on imaging of concurrent thrombus and hemorrhage. The authors of this chapter recently published radiographic documentation of an acute draining vein thrombus immediately preceding AVM hemorrhage and evidence of arterial inflow alterations (dilated internal carotid and middle cerebral arteries) in the setting of venous outflow obstruction. Based on both the current understanding of the tissue effect of radiation and the evidence to support the hemodynamic alterations that link acute venous obstruction and intracranial hemorrhage, we postulate that one cause of AVM hemorrhage in the early period following radiosurgery may be acute venous thrombus formation, not due to early or accelerated radiation-induced changes that result in eventual vessel obliteration, but, rather, due to the acute inflammatory response of irradiated tissue.

6. Acute inflammatory response after radiation exposure

Radiation is a known stimulus for the acute inflammatory reaction, and vascular changes play a central role in the acute inflammatory response. Initiation of the acute inflammatory reaction results in the release of a variety of cytokines, especially thromboxane and prostaglandins, with vascular effects. Characteristic alterations in vessel caliber and endothelial permeability are hallmarks of the acute inflammatory response. (Acute and Chronic Inflammation 2005) Vasodilation and a leaky vasculature cause a slowing of blood flow and perivascular edema, and these hemodynamic changes may predispose to stasis and thrombus formation. Cytokine-mediated vascular changes and the hemodynamic consequences in various tissues, including the central nervous system (CNS), have been studied and the time course of pathogenic processes documented. (Nieder et al. 2002) Animal models of CNS irradiation have shown cytokine-mediated vascular changes resulting in vasodilation and endothelial permeability can occur within the first few hours after irradiation. (Siegal and Pfeffer 1995) The levels of vasoactive cytokines variably change in the weeks following irradiation with simultaneous increasing and decreasing levels of different cytokines resulting in phasic changes in vessel caliber and vascular permeability. (Mildenberger et al. 1990; Siegal and Pfeffer 1995; Siegal et al. 1996)

Functional vascular changes related to radiation-induced cytokine release are accompanied by structural alterations following irradiation. Endothelial cells are highly radiosensitive (Fajardo and Berthrong 1988) and even low doses of radiation can cause endothelial cell injury and death. Histopathological studies documenting endothelial cell death after irradiation have shown endothelial cell swelling leading to a narrowed vessel lumen followed by platelet and fibrin thrombi during the course of progressive capillary damage in an animal model. (Fajardo and Stewart 1973) Additional animal studies provide evidence for a dose-dependent reduction in the number of endothelial cells in rat CNS within one week following irradiation. (Hopewell et al. 1989) More recent studies have shown that endothelial cells in the CNS of mice undergo time- and dose-dependent apoptosis beginning within a few hours after irradiation. (Pena, Fuks, and Kolesnick 2000) Vessel smooth muscle cell atrophy is also a time- and dose-dependent phenomenon following irradiation. (Hopewell et al. 1989) With increasing radiation dose the severity of vascular damage in rat CNS increases while the latency decreases. (Kamiryo et al. 1996)

While highly radiosensitive, endothelial cells do not respond homogeneously after radiation exposure, (Brown, Farjardo, and Stewart 1973) and the response of the vasculature to radiation is not only time- and dose-dependent, but varies by tissue and vessel type. (Fajardo and Berthrong 1988) In human tissue, capillaries are the most sensitive to irradiation, while large arteries are less affected and medium-sized and large veins are even more resistant to radiation injury. Veins are generally radioresistant, but small veins in the submucosa of the intestinal tract and the centrilobular veins of the liver have been shown to be susceptible to significant acute and chronic radiation injury, (Berthrong and Fajardo 1981; Fajardo and Colby 1980) demonstrating the variable tissue effect of irradiation.

Endothelial cell damage and functional changes of the vasculature can cause hemodynamic alterations that result in slowed blood flow and perivascular edema and predispose to stasis and thrombus formation. Independent of this pathway, whereby inflammation-induced vascular changes can lead to thrombosis, inflammation and thrombosis are directly linked. Specific cytokines, such as tumor necrosis factor (TNF) and interleukin-1 (IL-1), are important mediators of both the inflammatory and coagulation pathways. Tumor necrosis factor is activated during the inflammatory process and functions to activate the inflammatory pathway. It also plays a role in initiation of the coagulation cascade. (Conway et al. 1989; Nawroth and Stern 1986; van der Poll et al. 1990) Interleukin-1 is another cytokine with pro-inflammatory and pro-coagulant effects. (Bevilacqua et al. 1986; Le and Vilcek 1987) In the central nervous system, animal studies of cytokine production after CNS irradiation provide evidence for radiation-induced production of TNF-α and IL-1 by microglia and astrocytes. (Chiang and McBride 1991; Hong et al. 1995; Merrill 1991) Models for the direct interactions between inflammation and thrombosis have been proposed to explain the association of endothelial injury, the inflammatory response, and thrombus formation. (Furie and Furie 1992; Stewart 1993)

Complications of the increased endothelial permeability and altered vessel caliber that characterize the acute inflammatory reaction following SRS are most commonly manifest through the development of vasogenic cerebral edema rather than thrombus formation. Vasogenic edema begins within hours after irradiation, but symptomatic edema may not be evident for days, or the edema may never become symptomatic. At our institution, this known acute complication of radiosurgery is treated prophylactically with the glucocorticoid dexamethasone beginning prior to SRS and continuing for 5 days following treatment. Corticosteroids function to reduce the manifestations of the acute inflammatory reaction by inhibiting the production of inflammatory mediators and reversing the permeability of the vascular endothelium. (Yamada K 1989; Hedley-Whyte and Hsu 1986; Jarden et al. 1989; Shapiro et al. 1990) Reduced endothelial permeability results in decreased tissue edema and improved microvascular circulation. (Hartman and Goode 1987; Zarem and Soderberg 1982)

The acute inflammatory response provides a mechanism for both direct and indirect thrombus formation following irradiation that could result in AVM rupture in the early period following SRS, and the variable response of vessels to radiation may explain the rare occurrence of AVM hemorrhage during the early period. Stereotactic radiosurgery can induce an acute inflammatory reaction in the AVM vessels that causes endothelial cell injury and vessel thrombosis. Due to the decreased radiosensitivity of veins, venous thrombosis and outflow obstruction resulting from radiation-induced acute inflammatory reaction is likely a rare event with clinical consequences that can range from none to edema and neurological deficits to devastating hemorrhage.

7. Conclusion

A risk of AVM hemorrhage following SRS persists during the latency interval. There is evidence on the role of inflammation in the pathophysiology of AVM rupture, and the association between inflammation and AVM hemorrhage has been established. Arteriovenous malformation hemorrhage in the early period following radiosurgery may be related to the acute inflammatory response of irradiated vessels resulting in venous thrombus formation. There is an acute inflammatory response following tissue irradiation, resulting in structural and functional vascular changes that can lead to vessel thrombosis. The proposed mechanism of venous outflow obstruction leading to early AVM hemorrhage following radiosurgery is supported by laboratory evidence and suggested by clinical evidence. Radiographic evidence of the time course of thrombosis and hemorrhage supports the hypothesis that acute venous outflow obstruction immediately precedes AVM hemorrhage in this setting. The pathophysiology of AVM hemorrhage in the early period following SRS is different from that of AVM hemorrhage occurring months to years following radiosurgery.

8. Acknowledgements

Portions of this chapter were originally published in an abridged form in a case report in The Journal of Neurosurgery.

9. References

Acute and Chronic Inflammation. 2005. In *Robbins and Cotran Pathologic Basis of Disease*, edited by V. Kumar, A. K. Abbas and N. Fausto. Philadelphia: Elsevier Saunders.

Adams, R. D. 1991. The neuropathology of radiosurgery. *Stereotact Funct Neurosurg* 57 (1-2):82-6.

al-Rodhan, N. R. , T. M. Sundt, Jr. , D. G. Piepgras, D. A. Nichols, D. Rufenacht, and L. N. Stevens. 1993. Occlusive hyperemia: a theory for the hemodynamic complications following resection of intracerebral arteriovenous malformations. *J Neurosurg* 78 (2):167-75.

Al-Shahi, R. , J. S. Fang, S. C. Lewis, and C. P. Warlow. 2002. Prevalence of adults with brain arteriovenous malformations: a community based study in Scotland using capture-recapture analysis. *J Neurol Neurosurg Psychiatry* 73 (5):547-51.

Albert, P. 1982. Personal experience in the treatment of 178 cases of arteriovenous malformations of the brain. *Acta Neurochir (Wien)* 61 (1-3):207-26.

Albert, P. , H. Salgado, M. Polaina, F. Trujillo, A. Ponce de Leon, and F. Durand. 1990. A study on the venous drainage of 150 cerebral arteriovenous malformations as related to haemorrhagic risks and size of the lesion. *Acta Neurochir (Wien)* 103 (1-2):30-4.

Barrow, D. L. , and A. Reisner. 1993. Natural history of intracranial aneurysms and vascular malformations. *Clin Neurosurg* 40:3-39.

Berman, M. F. , R. R. Sciacca, J. Pile-Spellman, C. Stapf, E. S. Connolly, Jr. , J. P. Mohr, and W. L. Young. 2000. The epidemiology of brain arteriovenous malformations. *Neurosurgery* 47 (2):389-96; discussion 397.

Berthrong, M. , and L. F. Fajardo. 1981. Radiation injury in surgical pathology. Part II. Alimentary tract. *Am J Surg Pathol* 5 (2):153-78.

Bevilacqua, M. P. , R. R. Schleef, M. A. Gimbrone, Jr. , and D. J. Loskutoff. 1986. Regulation of the fibrinolytic system of cultured human vascular endothelium by interleukin 1. *J Clin Invest* 78 (2):587-91.

Brown, J. M. , L. F. Farjardo, and J. R. Stewart. 1973. Mural thrombosis of the heart induced by radiation. *Arch Pathol* 96 (1):1-4.

Brown, R. D. , Jr. , D. O. Wiebers, G. Forbes, W. M. O'Fallon, D. G. Piepgras, W. R. Marsh, and R. J. Maciunas. 1988. The natural history of unruptured intracranial arteriovenous malformations. *J Neurosurg* 68 (3):352-7.

Celix, J. M. , J. G. Douglas, D. Haynor, and R. Goodkin. 2009. Thrombosis and hemorrhage in the acute period following Gamma Knife surgery for arteriovenous malformation. Case report. *J Neurosurg* 111 (1):124-31.

Chang, S. D. , D. L. Shuster, G. K. Steinberg, R. P. Levy, and K. Frankel. 1997. Stereotactic radiosurgery of arteriovenous malformations: pathologic changes in resected tissue. *Clin Neuropathol* 16 (2):111-6.

Chang, T. C. , H. Shirato, H. Aoyama, S. Ushikoshi, N. Kato, S. Kuroda, T. Ishikawa, K. Houkin, Y. Iwasaki, and K. Miyasaka. 2004. Stereotactic irradiation for intracranial arteriovenous malformation using stereotactic radiosurgery or hypofractionated stereotactic radiotherapy. *Int J Radiat Oncol Biol Phys* 60 (3):861-70.

Chapman, P. H. , C. S. Ogilvy, and J. S. Loeffler. 2004. The relationship between occlusive hyperemia and complications associated with the radiosurgical treatment of arteriovenous malformations: report of two cases. *Neurosurgery* 55 (1):228-33; discussion 233-4.

Chiang, C. S. , and W. H. McBride. 1991. Radiation enhances tumor necrosis factor alpha production by murine brain cells. *Brain Res* 566 (1-2):265-9.

Coffey, R. J. , D. A. Nichols, and E. G. Shaw. 1995. Stereotactic radiosurgical treatment of cerebral arteriovenous malformations. Gamma Unit Radiosurgery Study Group. *Mayo Clin Proc* 70 (3):214-22.

Colombo, F. , F. Pozza, G. Chierego, L. Casentini, G. De Luca, and P. Francescon. 1994. Linear accelerator radiosurgery of cerebral arteriovenous malformations: an update. *Neurosurgery* 34 (1):14-20; discussion 20-1.

Conway, E. M. , R. Bach, R. D. Rosenberg, and W. H. Konigsberg. 1989. Tumor necrosis factor enhances expression of tissue factor mRNA in endothelial cells. *Thromb Res* 53 (3):231-41.

Crawford, P. M. , C. R. West, D. W. Chadwick, and M. D. Shaw. 1986. Arteriovenous malformations of the brain: natural history in unoperated patients. *J Neurol Neurosurg Psychiatry* 49 (1):1-10.

da Costa, L. , M. C. Wallace, K. G. Ter Brugge, C. O'Kelly, R. A. Willinsky, and M. Tymianski. 2009. The natural history and predictive features of hemorrhage from brain arteriovenous malformations. *Stroke* 40 (1):100-5.

Davis, C. , and L. Symon. 1985. The management of cerebral arteriovenous malformations. *Acta Neurochir (Wien)* 74 (1-2):4-11.

Dias, M. S. , and L. N. Sekhar. 1990. Intracranial hemorrhage from aneurysms and arteriovenous malformations during pregnancy and the puerperium. *Neurosurgery* 27 (6):855-65; discussion 865-6.

Duong, D. H. , W. L. Young, M. C. Vang, R. R. Sciacca, H. Mast, H. C. Koennecke, A. Hartmann, S. Joshi, J. P. Mohr, and J. Pile-Spellman. 1998. Feeding artery pressure and venous drainage pattern are primary determinants of hemorrhage from cerebral arteriovenous malformations. *Stroke* 29 (6):1167-76.

Fabrikant, J. I. , R. P. Levy, G. K. Steinberg, M. H. Phillips, K. A. Frankel, J. T. Lyman, M. P. Marks, and G. D. Silverberg. 1992. Charged-particle radiosurgery for intracranial vascular malformations. *Neurosurg Clin N Am* 3 (1):99-139.
Fajardo, L. F. 1982. *Pathology of Radiation Injury*. New York: Masson.
Fajardo, L. F. , and M. Berthrong. 1988. Vascular lesions following radiation. *Pathol Annu* 23 Pt 1:297-330.
Fajardo, L. F. , and T. V. Colby. 1980. Pathogenesis of veno-occlusive liver disease after radiation. *Arch Pathol Lab Med* 104 (11):584-8.
Fajardo, L. F. , and J. R. Stewart. 1973. Pathogenesis of radiation-induced myocardial fibrosis. *Lab Invest* 29 (2):244-57.
Field, L. R. , and E. J. Russell. 1995. Spontaneous hemorrhage from a cerebral venous malformation related to thrombosis of the central draining vein: demonstration with angiography and serial MR. *AJNR Am J Neuroradiol* 16 (9):1885-8.
Forster, D. M. , I. H. Kunkler, and P. Hartland. 1993. Risk of cerebral bleeding from arteriovenous malformations in pregnancy: the Sheffield experience. *Stereotact Funct Neurosurg* 61 Suppl 1:20-2.
Forster, D. M. , L. Steiner, and S. Hakanson. 1972. Arteriovenous malformations of the brain. A long-term clinical study. *J Neurosurg* 37 (5):562-70.
Franco-Vidal, V. , M. Songu, H. Blanchet, X. Barreau, and V. Darrouzet. 2007. Intracochlear hemorrhage after gamma knife radiosurgery. *Otol Neurotol* 28 (2):240-4.
Friedman, W. A. , D. L. Blatt, F. J. Bova, J. M. Buatti, W. M. Mendenhall, and P. S. Kubilis. 1996. The risk of hemorrhage after radiosurgery for arteriovenous malformations. *J Neurosurg* 84 (6):912-9.
Friedman, W. A. , and F. J. Bova. 1992. Linear accelerator radiosurgery for arteriovenous malformations. *J Neurosurg* 77 (6):832-41.
Friedman, W. A. , F. J. Bova, and W. M. Mendenhall. 1995. Linear accelerator radiosurgery for arteriovenous malformations: the relationship of size to outcome. *J Neurosurg* 82 (2):180-9.
Fults, D. , and D. L. Kelly, Jr. 1984. Natural history of arteriovenous malformations of the brain: a clinical study. *Neurosurgery* 15 (5):658-62.
Furie, B. , and B. C. Furie. 1992. Molecular and cellular biology of blood coagulation. *N Engl J Med* 326 (12):800-6.
Garcia Monaco, R. , H. Alvarez, A. Goulao, P. Pruvost, and P. Lasjaunias. 1990. Posterior fossa arteriovenous malformations. Angioarchitecture in relation to their hemorrhagic episodes. *Neuroradiology* 31 (6):471-5.
Graf, C. J. , G. E. Perret, and J. C. Torner. 1983. Bleeding from cerebral arteriovenous malformations as part of their natural history. *J Neurosurg* 58 (3):331-7.
Guidetti, B. , and A. Delitala. 1980. Intracranial arteriovenous malformations. Conservative and surgical treatment. *J Neurosurg* 53 (2):149-52.
Guo, W. Y. , C. Lindquist, B. Karlsson, L. Kihlstrom, and L. Steiner. 1993. Gamma knife surgery of cerebral arteriovenous malformations: serial MR imaging studies after radiosurgery. *Int J Radiat Oncol Biol Phys* 25 (2):315-23.
Hademenos, G. J. , and T. F. Massoud. 1996. An electrical network model of intracranial arteriovenous malformations: analysis of variations in hemodynamic and biophysical parameters. *Neurol Res* 18 (6):575-89.

———. 1996. Risk of intracranial arteriovenous malformation rupture due to venous drainage impairment. A theoretical analysis. *Stroke* 27 (6):1072-83.

Hademenos, G. J. , T. F. Massoud, and F. Vinuela. 1996. A biomathematical model of intracranial arteriovenous malformations based on electrical network analysis: theory and hemodynamics. *Neurosurgery* 38 (5):1005-14; discussion 1014-5.

Halim, A. X. , S. C. Johnston, V. Singh, C. E. McCulloch, J. P. Bennett, A. S. Achrol, S. Sidney, and W. L. Young. 2004. Longitudinal risk of intracranial hemorrhage in patients with arteriovenous malformation of the brain within a defined population. *Stroke* 35 (7):1697-702.

Hartman, D. F. , and R. L. Goode. 1987. Pharmacologic enhancement of composite graft survival. *Arch Otolaryngol Head Neck Surg* 113 (7):720-3.

Hecht, S. T. , J. A. Horton, and C. W. Kerber. 1991. Hemodynamics of the central nervous system arteriovenous malformation nidus during particulate embolization. A computer model. *Neuroradiology* 33 (1):62-4.

Hedley-Whyte, E. T. , and D. W. Hsu. 1986. Effect of dexamethasone on blood-brain barrier in the normal mouse. *Ann Neurol* 19 (4):373-7.

Hong, J. H. , C. S. Chiang, I. L. Campbell, J. R. Sun, H. R. Withers, and W. H. McBride. 1995. Induction of acute phase gene expression by brain irradiation. *Int J Radiat Oncol Biol Phys* 33 (3):619-26.

Hopewell, J. W. , W. Calvo, D. Campling, H. S. Reinhold, M. Rezvani, and T. K. Yeung. 1989. Effects of radiation on the microvasculature. Implications for normal-tissue damage. *Front Radiat Ther Oncol* 23:85-95.

Horton, J. C. , W. A. Chambers, S. L. Lyons, R. D. Adams, and R. N. Kjellberg. 1990. Pregnancy and the risk of hemorrhage from cerebral arteriovenous malformations. *Neurosurgery* 27 (6):867-71; discussion 871-2.

Inoue, H. K. , and C. Ohye. 2002. Hemorrhage risks and obliteration rates of arteriovenous malformations after gamma knife radiosurgery. *J Neurosurg* 97 (5 Suppl):474-6.

Itoyama, Y. , S. Uemura, Y. Ushio, J. Kuratsu, N. Nonaka, H. Wada, Y. Sano, A. Fukumura, K. Yoshida, and T. Yano. 1989. Natural course of unoperated intracranial arteriovenous malformations: study of 50 cases. *J Neurosurg* 71 (6):805-9.

Izawa, M. , M. Chernov, M. Hayashi, Y. Kubota, H. Kasuya, and T. Hori. 2006. Fatal intratumoral hemorrhage immediately after gamma knife radiosurgery for brain metastases: case report. *Minim Invasive Neurosurg* 49 (4):251-4.

Izawa, M. , M. Hayashi, M. Chernov, K. Nakaya, T. Ochiai, N. Murata, Y. Takasu, O. Kubo, T. Hori, and K. Takakura. 2005. Long-term complications after gamma knife surgery for arteriovenous malformations. *J Neurosurg* 102 Suppl:34-7.

Jarden, J. O. , V. Dhawan, J. R. Moeller, S. C. Strother, and D. A. Rottenberg. 1989. The time course of steroid action on blood-to-brain and blood-to-tumor transport of 82Rb: a positron emission tomographic study. *Ann Neurol* 25 (3):239-45.

Kader, A. , W. L. Young, J. Pile-Spellman, H. Mast, R. R. Sciacca, J. P. Mohr, and B. M. Stein. 1994. The influence of hemodynamic and anatomic factors on hemorrhage from cerebral arteriovenous malformations. *Neurosurgery* 34 (5):801-7; discussion 807-8.

Kamiryo, T. , N. F. Kassell, Q. A. Thai, M. B. Lopes, K. S. Lee, and L. Steiner. 1996. Histological changes in the normal rat brain after gamma irradiation. *Acta Neurochir (Wien)* 138 (4):451-9.

Karlsson, B. , I. Lax, and M. Soderman. 2001. Risk for hemorrhage during the 2-year latency period following gamma knife radiosurgery for arteriovenous malformations. *Int J Radiat Oncol Biol Phys* 49 (4):1045-51.

Karlsson, B. , C. Lindquist, A. Johansson, and L. Steiner. 1997. Annual risk for the first hemorrhage from untreated cerebral arteriovenous malformations. *Minim Invasive Neurosurg* 40 (2):40-6.

Karlsson, B. , C. Lindquist, and L. Steiner. 1996. Effect of Gamma Knife surgery on the risk of rupture prior to AVM obliteration. *Minim Invasive Neurosurg* 39 (1):21-7.

———. 1997. Prediction of obliteration after gamma knife surgery for cerebral arteriovenous malformations. *Neurosurgery* 40 (3):425-30; discussion 430-1.

Kjellberg, R. N. 1986. Stereotactic Bragg peak proton beam radiosurgery for cerebral arteriovenous malformations. *Ann Clin Res* 18 Suppl 47:17-9.

Kjellberg, R. N. , T. Hanamura, K. R. Davis, S. L. Lyons, and R. D. Adams. 1983. Bragg-peak proton-beam therapy for arteriovenous malformations of the brain. *N Engl J Med* 309 (5):269-74.

Langer, D. J. , T. M. Lasner, R. W. Hurst, E. S. Flamm, E. L. Zager, and J. T. King, Jr. 1998. Hypertension, small size, and deep venous drainage are associated with risk of hemorrhagic presentation of cerebral arteriovenous malformations. *Neurosurgery* 42 (3):481-6; discussion 487-9.

Le, J. , and J. Vilcek. 1987. Tumor necrosis factor and interleukin 1: cytokines with multiple overlapping biological activities. *Lab Invest* 56 (3):234-48.

Levy, R. P. , J. I. Fabrikant, K. A. Frankel, M. H. Phillips, and J. T. Lyman. 1989. Stereotactic heavy-charged-particle Bragg peak radiosurgery for the treatment of intracranial arteriovenous malformations in childhood and adolescence. *Neurosurgery* 24 (6):841-52.

Lindquist, C. , W. Y. Guo, B. Karlsson, and L. Steiner. 1993. Radiosurgery for venous angiomas. *J Neurosurg* 78 (4):531-6.

Lindqvist, M. , B. Karlsson, W. Y. Guo, L. Kihlstrom, B. Lippitz, and M. Yamamoto. 2000. Angiographic long-term follow-up data for arteriovenous malformations previously proven to be obliterated after gamma knife radiosurgery. *Neurosurgery* 46 (4):803-8; discussion 809-10.

Lo, E. H. 1993. A haemodynamic analysis of intracranial arteriovenous malformations. *Neurol Res* 15 (1):51-5.

———. 1993. A theoretical analysis of hemodynamic and biomechanical alterations in intracranial AVMs after radiosurgery. *Int J Radiat Oncol Biol Phys* 27 (2):353-61.

Lo, E. H. , J. I. Fabrikant, R. P. Levy, M. H. Phillips, K. A. Frankel, and E. L. Alpen. 1991. An experimental compartmental flow model for assessing the hemodynamic response of intracranial arteriovenous malformations to stereotactic radiosurgery. *Neurosurgery* 28 (2):251-9.

Lunsford, L. D. , D. Kondziolka, J. C. Flickinger, D. J. Bissonette, C. A. Jungreis, A. H. Maitz, J. A. Horton, and R. J. Coffey. 1991. Stereotactic radiosurgery for arteriovenous malformations of the brain. *J Neurosurg* 75 (4):512-24.

Maesawa, S. , J. C. Flickinger, D. Kondziolka, and L. D. Lunsford. 2000. Repeated radiosurgery for incompletely obliterated arteriovenous malformations. *J Neurosurg* 92 (6):961-70.

Marks, M. P. , B. Lane, G. K. Steinberg, and P. J. Chang. 1990. Hemorrhage in intracerebral arteriovenous malformations: angiographic determinants. *Radiology* 176 (3):807-13.

Maruyama, K. , N. Kawahara, M. Shin, M. Tago, J. Kishimoto, H. Kurita, S. Kawamoto, A. Morita, and T. Kirino. 2005. The risk of hemorrhage after radiosurgery for cerebral arteriovenous malformations. *N Engl J Med* 352 (2):146-53.

Maruyama, K. , M. Shin, M. Tago, J. Kishimoto, A. Morita, and N. Kawahara. 2007. Radiosurgery to reduce the risk of first hemorrhage from brain arteriovenous malformations. *Neurosurgery* 60 (3):453-8; discussion 458-9.

Mast, H. , W. L. Young, H. C. Koennecke, R. R. Sciacca, A. Osipov, J. Pile-Spellman, L. Hacein-Bey, H. Duong, B. M. Stein, and J. P. Mohr. 1997. Risk of spontaneous haemorrhage after diagnosis of cerebral arteriovenous malformation. *Lancet* 350 (9084):1065-8.

Matsumoto, H. , T. Takeda, K. Kohno, Y. Yamaguchi, K. Kohno, A. Takechi, D. Ishii, M. Abiko, and U. Sasaki. 2006. Delayed hemorrhage from completely obliterated arteriovenous malformation after gamma knife radiosurgery. *Neurol Med Chir (Tokyo)* 46 (4):186-90.

Merrill, J. E. 1991. Effects of interleukin-1 and tumor necrosis factor-alpha on astrocytes, microglia, oligodendrocytes, and glial precursors in vitro. *Dev Neurosci* 13 (3):130-7.

Merten, C. L. , H. O. Knitelius, J. P. Hedde, J. Assheuer, and H. Bewermeyer. 1998. Intracerebral haemorrhage from a venous angioma following thrombosis of a draining vein. *Neuroradiology* 40 (1):15-8.

Mildenberger, M. , T. G. Beach, E. G. McGeer, and C. M. Ludgate. 1990. An animal model of prophylactic cranial irradiation: histologic effects at acute, early and delayed stages. *Int J Radiat Oncol Biol Phys* 18 (5):1051-60.

Miyasaka, Y. , A. Kurata, K. Tokiwa, R. Tanaka, K. Yada, and T. Ohwada. 1994. Draining vein pressure increases and hemorrhage in patients with arteriovenous malformation. *Stroke* 25 (2):504-7.

Miyasaka, Y. , K. Yada, T. Ohwada, T. Kitahara, A. Kurata, and K. Irikura. 1992. An analysis of the venous drainage system as a factor in hemorrhage from arteriovenous malformations. *J Neurosurg* 76 (2):239-43.

Miyawaki, L. , C. Dowd, W. Wara, B. Goldsmith, N. Albright, P. Gutin, V. Halbach, G. Hieshima, R. Higashida, B. Lulu, L. Pitts, M. Schell, V. Smith, K. Weaver, C. Wilson, and D. Larson. 1999. Five year results of LINAC radiosurgery for arteriovenous malformations: outcome for large AVMS. *Int J Radiat Oncol Biol Phys* 44 (5):1089-106.

Nagasawa, S. , M. Kawanishi, S. Kondoh, S. Kajimoto, K. Yamaguchi, and T. Ohta. 1996. Hemodynamic simulation study of cerebral arteriovenous malformations. Part 2. Effects of impaired autoregulation and induced hypotension. *J Cereb Blood Flow Metab* 16 (1):162-9.

Nataf, F. , M. Ghossoub, M. Schlienger, R. Moussa, J. F. Meder, and F. X. Roux. 2004. Bleeding after radiosurgery for cerebral arteriovenous malformations. *Neurosurgery* 55 (2):298-305; discussion 305-6.

Nawroth, P. P. , and D. M. Stern. 1986. Modulation of endothelial cell hemostatic properties by tumor necrosis factor. *J Exp Med* 163 (3):740-5.

Nicolato, A. , F. Lupidi, M. F. Sandri, R. Foroni, P. Zampieri, C. Mazza, S. Maluta, A. Beltramello, and M. Gerosa. 2006. Gamma knife radiosurgery for cerebral arteriovenous malformations in children/adolescents and adults. Part I: Differences in epidemiologic, morphologic, and clinical characteristics, permanent complications, and bleeding in the latency period. *Int J Radiat Oncol Biol Phys* 64 (3):904-13.

Nieder, C. , N. Andratschke, R. E. Price, B. Rivera, and K. K. Ang. 2002. Innovative prevention strategies for radiation necrosis of the central nervous system. *Anticancer Res* 22 (2A):1017-23.

O'Connor, M. M. , and M. R. Mayberg. 2000. Effects of radiation on cerebral vasculature: a review. *Neurosurgery* 46 (1):138-49; discussion 150-1.

Ondra, S. L. , H. Troupp, E. D. George, and K. Schwab. 1990. The natural history of symptomatic arteriovenous malformations of the brain: a 24-year follow-up assessment. *J Neurosurg* 73 (3):387-91.

Ornstein, E. , W. B. Blesser, W. L. Young, and J. Pile-Spellman. 1994. A computer simulation of the haemodynamic effects of intracranial arteriovenous malformation occlusion. *Neurol Res* 16 (5):345-52.

Park, C-K. , D. G. Kim, H-S. Gwak, H-T. Chung, and S. H. Paek. 2000. Intracerebral Hemorrhage After Gamma-Knife Surgery for Metastatic Brain Tumor. *Journal of Radiosurgery* 3 (1):17-20.

Parkinson, D. , and G. Bachers. 1980. Arteriovenous malformations. Summary of 100 consecutive supratentorial cases. *J Neurosurg* 53 (3):285-99.

Pena, L. A. , Z. Fuks, and R. N. Kolesnick. 2000. Radiation-induced apoptosis of endothelial cells in the murine central nervous system: protection by fibroblast growth factor and sphingomyelinase deficiency. *Cancer Res* 60 (2):321-7.

Pollock, B. E. 2000. Occlusive hyperemia: a radiosurgical phenomenon? *Neurosurgery* 47 (5):1178-82; discussion 1182-4.

Pollock, B. E. , J. C. Flickinger, L. D. Lunsford, D. J. Bissonette, and D. Kondziolka. 1996. Factors that predict the bleeding risk of cerebral arteriovenous malformations. *Stroke* 27 (1):1-6.

———. 1996. Hemorrhage risk after stereotactic radiosurgery of cerebral arteriovenous malformations. *Neurosurgery* 38 (4):652-9; discussion 659-61.

Pollock, B. E. , L. D. Lunsford, D. Kondziolka, A. Maitz, and J. C. Flickinger. 1994. Patient outcomes after stereotactic radiosurgery for "operable" arteriovenous malformations. *Neurosurgery* 35 (1):1-7; discussion 7-8.

Prat, R. , I. Galeano, R. Conde, J. A. Simal, and E. Cardenas. 2009. Surgical removal after first bleeding of an arteriovenous malformation previously obliterated with radiosurgery: case report. *Surg Neurol* 71 (2):211-4; discussion 214-5.

Quisling, R. G. , K. R. Peters, W. A. Friedman, and R. P. Tart. 1991. Persistent nidus blood flow in cerebral arteriovenous malformation after stereotactic radiosurgery: MR imaging assessment. *Radiology* 180 (3):785-91.

Robinson, J. L. , C. S. Hall, and C. B. Sedzimir. 1974. Arteriovenous malformations, aneurysms, and pregnancy. *J Neurosurg* 41 (1):63-70.

Schneider, B. F. , D. A. Eberhard, and L. E. Steiner. 1997. Histopathology of arteriovenous malformations after gamma knife radiosurgery. *J Neurosurg* 87 (3):352-7.

Shapiro, W. R. , E. M. Hiesiger, G. A. Cooney, G. A. Basler, L. E. Lipschutz, and J. B. Posner. 1990. Temporal effects of dexamethasone on blood-to-brain and blood-to-tumor

transport of 14C-alpha-aminoisobutyric acid in rat C6 glioma. *J Neurooncol* 8 (3):197-204.
Shimizu, S. , K. Irikura, Y. Miyasaka, T. Mochizuki, A. Kurata, S. Kan, and K. Fujii. 2001. Rupture of pial arteriovenous malformation associated with early thrombosis of the draining system following stereotactic radiosurgery--case report. *Neurol Med Chir (Tokyo)* 41 (12):599-602.
Shin, M. , N. Kawahara, K. Maruyama, M. Tago, K. Ueki, and T. Kirino. 2005. Risk of hemorrhage from an arteriovenous malformation confirmed to have been obliterated on angiography after stereotactic radiosurgery. *J Neurosurg* 102 (5):842-6.
Shin, M. , K. Maruyama, H. Kurita, S. Kawamoto, M. Tago, A. Terahara, A. Morita, K. Ueki, K. Takakura, and T. Kirino. 2004. Analysis of nidus obliteration rates after gamma knife surgery for arteriovenous malformations based on long-term follow-up data: the University of Tokyo experience. *J Neurosurg* 101 (1):18-24.
Siegal, T. , and M. R. Pfeffer. 1995. Radiation-induced changes in the profile of spinal cord serotonin, prostaglandin synthesis, and vascular permeability. *Int J Radiat Oncol Biol Phys* 31 (1):57-64.
Siegal, T. , M. R. Pfeffer, A. Meltzer, E. Shezen, A. Nimrod, N. Ezov, and H. Ovadia. 1996. Cellular and secretory mechanisms related to delayed radiation-induced microvessel dysfunction in the spinal cord of rats. *Int J Radiat Oncol Biol Phys* 36 (3):649-59.
Spetzler, R. F. , R. W. Hargraves, P. W. McCormick, J. M. Zabramski, R. A. Flom, and R. S. Zimmerman. 1992. Relationship of perfusion pressure and size to risk of hemorrhage from arteriovenous malformations. *J Neurosurg* 76 (6):918-23.
Spetzler, R. F. , C. B. Wilson, P. Weinstein, M. Mehdorn, J. Townsend, and D. Telles. 1978. Normal perfusion pressure breakthrough theory. *Clin Neurosurg* 25:651-72.
Stapf, C. , H. Mast, R. R. Sciacca, A. Berenstein, P. K. Nelson, Y. P. Gobin, J. Pile-Spellman, and J. P. Mohr. 2003. The New York Islands AVM Study: design, study progress, and initial results. *Stroke* 34 (5):e29-33.
Stefani, M. A. , P. J. Porter, K. G. terBrugge, W. Montanera, R. A. Willinsky, and M. C. Wallace. 2002. Angioarchitectural factors present in brain arteriovenous malformations associated with hemorrhagic presentation. *Stroke* 33 (4):920-4.
———. 2002. Large and deep brain arteriovenous malformations are associated with risk of future hemorrhage. *Stroke* 33 (5):1220-4.
Steinberg, G. K. , J. I. Fabrikant, M. P. Marks, R. P. Levy, K. A. Frankel, M. H. Phillips, L. M. Shuer, and G. D. Silverberg. 1990. Stereotactic heavy-charged-particle Bragg-peak radiation for intracranial arteriovenous malformations. *N Engl J Med* 323 (2):96-101.
Steiner, L. , C. Lindquist, J. R. Adler, J. C. Torner, W. Alves, and M. Steiner. 1992. Clinical outcome of radiosurgery for cerebral arteriovenous malformations. *J Neurosurg* 77 (1):1-8.
Stewart, G. J. 1993. Neutrophils and deep venous thrombosis. *Haemostasis* 23 Suppl 1:127-40.
Suzuki, H. , S. Toyoda, M. Muramatsu, T. Shimizu, T. Kojima, and W. Taki. 2003. Spontaneous haemorrhage into metastatic brain tumours after stereotactic radiosurgery using a linear accelerator. *J Neurol Neurosurg Psychiatry* 74 (7):908-12.

Szeifert, G. T. , A. A. Kemeny, W. R. Timperley, and D. M. Forster. 1997. The potential role of myofibroblasts in the obliteration of arteriovenous malformations after radiosurgery. *Neurosurgery* 40 (1):61-5; discussion 65-6.

Szeifert, G. T. , O. Major, and A. A. Kemeny. 2005. Ultrastructural changes in arteriovenous malformations after gamma knife surgery: an electron microscopic study. *J Neurosurg* 102 Suppl:289-92.

Tu, J. , M. A. Stoodley, M. K. Morgan, and K. P. Storer. 2006. Responses of arteriovenous malformations to radiosurgery: ultrastructural changes. *Neurosurgery* 58 (4):749-58; discussion 749-58.

Turjman, F. , T. F. Massoud, F. Vinuela, J. W. Sayre, G. Guglielmi, and G. Duckwiler. 1995. Correlation of the angioarchitectural features of cerebral arteriovenous malformations with clinical presentation of hemorrhage. *Neurosurgery* 37 (5):856-60; discussion 860-2.

Uchino, M. , S. Kitajima, C. Miyazaki, T. Otsuka, Y. Seiki, and I. Shibata. 2003. [Peritumoral hemorrhage immediately after radiosurgery for metastatic brain tumor]. *No Shinkei Geka* 31 (8):911-6.

van der Poll, T. , H. R. Buller, H. ten Cate, C. H. Wortel, K. A. Bauer, S. J. van Deventer, C. E. Hack, H. P. Sauerwein, R. D. Rosenberg, and J. W. ten Cate. 1990. Activation of coagulation after administration of tumor necrosis factor to normal subjects. *N Engl J Med* 322 (23):1622-7.

Vinuela, F. , L. Nombela, M. R. Roach, A. J. Fox, and D. M. Pelz. 1985. Stenotic and occlusive disease of the venous drainage system of deep brain AVM's. *J Neurosurg* 63 (2):180-4.

Waltimo, O. 1973. The relationship of size, density and localization of intracranial arteriovenous malformations to the type of initial symptom. *J Neurol Sci* 19 (1):13-9.

Willinsky, R. , P. Lasjaunias, K. Terbrugge, and P. Pruvost. 1988. Brain arteriovenous malformations: analysis of the angio-architecture in relationship to hemorrhage (based on 152 patients explored and/or treated at the hopital de Bicetre between 1981 and 1986). *J Neuroradiol* 15 (3):225-37.

Wilson, C. B. , and G. Hieshima. 1993. Occlusive hyperemia: a new way to think about an old problem. *J Neurosurg* 78 (2):165-6.

Yamada K, Ushio Y, Hayakawa T. 1989. Effects of steroids on the blood–brain barrier. In *Implications of the Blood–Brain Barrier and Its Manipulation*, edited by N. EA. New York: Plenum Press.

Yamamoto, M. , T. Inagawa, K. Kamiya, H. Ogasawara, S. Monden, and T. Yano. 1989. Intracerebral hemorrhage due to venous thrombosis in venous angioma--case report. *Neurol Med Chir (Tokyo)* 29 (11):1044-6.

Yamamoto, M. , M. Jimbo, M. Ide, C. Lindquist, and L. Steiner. 1993. Postradiation volume changes in gamma unit-treated cerebral arteriovenous malformations. *Surg Neurol* 40 (6):485-90.

Yamamoto, M. , M. Jimbo, M. Kobayashi, C. Toyoda, M. Ide, N. Tanaka, C. Lindquist, and L. Steiner. 1992. Long-term results of radiosurgery for arteriovenous malformation: neurodiagnostic imaging and histological studies of angiographically confirmed nidus obliteration. *Surg Neurol* 37 (3):219-30.

Yamamoto, Y. , R. J. Coffey, D. A. Nichols, and E. G. Shaw. 1995. Interim report on the radiosurgical treatment of cerebral arteriovenous malformations. The influence of size, dose, time, and technical factors on obliteration rate. *J Neurosurg* 83 (5):832-7.

Yen, C. P. , P. Varady, J. Sheehan, M. Steiner, and L. Steiner. 2007. Subtotal obliteration of cerebral arteriovenous malformations after gamma knife surgery. *J Neurosurg* 106 (3):361-9.

Young, W. L. , A. Kader, J. Pile-Spellman, E. Ornstein, and B. M. Stein. 1994. Arteriovenous malformation draining vein physiology and determinants of transnidal pressure gradients. The Columbia University AVM Study Project. *Neurosurgery* 35 (3):389-95; discussion 395-6.

Zabel, A. , S. Milker-Zabel, P. Huber, D. Schulz-Ertner, W. Schlegel, and J. Debus. 2005. Treatment outcome after linac-based radiosurgery in cerebral arteriovenous malformations: retrospective analysis of factors affecting obliteration. *Radiother Oncol* 77 (1):105-10.

Zabel-du Bois, A. , S. Milker-Zabel, P. Huber, W. Schlegel, and J. Debus. 2007. Risk of Hemorrhage and Obliteration Rates of LINAC-Based Radiosurgery for Cerebral Arteriovenous Malformations Treated After Prior Partial Embolization. *Int J Radiat Oncol Biol Phys* 68 (4):999-1003.

Zarem, H. A. , and R. Soderberg. 1982. Tissue reaction to ischemia in the rabbit ear chamber: effects of prednisolone on inflammation and microvascular flow. *Plast Reconstr Surg* 70 (6):667-76.

Zipfel, G. J. , P. Bradshaw, F. J. Bova, and W. A. Friedman. 2004. Do the morphological characteristics of arteriovenous malformations affect the results of radiosurgery? *J Neurosurg* 101 (3):393-401.

Part 3

Basic Science

9

Applications of Gamma Knife Radiosurgery for Experimental Investigations in Small Animal Models

Gabriel Charest, Benoit Paquette and David Mathieu
Department of Nuclear Medicine and Radiobiology, Sherbrooke University
Canada

1. Introduction

The Gamma Knife (GK) was not originally designed for experimentations in small animals. In fact, there are no compatible custom accessories or stereotactic frames on the market for the spatial positioning of small animals in the GK. In addition, the GK is intensively used for patient treatments, and consequently the access for research with small animals is limited. On the other hand, devices specially designed for the irradiation of small animals are available on the market. For examples, small animal irradiators can be purchasable from Best Theratronics (Theratronics, 2011), Rad Source Technologies (Rad Source Technologies, 2011), Precision X-Ray Inc. (Precision X-Ray, 2011) and Xstrahl-Gulmay Medical Inc. (Xstrahl, 2011). Compared to the GK, these small animal irradiators have the following advantages: lower cost, smaller size, some are shielded and thus don't require a special shielded room, some can be combined with an imaging device that allows to image the animal and immediately irradiate the region of interest and, if needed, repeat imaging. Then, since irradiators designed for small animal already exist, why use a GK for animal experimentations? The answer should include technical as well as conceptual aspects. The most important benefit of using the GK for small animals is related to the difference between conventional external radiotherapy and GK radiosurgery (GKRS). Radiation deposition with a GK is produced by multiple concentric beams that allow high dose deposition in a very small volume. These converging beams of ionizing radiation in a precise volume allow a rapid fall-off of dose near the edges which limit adverse effects on the surrounding adjacent tissue.

This chapter is devoted to a review of some characteristics of "homemade" stereotactic frames allowing small animal fixation in the Gamma Knife, and explores small animal researches done with a Gamma Knife published in the literature.

2. In-house designed stereotactic frame for use with the Gamma Knife for small animals

Even if GK is reported to be used for irradiation of large animals like cat and baboon (Kondziolka et al., 2002; Kondziolka et al., 2000; Lunsford et al., 1990; Nilsson et al., 1978), this chapter is focused on small animals (mouse, rat) because of their frequent uses in translational research, which is justified by their low cost, availability and reliable mimic of healthy or diseased human tissues/organs. When research groups plan to use the GK for experimental irradiations with small animals, the first step is to create a stereotactic device to hold the animals. These new devices need to show their efficiency and functionality and their approbation from the scientific community usually requires a publication that is peer-reviewed. For clinical application, GK radiosurgery is roughly separated in three steps: 1- imaging, 2- dose and localization planning with appropriate software and 3- positionning and irradiation. To mimic this, the animal stereotactic devices are generally designed to allow excellent transition from the imaging facility (MRI, CT-scan or X-ray radiography) to the planning software (i.e. Leksell Gamma Plan). After dose planning, the small animal stereotactic device must dock perfectly with the automatic positioning system (APS) of the GK, which is the part of the GK that allows movements in three dimensions to place the target at the exact irradiation coordinates. This is the basis for a stereotactic frame but, as we will see, some groups designed their device to bypass the conventional clinical stages or added features not related to radiosurgery to allow more functions. Fifteen articles concerning the use of new stereotactic frames for small animals were found in the literature (see Table 1).

Unfortunately, some of these articles do not mention clearly the details of their new devices, but they are suspected to be used as the first time in a series of experiments (Kouyama et al., 2003; Major et al., 2006; Pellerin et al., 2006; Rao et al., 1998; Takahashi et al., 1996; Xu et al., 2006; Zerris et al., 2002). The first mention of a stereotactic frame for small animals was reported by Kondziolka (Kondziolka et al., 1992b) in 1992. This device was a simple plate held by a modified Leksell model G stereotactic frame where the rat was maintained with adhesive restraints. This device allowed to be imaged by plain radiography and images are expected to be exported to a treatment planning software to assess the stereotactic coordinates. The Kondziolka device was subsequently used in other experiments (Kondziolka et al., 1992b; Kondziolka et al., 1996; Kondziolka et al., 1997; Mori et al., 2000; Niranjan et al., 2000; Niranjan et al., 2003) by the research group of the University of Pittsburgh. One year later, in 1993, Kamiryo *et al.* (Kamiryo et al., 1993) constructed a rat stereotactic device consisting of plate with earplugs and incisor bar to immobilize the animal, and a sliding Y and Z scales. This device has holes that adapt to the manual positioning system (trunnion) of the Gamma Knife. The coordinates of the target were "atlas-guided" using "the rat brain in stereotaxis coordinates" by Paxinos and Watson (Paxinos & Watson, 1986). A removable brain cutter and stereotactic arc to be used for surgical positioning according to the same coordinate system could be added to this device. In 1995, Kamiryo's group built another device to be used with magnetic resonance imaging (MRI). These two devices from Kamiryo's group were used in a few publications of the University of Virginia (Chen et al., 2001; Kamiryo et al., 1996; Kamiryo et al., 1996; Omary et al., 1995; Vincent et al., 2005). A similar atlas-guided stereotactic frame, known as the "Régis-Valliccioni stereotactic frame", was developed in 1996 (Rey et al., 1996) and used for research in Marseille (Bartolomei et al., 1998; Regis et al., 1996).

In 2002, a group from Czech Republic designed a rat stereotactic device compatible for GKRS and MR imaging (Liscak et al., 2002). This device has earplugs and incisor bar, and is used with the APS of the GK. Few publications are reported using this device (Herynek et al., 2004; Jirak et al., 2007b; Novotny et al., 2002a; Novotny et al., 2002b). In 2003, a new Régis-Valliccioni frame was used by a group from Tokyo (Kouyama et al., 2003; Tokumaru

First author	Location	Publication year	Objective	Target	Doses (Gy)	Positioning Methods
D. Kondziolka	Pittsburgh, USA	1992	Dose-response relationship and temporal effect of GKRS of the normal rat brain	Rat Brain: Right frontal lobe	30, 40, 50, 60, 70, 80, 100, 150, 200	Lateral and anterior-posterior radiography
T. Kamiryo	Charlottesville, USA	1993 1995	Technical note of new stereotactic device: Evaluation of geometric and dosimetric inaccuracies during GKRS. The device is built to accept a brain cutting system and an open stereotactic surgery system. In 1995 a new MRI device was developed to fit the same frame	Rat Brain: Right parietal cortex and phantom of thermoluminescence dosimetry (TLD) implanted in rat brain	4, 200, 300	Atlas-guided protocol and/or MRI
M. Rey	Marseille France	1996	Development of a stereotactic device for rat for use with GK. (Regis-Valliccioni model)	Rat Brain: Left striatum	100, 200	Atlasguided protocol
Z-R, Rao	Xi'an, China	1998	Expression and changes of GFAP after GKRS	Rat Brain: right caudate nucleus	100	MRI prior to GK
J. Novotny	Prague, Czech Republic	2002	Use of polymer gel dosimeter for evaluation of geometric and dosimetric inaccuracies during GKRS	Rat phantom	8	MRI prior to GK
N. Kouyama	Tokyo, Japan	2003	Survey of functional alteration in the rat striatum after GKRS. Preliminary results	Rat Brain: Unilateral striatum	150	?
C. DesRosiers	Indianapolis, USA	2003	Technical note about rat platform for GKRS and study of eye lens irradiation.	Rat eye: right eye lens of phantom and living rat	5, 10, 15	Observation through 4 mm collimator
Y-S, Im	Seoul, Korea	2006	Technical note: Stereotactic device for rats for GK model B and C. Testing for accuracy with phantom and normal and C6-glioma-inoculated rats	Film. Ionization chamber	150	Beam direction indicator

Table 1. Publications of new small animal stereotactic devices.

First author	Location	Publication year	Objective	Target	Doses (Gy)	Positioning Methods
D. Xu	Tianjin, China	2006	GKRS on C6 glioma in combination with adenoviral p53	Rat right frontal lobe: Tumor volume	15	MRI prior to GK
H-T. Chung	Goyang, Korea	2008	Development of a stereotactic device for rat for use with GK.	Phantom, ion chamber, radiochromic films, glioma bearing rat	30	X ray imaging
S. Takahashi	Sapporo, Japan	1996	Study of relaxation and contraction responses on common carotid artery following GKRS	Rat common carotid artery	100	Lateral and anterior-posterior radiogram
O. Major	Budapest, Hungary	2006	Modulation of blood vessel obliteration after GKRS and combination of paclitaxel.	Rat common carotid artery	15, 20, 25, 50, 80, 200	Atlasguided protocol
D. Wiant	Winston-Salem, USA	2009	High resolution treatment planning by MRi for GKRS	Radiographic film inserted in phantom and dead rat.	35	High resolution MRi prior to GK
G. Charest	Sherbrooke, Canada	2009	Technique evaluation: Stereotactic frame for GK model 4C docking with APS, Angiographic box and Bubble head measurement	Phantom: Polymer gel poured into skull of dead rats.	15	Radiography and recurrent position
G. Charest	Sherbrooke, Canada	Reported here	Stereotactic device (sarcophagus) for mice to use with GK 4C and Perfexion. For irradiation of mammary gland (breast cancer model) and hips (colorectal cancer model)	Gafchromic film. Ionization chamber	15	CT scan and recurrent positions
M. Pellerin	Sherbrooke, Canada	2006	Monitoring micro-vasculature damage of breast carcinoma induced by GKRS	Mice: breast cancer implanted in left hind limb	40	Direct measurement from the frame

Table 1. (Continued)

et al., 2005b). As the older version, this model uses earplugs and an incisor bar to fix the animal and enable target planning directly on the MR images. This new device appear in few publications (Hirano et al., 2009; Tokumaru et al., 2007a). In the series of devices equipped with earplugs and incisor bar, the most recent one from Chung *et al.* in 2008 (Chung et al., 2008) is a combination of a Leksell G-frame and KOPF rat adaptor. No publication that uses this tool has been found in the literature at the time of writing this chapter. One of the most simple device is reported in a publication of DesRosiers in 2003 (DesRosiers et al., 2003). This device is simply an 8" X 10" wood platform with holes to allow reproducible docking onto the GK manual positioning system. The rats were placed on another 6" X 8" wood resting plate that could be moved by hand in the X and Z direction and a leveling screw was set into the platform to allow motion in the Y direction. The targeting was performed by direct observation through 4 mm collimators. This visual targeting was deemed adequate because the target was the external eye of the animal, but could not be used for internal organ targeting. This device and method are reported elsewhere (Dynlacht et al., 2006; Dynlacht et al., 2008) and the coordinates were finally confirmed by CT scan (Tinnel et al., 2007). Im et al. (Im et al., 2006) also created a stereotactic device for rat consisting of a plate with ear plugs, incisor bar and a sliding Y and Z scales. The target was atlas-guided and a metallic bar that fitted exactly with one of the collimator holes of the collimator helmet was used as a beam direction indicator. This system is suspected to be used later by Lee et al. (Lee et al., 2006). It is to note that the positioning methods reported for the devices of DesRosiers (DesRosiers et al., 2003) and Im (Im et al., 2006) cannot be used with the newer Leksell Gamma Knife model Perfexion, because in this latest model, the internal collimators are inaccessible, which prevents their use as beam direction indicators. In 2009, the group of Wiant *et al.* (Wiant et al., 2009) developed a restrain jig with fiducial system small enough to be compatible with a small-bore 7T MR scanner aperture. This jig provides repeatability, accuracy, and interchangeability with MR scanner and the Gamma Knife headframe. This device was developed to gain a very high-resolution of MRI with a field of view of 50 mm^2 compare to 250 mm^2 with a clinical 3T MRI.

Our group at the University of Sherbrooke built three small animal stereotactic devices for GK. In 2006 Pellerin *et al.* (Pellerin et al., 2006) constructed a mouse frame where the animal was held in a 50 ml Falcon tube. The tube containing the mouse was positioned in relation to a mark onto the stereotactic frame. The use of this device is reported by Lemay *et al.* in 2011 (Lemay et al., 2011). In a long-term project that uses several animals, Charest *et al.* developed in 2009 a stereotactic frame for rat that allows constant and reproducible positioning using the same target coordinates (Charest et al., 2009). This device is a resin mold mimicking the rat body equipped with a silicon absorber on the sides to better fit the contour of the rat head. There is no metallic part in this frame, allowing MR imaging and radiographic imaging without interference. This frame was built to be used with clinical devices, such as the angiographic fiducial box, the bubble head measurement device and the APS. To test the accuracy of the coordinates of the focused radiation, the rat brain was removed and the intracranial cavity was washed and filled with a radiation sensitive polymer gel. After irradiation, the gel was removed, the polymerized area was measured and the coordinates were compiled to ensure the reproducible and accurate positioning of the rat head for GK radiosurgery. This project will be discussed in section 3 of this chapter, but briefly, our preclinical research effort focuses on the development or improvement of therapeutic modalities for malignant glioma. Our rat glioma model was extensively characterized and showed that the implanted tumors always grow in the same position (Blanchard et al., 2006; Mathieu et al., 2007). Thus, after preliminary testing which showed reproducible and accurate positioning, we were able to use the same coordinates of irradiation for each animal with implanted tumor, bypassing the time-consuming step of imaging and planning. This frame was used for radioprotection (Belzile et al., 2009) and radiosensitizing (Charest et al., 2011; Charest et al., Article in preparation) experiments, and investigations on tumor invasion in irradiated brain are in progress. We recently upgraded our GK unit to the Perfexion model, and the reproducible and accurate positioning of our frame in this new model of GK was confirmed by intracranial polymer gel irradiation, ionic chamber measurement and Gafchromic film irradiation. Our rat frame fitting in the frame holder of the GK Perfexion is shown in figure 1. The department of Nuclear Medicine and Radiobiology of the University of Sherbrooke also conducts experiment using a mouse model. The mouse model is used for research on colorectal cancer, breast cancer and metastasis (details in section 3). As for rat glioblastoma experiments, the irradiation coordinates with mice are recurrent, focusing on the posterior thigh or the anterior mammary gland of the mouse. The stereotactic frame was built as a sarcophagus, to prevent movement of the animal (figure 2). Because some of these protocols require fractionated irradiation and because mice do not tolerate successive anaesthesias by i.v. injection, an isoflurane delivery system was also introduced in the design of this device. As with the rat frame, the mouse frame was tested for reproducible and accurate positioning, confirmed by ionic chamber measurements and Gafchromic film irradiations.

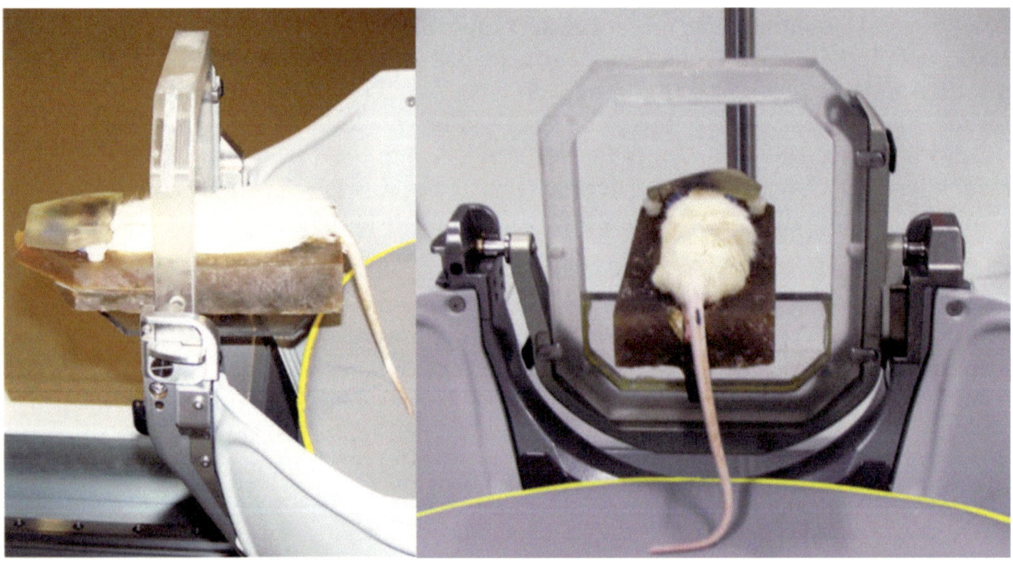

Fig. 1. Rat stereotactic frame held by the frame adaptator of the Gamma Knife Perfexion.

In this section, we described different devices that use various methods of positioning in the GK, from a simple visual confirmation of the target through the collimators, atlas-guided protocol, recurrent positioning and precise planning using MR or radiography imaging. In addition, some devices were not described clearly in the literature and we should assume that the efficiency is good enough to do GK radiosurgery. The design of these devices comes from the need of precise small animal stereotactic radiosurgery for different kind of researches that are reported in the next section.

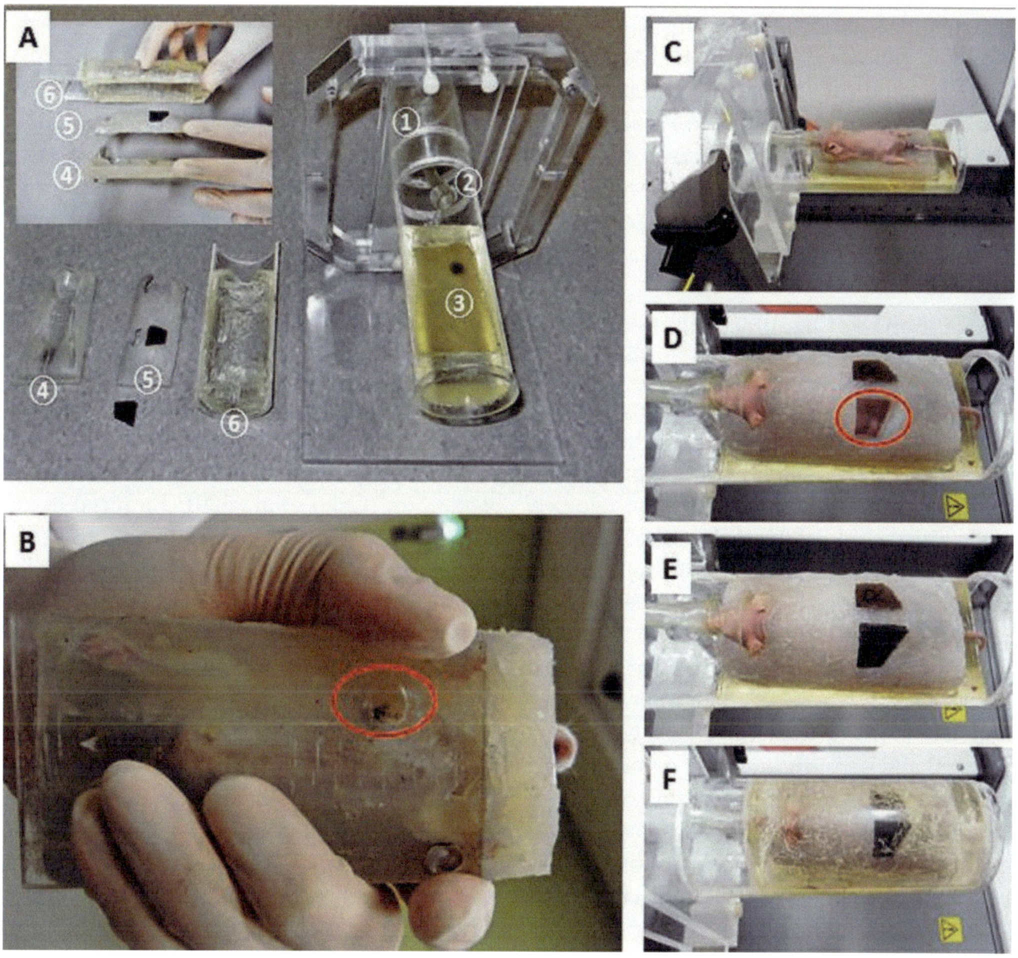

Fig. 2. Mouse sarcophagus stereotactic device.
A) Disassembled device. The numbers correspond to the following parts; 1: Compatible APS frame holding the tubular mouse platform, 2: Tubing for isoflurane delivery, 3: Bolus skin-equivalent layer, 4: lower part of mouse mold, 5: upper part of mouse mold with windows allowing fine positioning, 6:Top of the outer frame. B) Positioning window for mammary gland (red circle) under the lower part of the mouse mold (4). C) Nu/Nu nude mouse bearing colorectal cancer positioned on parts # 1, 2, 3, 4. D) Part #5 with open window for fine positioning of the subcutaneous cancer implanted into the thigh. E) Positioning windows closed with bolus skin-equivalent pieces. F) The sarcophagus is completed with part #6 and the mouse is ready for GKRS.

3. Experimental investigations using gamma knife technique with small animals

Five decades ago, Lars Leksell invented the Gamma Knife as a non-invasive method of delivering high-dose radiation to destroy discrete anatomical regions within the brain while minimizing the radiation effect on the surrounding tissues. Since 1991, over half a million patients had radiosurgery using the Gamma Knife to treat malignant and benign tumors, vascular, functional and ocular disorders (ELEKTA, 2011). On the other hand, in the last 20 years, around fifty publications reporting small animal radiosurgery by GK were found in the literature (Table 2). These *in vivo* GK radiosurgery (GKRS) experiments were designed to evaluate the dose-response relationship and temporal effect of GKRS in normal and pathologic brain tissue. For more clarity, this section about experimental *in vivo* investigation is divided in the following subsections: healthy brain matter, functional disorders, target outside the brain and cancer.

3.1 Response of healthy brain to focused radiation

Radiation treatments affect all cells. When tumors or other brain pathologies are targeted by GKRS, inevitably some surrounding normal healthy cells are also irradiated in the dose fall-off volume around the target. The most basic irradiated brain tissue experiments were conducted to correlated the position planning of high dose of radiation with a necrotic area into the rat brain visualized by pathological observation (Chen et al., 2001; Kamiryo et al., 1993; Regis et al., 1996; Rey et al., 1996; Tokumaru et al., 2005a) or by MRi (Kamiryo et al., 1995; Kamiryo et al., 1996). The evolution of the histological changes after GKRS were also monitored in function of time (1-60 days) for the targeted volume and surrounding brain tissue (2 mm) (Kondziolka et al., 1992a). It was shown that at 90 days, no histological changes were observed for a dose lower than 70 Gy. At 70 Gy, shrunken neurons were observed, and vascular changes were reported to occur after a radiation dose between 80 and 100 Gy. A dose of 150 to 200 Gy generated necrosis and cavitation of the targeted area whereas the surrounding area demonstrated reactive astrocytosis, edema, microhemorrhage and thickened vessels. The same group has shown that the edema and vasculopathy caused by a high dose of radiation (100 Gy) can be prevented with high doses of a radio protective agent (Kondziolka et al., 1997). Subsequently, edema and metabolite changes were analyzed in the early stage (months) after irradiation. Researches on the levels of n-acethylaspartate (NAA), creatin and choline compounds (Cr/Cho) and lactate (Lac) did not detect any changes four weeks after GKRS by using ^{1}H magnetic resonance spectroscopy (MRS), but edema was observed using MRI (Omary et al., 1995). Another group using the same technique has shown that at 8 months after GKRS an increase of Lac and Cho was seen, whereas the level of Cr and NAA decreased (Herynek et al., 2004). These changes in metabolite levels were accompanied by edema.

A study conducted on expression of the proto-oncogene c-fos showed that a specific stress response following GKRS appears with two peaks (12-24h and at one month) in the target region but also in the surrounding forebrain regions (Duan et al., 1999a). The same group found that there are three types of Fos-immunoreactive cells induced after GKRS (Duan et al., 1999b). GKRS also upregulates the N-methyl-D-aspatate receptor (NMDARs) subunits NR1 and NR2A, which might represent a possible explanation for the therapeutic effect of GKRS on many neurological diseases because of the crucial roles of NMDARs in synaptic transmission, plasticity and neurodegeneration (Liang et al., 2008). The heat shock proteins (HSPs) are a group of stress proteins whose synthesis of some can be inducted and are suggested to play a role in neuron protection. The group of Rao has shown that from 3 hours to 30 days after GKRS, the expression of HSP70 changed in function of time and according to the cell types (Rao et al., 2000). This animal model was useful to perform assays

First author	Location	Publication year	Objective	Target	Doses (Gy)
Response of healthy brain matter to focused radiation					
D. Kondziolka	Pittsburgh, USA	1992a	Dose-response relationship and temporal effect of focused single dose irradiation of the normal rat brain.	Rat Brain: Right frontal lobe	30, 40, 50, 60, 70, 80, 100, 150, 200
D. Kondziolka	Pittsburgh, USA	1997	Evaluation of a radioprotector on brain tissue.	Rat Brain: Frontal lobe	50, 100, 150
T. Kamiryo	Charlottesville, USA	1993 1995 1996	Technical note of new stereotactic device: Evaluation of geometric and dosimetric inaccuracies during GKRS. The device is built to accept a brain cutting system and an open stereotactic surgery system. In 1995 a new MRI device were developed to fit the same frame.	Rat Brain: Right parietal cortex	4, 200, 300
R.A. Omary	Charlottesville, USA	1995	Study on blood-brain barrier breakdown caused by GKRS.	Rat Brain: Frontoparietal cortex	120
J. Régis	Marseille, France	1996	Effect on GKRS for epilepsy on biochemical differential functional effects for glutamate decarboxylase and choline acetyltransferase, excitatory amino acids (AAs) and non-excitatory AAs and gamma-aminobutyric acid.	Rat Brain: Left striatum.	50, 200
Z-F, Chen	Charlottesville, USA	2001	Anticonvulsant effect of GK for epilepsy.	Rat Brain: Bilateral irradiation of the ventral hippocampal formation.	10, 20, 40
D. A. Vincent	Plymouth, UK	2005	Evaluation of the effect on body weight after GKRS.	Obese Zucker rat brain: hypothalamus	40
M. Rey	Marseille France	1996	Development of a stereotactic device for rat for use with GK. (Régis-Valliccioni model).	Rat Brain: Left striatum.	100, 200
X.Q. Duan	Xi'an and Guangzhou, China	1999a 1999b	Expression and change of Fos protein after GK irradiation.	Rat Brain: Caudate putamen, whole left forebrain.	100

Table 2. Radio-biological experiments with small animals.

Table 2. (Continued)

First author	Location	Publication year	Objective	Target	Doses (Gy)
Z-R, Rao	Xi'an, China	2000	Expression and changes of HSP70 after GK irradiation and survival.	Rat Brain: Right caudate putamen nucleus.	100
V. Herynek	Prague, Czech Republic	2004	Metabolite (Lac, Cho, Cr, NAA) and diffusion coefficient after GK irradiation.	Rat Brain: Bilateral irradiation of the hippocampus.	35
D. Jirak	Usti nad Labem, Czech Republic	2007	Lesion evolution after GKRS observed by MRI.	Rat Brain: Whole hippocampus	25, 50, 75
N. Kouyama	Tokyo, Japan	2003	Survey of functional alteration in the rat striatum after GK irradiation. Preliminary results.	Rat Brain: Unilateral striatum.	150
O. Tokumaru	Tokyo, Japan	2005a 2007	Survey of functional alteration in the rat striatum after GK irradiation.	Rat Brain: Left striatum.	150
M. Hirano	Tokyo, Japan	2009	Transcriptomic analysis of rat brain after GKRS.	Rat Brain: Striatum	60
C-d, Liang.	Shijiazhuang, China	2008	Effect of radiation on the expression of NMDAR subunits (NR1, NR2A, NR2B).	Rat Brain: Center at caudate putamen, whole left forebrain.	60
R. Liscak	Prague, Czech Republic	2002	Evaluation of changes in behavior (memory, orientation) and structural damage after GKRS.	Rat Brain: Bilateral irradiation of the hippocampus.	25, 50, 75, 100, 150
Epilepsy & Parkinson					
J. Régis	Marseille, France	1996	Effect on GKRS for epilepsy on biochemical differential functional effects for glutamate decarboxylase and choline acetyltransferase, excitatory amino acids (AAs) and non-excitatory AAs and gamma-aminobutyric acid.	Rat Brain: Left striatum.	50, 200
Y. Mori	Pittsburgh, USA	2000	Effect of GKRS on animal model of hippocampal epilepsy.	Rat Brain: hippocampus	20, 40, 60, 100
F. Bartolomei	Marseille, France	1998	Effect of GKRS on rat brain sodium channel subunit mRNA expression.	Rat Brain: Left dentate gyrus and upper thalamic region	100
Z-F, Chen	Charlottesville, USA	2001	Anticonvulsant effect of GK for epilepsy.	Rat Brain: Bilateral irradiation of the ventral hippocampal formation.	10, 20, 40

First author	Location	Publication year	Objective	Target	Doses (Gy)
Outside the brain matter					
C. DesRosiers	Indianapolis, USA	2003	Technical note about rat platform for GKRS and study of eye lens irradiation.	Rat eye: right eye lens of phantom and living rat	5, 10, 15
J. R. Dynlacht	Indianapolis, USA	2006 2008	Evaluation of estrogen as a radioprotector against cataractogenesis.	Rat right eye	10, 15
R.A. Omary	Charlottesville, USA	1995	Study on blood-brain barrier breakdown caused by GKRS.	Rat Brain: Frontoparietal cortex	120
S. Takahashi	Sapporo, Japan	1996	Study of relaxation and contraction responses on common carotid artery following GKRS.	Rat common carotid artery	100
O. Major	Budapest, Hungary	2006	Modulation of blood vessel obliteration after GKRS and combination of paclitaxel.	Rat common carotid artery	15, 20, 25, 50, 80, 200
B. Tinnel	Indianapolis, USA	2007	Evaluation of lung toxicity after GKRS in rat.	Rat right bronchus, GAF-chromic film	20, 40, 80
M. Pellerin	Sherbrooke, Canada	2006	Monitoring micro-vasculature damage of breast carcinoma induced by GKRS.	Mice: breast cancer implanted in left hind limb	40
M. Belzile	Sherbrooke, Canada	2009	Octreotide can be considered for prevention of radiation-induced salivary gland damage.	Rat parotid glands	30
CANCER **Brain cancer**					
D. Kondziolka	Pittsburgh, USA	1992b	Evaluation of tumoricidal effect of focused single dose irradiation of the rat C6 glioma model.	Rat Brain: Tumor in the right frontal lobe	30, 40, 50, 70, 100
D. Kondziolka	Pittsburgh, USA	1996	Evaluation of different techniques for irradiation of the rat C6 glioma model.	Rat Brain: Tumor in the right frontal lobe and WBRT	20, 35, 85
A. Niranjan	Pittsburgh, USA	2000	Treatment of mice glioblastoma by combination of TNF-alpha and HSV-tk gene transfer and GKRS.	Hsd nu/nu mice brain: Tumor in the right frontal lobe	21.4
A. Niranjan	Pittsburgh, USA	2003	Treatment of rat gliosarcoma by combination of HSV-based multigene therapy and GKRS.	Rat Brain: Tumor in the right frontal lobe	21.4

Table 2. (Continued)

First author	Location	Publication year	Objective	Target	Doses (Gy)
Y-S, Im	Seoul, Korea	2006	Technical note: Stereotactic device for rats for GK model B and C. Testing for accuracy with phantom and normal and C6-glioma-inoculated rats.	Film. Ionization chamber	150
J-I, Lee	Kyoto, Japan	2006	Combination of GKRS and antiangiogenic agent in treatment of glioma.	Rat right frontal lobe: Tumor volume	5, 10, 20, 40, 80, 160
D. Xu	Tianjin, China	2006	GKRS on C6 glioma in combination with adenoviral p53.	Rat right frontal lobe: Tumor volume	15
Y. Li	Tianjin, China	2010	Combination therapy with GKRS and antisense EGFR for malignant glioma.	Rat right frontal lobe: Tumor volume	15
Q. Jia	Tianjin, China	2010	Radio sensitivity enhanced by RNA Ku70 for glioma treatment prior to GKRS.	Rat right frontal lobe: Tumor volume	15
H-T. Chung	Goyang, Korea	2008	Development of a stereotactic device for rat for use with GK.	Phantom, ion chamber, radiochromic films, glioma bearing rat	30
G. Desmarrais	Sherbrooke, Canada	submitted	Ongoing research on glioma (invasion, migration).	Rat brain	
G. Charest	Sherbrooke, Canada	2011 ongoing	Ongoing research on glioma (chemo-radio therapy).	Rat right frontal lobe: Tumor volume	15
Breast cancer					
R. Lemay	Sherbrooke, Canada	2011	Study of invasiveness of mammary cancer cells after irradiation.	Mice: thigh prior to cancer cells implantation.	30
G. Bouchard	Sherbrooke, Canada	ongoing	Ongoing research on breast cancer.	Mice: mammary gland	
Colorectal cancer					
T. Tippayamontri	Sherbrooke, Canada	ongoing	Ongoing research on colorectal cancer (radio-chemo therapy).	Mice: thigh implanted with colorectal tumor cells	15

Table 2. (Continued)

at protein and metabolite level in brain tissue after GKRS. In fact, this field is probably just at its infancy. A recent study with rats (Hirano et al., 2009) showed that only 16 hours after a dose of 60 Gy, there are 230 induced and 144 repressed genes in the irradiated striatum and 432 induced and 239 repressed genes in the contralateral unirradiated striatum.

Interestingly, the biochemical changes of the brain following GKRS can be explored using behavioral experiments with the apomorphine test. Apomorphine is a dopamine agonist that stimulates dopamine receptors. After injection of apomorphine, a temporal increase of physical activity for about 30 minutes is observed. When the striatum is unilaterally irradiated, the dopaminergic function is then impaired on the irradiated site resulting in unbalanced dopaminergic activity between left and right striatum that results in a circling behavior (Kouyama et al., 2003; Tokumaru et al., 2005a; Tokumaru et al., 2007b). These studies emphasized the extreme precision of the GK and described how GKRS to the striatum can affect the behavior of small animals. The striatum is one site of dopaminergic function and the hippocampus is implicated in memory. In fact, irradiation of the rat hippocampus has been shown to affect memory (measured with the Morris water maze test) and the dose is correlated in function of time and size to the occurrence of edema following GKRS (Jirak et al., 2007a; Liscak et al., 2002). Finally, a pilot study of 40 Gy irradiation of the hypothalamus of obese Zucker rats produced an effect on weight control comparable to drug therapy with a metalloporphyrin. The authors hypothesized that this GKRS treatment leads to a resetting of the hypothalamic set point for body weight (Vincent et al., 2005).

In summary, small animal experiments have demonstrated that the effects of GK radiation onto the healthy brain tissue can appear a few hours to a few months after irradiation. The changes in the brain are observed not only at the dose deposition area but can be detected in the non-irradiated contralateral part of the brain. These changes were monitored by histological essays, external imaging and behavioral tests.

3.2 Focused radiation for epilepsy and Parkinson disease

We denoted only four studies using GKRS treatment for epilepsy in small animals. In 1996, Régis et al. showed that the biochemical effect on brain tissue obtained by GKRS could translate into a therapeutic effect for epilepsy. These biochemical changes were observed for glutamate decarboxylase, choline acetyl transferase, excitatory amino acids and non-excitatory amino acids as γ-aminobutyric acid (Regis et al., 1996) but no modification was observed in mRNA expression for the sodium channel subunit II and III up to 60 days following 100 Gy to the left dental gyrus and thalamus (Bartolomei et al., 1998). Thereafter GKRS was used in an epilepsy rat experiments. An animal model of hippocampal epileptic rat was produced by injection of kainic acid into the rat hippocampus and confirmed by electroencephalography (EEG). Different animal groups received doses of 20, 40, 60 or 100 Gy to the hippocampus and a significant dose-dependent reduction in the frequency of observed and EEG-defined seizures was reported (Mori et al., 2000). Another epileptic rat model was developed by repetitive electrical stimulations of the hippocampus in rats. The ventral hippocampus was irradiated and it is reported that a single dose of 20 or 40 Gy, but not 10 Gy, reduced substantially or eliminated the behavioral and EEG recognized seizures (Chen et al., 2001). These models of epileptic rats have improved our understanding of the fundamental mechanisms in epilepsy treatment by GKRS.

Parkinson's disease is another functional disorder for which GKRS experiments were performed. Only one rodent model of hemi-Parkinson was found in the literature. This animal model was developed by injection of 6-hydroxy-dopamine (6-OHDA) and the effect of unilateral dopaminergic loss was confirmed. The unilateral 6-OHDA lesion on rats showed ipsilateral rotation with the apomorphine test. A highly statistical reduction of apomorphine-induced rotation was observed at 2, 3 and 4 months after administration of 140 Gy to the striatum of these hemi-parkinsonian animals. The authors concluded that the focused radiation is potentially capable of inducing regeneration of dopaminergic pathway in the adult CNS.

3.3 Focused radiation targeted outside the brain

Few researches on irradiated organs and tissues located outside the brain using GKRS were reported. Eye cataractogenesis is a complication observed in patient receiving total-body irradiation prior to bone marrow transplantation, head and neck radiotherapy and for astronauts that receive low dose of densely ionizing space radiation. To study the effect of radiation on the eye, a research group at Indiana University (Indiana, IN) irradiated a single rat eye and lens using GKRS. They reported that the GK was precise enough to create a cataract in the irradiated eye while keeping the contralateral eye intact (DesRosiers et al., 2003). Later, they have shown that the cataractogenesis of the irradiated eye can be modulated with estrogen. When estrogen is administrated one week before GKRS and continuously thereafter, the incidence of cataractogenesis is increased (Dynlacht et al., 2006). On the other hand, when estrogen is administrated continuously, but starting only after irradiation, a decrease of incidence of cataractogenese is observed (Dynlacht et al., 2008). These researches have important implication for the management of astronauts and patient receiving radiotherapy.

The effect of ionizing radiation on vascular tissue was also studied. In 1996, a study on the relaxation and contraction response of the carotid artery after GKRS was conducted. The authors mentioned that the irradiated carotid artery had a reduction in the vasoconstriction response induced by norepinephrine, endothelin-1 and phorbol dibuthyrate. This impairment is biphasic and peaks one day and one month after irradiation. This phenomenon is apparently caused by alterations of both the vascular endothelial and smooth muscle cells (Takahashi et al., 1996). Other researchers experimented on the reaction of the middle cerebral artery to GKRS. Briefly, two groups of animal were studied: animals that received only irradiation and animals that received paclitaxel prior to GKRS. The authors reported that the constriction responses were decreased in the paclitaxel treated group and that complete recovery was faster for the paclitaxel group (12 months compared to 18 month). It appears that paclitaxel causes acceleration in the time course of the late vascular effect of GKRS (Major et al., 2006).

Another group has studied the influence of the volume of the dose deposition on bronchus integrity. In their experiment, the mainstream bronchus was irradiated with 4 mm or 8 mm collimators. It was found that the bronchus well tolerated small volume (4 mm) of very high dose of radiotherapy but a bigger volume (8 mm) encompassing the surrounding support stroma and normal tissue produced cellular atypia, interstitial pneumonitis, bronchial and vascular damages (Tinnel et al., 2007). Finally, Belzile et al. showed that administration of octreotide, a drug used in acromegaly and other types of digestive pathologies, prior to

GKRS acted as a radioprotective agent on rat parotid glands one month after irradiation (Belzile et al., 2009). Octreotide can then be considered for prevention of radiation-induced salivary gland damages. Other GKRS experiments outside the brain matter are included in the subchapter concerning cancer research.

3.4 Gamma knife for cancer research

Radiation for cancer therapy is widely used for many types of cancer. Brain cancer radiotherapy is certainly the main subject of research for GKRS. The emphasis on brain cancer research is easy to understand considering the clinical use of the Gamma Knife that is mainly limited to the head. However, with the new model PERFEXION, head and neck target are theoretically achievable and clinical research may eventually expand to these areas. However, in research with small animals, any regions of the animal can be targeted. This subchapter will discuss some animal models to study brain cancer but also models of breast and colorectal cancer.

3.4.1 Breast cancer

It has been reported that radiation treatment can enhance the invasiveness of many types of cancer by increasing the expression of matrix metalloproteinase type-2 (Ohuchida et al., 2004; Qian et al., 2002; Speake et al., 2005; Wang et al., 2000; Wild-Bode et al., 2001). It was also reported that the metastatic frequency was significantly higher in tumors implanted in pre-irradiated beds (Milas et al., 1988; Rofstad et al., 2005). The research group of Dr. Paquette of Sherbrooke University has studied whether irradiation of normal tissues could increase the invasiveness of breast cancer cells in a mouse model. They concluded that the implantation of non-irradiated mammary cancer cells in previously irradiated normal tissue enhanced the invasive capacity of the mammary cancer cells (Lemay et al., 2011). Another hypothesis from the same group is that there is an activation of transforming growth factor beta (TGF-β) from healthy tissues by radiation. Recent studies reported that the antiproliferative effect of TGF-β accompanied the stimulation of cancer cell migration. This phenomenon can lead to radioresistance since radiation mainly target dividing cells. These facts led them to believe that an inhibitor of TGF-β could reduce radio-induced invasion and promote a synergistic effect with radiotherapy treatments. Ongoing experiments are in progress to determine if an inhibitor of TGF-β maturation (chloroquin) can prevent radiation-enhancement of cancer cell invasion in a mouse model (Bouchard et al., Ongoing research).

3.4.2 Colorectal cancer

At the University of Sherbrooke, a study about the combination of platinum compounds and radiation to treat colorectal cancer in animal model is in progress. Nu/Nu nude mice implanted with colorectal cell cancer (HCT 116) are treated by intravenous injection of different platinum compounds prior to GKRS (see GKRS set up in figure 2). The investigators hope to show a potential synergistic effect of the combination of this chemo-radiotherapy (Tippayamontri et al., Ongoing research). One goal is to determine the optimal chemo-radiotherapy schedule to treat colorectal cancer in regards to pharmacokinetic properties of platinum-base drugs to obtain the best synergistic effects, by varying the time delays between administration of the drug and GKRS.

3.4.3 Brain cancer

A group of the University of Pittsburgh conducted a series of experiments involving small animals as models to study the treatment of brain cancer by GKRS. In 1992 Kondziolka et al. used the rat C6 glioma model to evaluate the potential role of GKRS for treatment of glial neoplasms. With a single fraction of focused irradiation to the tumor volume, they showed that the glioma bearing animals treated by GK had a longer mean survival compared to the control animals (39.2 days compared to 29.4 days respectively). At sacrifice, the mean tumor volume was smaller for the radiosurgery group (6.47 mm) compared to the control group (9.64 mm) and the tumors of the radiosurgery group showed significant hypocellular appearance and cellular edema (Kondziolka et al., 1992b). Later, using the same animal model, they tried different irradiation schemes resulting in a median survival time increasing as follows: control < single-fraction of 35 Gy hemibrain < whole brain radiation therapy (WBRT) 20 Gy in 5 fractions < radiosurgery to the margin of the tumor 35 Gy = radiosurgery to the margin of the tumor 35 Gy + WBRT 20 Gy in 5 fractions < fractioned hemibrain radiotherapy of 85 Gy in 10 fractions. They also reported edema after radiosurgery to the margin of the tumor 35 Gy and for combined treatment of radiosurgery to the margin of the tumor 35 Gy + WBRT 20 Gy in 5 fractions but not after fractionated radiotherapy or single-fraction of 35 Gy hemibrain (Kondziolka et al., 1996). After these studies about the effects of ionizing radiation on the C6 glioma model, the Pittsburgh research group published two articles about the combination of radiation and gene therapy. They used athymic nude mice in whom they implanted in the brain the U87MG human glioblastoma cell line. The mice were treated with different combinations of GKRS, herpes simplex virus thymidine kinase suicide gene therapy (SGT), tumor necrosis factor alpha (TNF-alpha) and ganciclovir (GCV). Compared to the median surviving time of the control animals (21 days), the combination therapies increased the median life span of the treated animal as follows: GKRS+TNF-alpha+GCV= 46 days < SGT+TNF-alpha+GCV= 60 days < GKRS+SGT+TNF-alpha+GCV = 75 days. The combination of conventional therapeutic methods and gene therapy was considered a promising treatment to improve the survival time of patients afflicted with glioblastoma (Niranjan et al., 2000). This group also reported the use of multigene therapy using the model of immunocompetent rats bearing 9L gliosarcoma. For these experiments, they used a new vector called NUREL-C2 that co-express TNF-alpha + gap-junction-forming protein connexin43 (Cx) + infected cell protein zero (ICP0) + viral thymidine kinase (HSV-tk) (Niranjan et al., 2003). The median survival time of GCV plus combined therapy and/or GKRS increases as follows: SGT+TNF-alpha = 39 days < SGT+TNF-alpha+Cx = 68 days < SGT+TNF-alpha+GKRS = 80 days < SGT+TNF-alpha+Cx+GKRS = 150 days. The results of this investigation on multigene therapy with NUREL-C2 have shown that this vector could be estimated as an efficient prototype vector in clinical trial in patient with recurrent malignant glioblastoma.

More recently, a group from Tianjin, of the Republic of China, also used gene therapy in two publications followed by lipofection of antisense therapy in a rat model bearing C6 glioma. Their first article mentioned the use of adenoviral therapy for expression of p53, this protein playing a role in improving radiosensitivity, cell cycle arrest and apoptosis. Their different therapies resulted in an increase of life survival from control < p53 < GKRS < p53 + GKRS (Xu et al., 2006). Their second study using lipofection tested the antisense EGFR (As-EGFR). EGFR the epidermal growth factor receptor is known to be associated with radioresistance of glioma and increased proliferation. Once again, the effects of their different therapies have shown an increase in survival from control < GKRS < As-EGFR < As-EGFR+GKRS (Li et al., 2010). The same group from Tianjin published in 2010 a study using a recombinant adenovirus for the inhibition of Ku70 which play an important role in DNA double strands breaks repair. As in their other publications, they showed an increase in survival from control < inhibited Ku70 < GKRS < Inhibited Ku70+GKRS (Jia et al., 2010). Combination therapy with drugs and radiation was also reported by researchers from Kyoto, Japan. In their study, the authors combined GKRS and the antiangiogenic agent thalidomide (THD) or the chemotherapeutic agent temozolomide (TMZ). No surviving essay was reported in their article but they mentioned a significant decrease in tumor volume in rats bearing C6/LacZ glioma treated with the combination of GKRS and THD. Two other different groups (Chung et al., 2008; Im et al., 2006) published a new stereotactic frame for GKRS in small animals bearing a glioma tumor in their brain. Both groups mentioned that the biological data will be discussed in another articles in preparation.

To end this chapter on brain tumor experiments, we will talk about ongoing research in our department at the University of Sherbrooke. Radiotherapy remains one of the most effective treatment for glioblastoma (GBM), resulting in at least transient disease control in most patients. Since cancer cells always infiltrate adjacent normal brain, the target volume irradiated is 2-3 cm larger than the tumour volume detected by current imaging tools. Unfortunately, the radiation dose is not intended to restrain all cancer cells scattered in the brain, but is rather aimed at optimizing the number of cancer cells eliminated with minimal adverse effects. Therefore, the tumour frequently recurs in the brain volume previously irradiated. This observation raises the following question: Can the migration and proliferation capacity of cancer cells which are not eliminated by radiotherapy (or other modalities) be influenced by the surrounding microenvironment? To answer part of this question, we irradiated healthy brain tissue prior to tumour implantation (F98/Fischer rat glioma model) to observe the characteristics of the tumour development into an irradiated tissue, and how this might differ compared to normal non-irradiated tissue. Immunogenic reaction to radiation is an important aspect dictating the tumour growth and consequently altering the migration abilities of tumour cells. This investigation will allow us to have a better understanding of the tumour development and, hopefully, to translate this knowledge into an improved survival for GBM patients (Desmarrais et al., Submitted). Another study by our group is devoted to the potential synergistic effects of the combination of platinum compounds and GKRS. Platinum compounds were chosen because they are already approved for clinical use and are widely available. Zheng et al. demonstrated that the efficiency of low energy electrons produced by ionizing radiation to induce DNA strand breaks is significantly increased in presence of cisplatin (Zheng et al., 2008). Different routes of drug administration were evaluated in our study (Charest et al., Article in preparation). Five different platinum compounds were administrated by intravenous injection, intraarterial injection (carotid artery), or intraarterial injection after osmotic blood-brain barrier disruption. The drug treatments were also tested in combination with 15 Gy of radiation delivered by the Gamma Knife to the tumor volume. Surviving essays and drug uptake measurements were done. The biological and radiobiological data will be discussed in another article in preparation.

4. Conclusion

We reported here the development of our stereotactic devices for rat and mouse irradiation with the Leksell Gamma Knife models 4C and PERFEXION. Sixteen different stereotactic devices for small animal irradiation by GK, and about fifty *in vivo* experiments were reviewed. This relatively small amount of *in vivo* experiments seems paradoxal compared to the half a million patients that received radiosurgery using the Gamma Knife. Nevertheless, the *in vivo* articles reported here are important because they are often the first publications in specific fields and have the potential to lead to significant clinical breakthroughs. In all these published articles, the GK was reported to be accurate and reliable for small animal irradiation experiments.

5. References

Bartolomei, F., Massacrier, A., Rey, M., Viale, M., Regis, J., Gastaldi, M & Cau, P. (1998). Effect of gamma knife radiosurgery on rat brain sodium channel subunit mRNA expression. *Stereotact Funct Neurosurg,* Vol. 70 Suppl 1, Oct, pp. 237-242, ISSN/ISBN: 1011-6125; 1011-6125.

Belzile, M., St-Amant, M., Mathieu, D., Doueik, AA., Fortier, PH & Dorion, D. (2009). Radiation-induced xerostomia: is octreotide the solution? *J Otolaryngol Head Neck Surg,* Vol. 38, No. 5, Oct, pp. 545-551, ISSN/ISBN: 1916-0216.

Blanchard, J., Mathieu, D., Patenaude, Y & Fortin, D. (2006). MR-pathological comparison in F98-Fischer glioma model using a human gantry. *Can J Neurol Sci,* Vol. 33, No. 1, Feb, pp. 86-91, ISSN/ISBN: 0317-1671.

Bouchard, G., Bujold, R., Saucier, C & Paquette, B. (Ongoing research). Ongoing research.

Charest, G., Mathieu, D., Lepage, M., Fortin, D., Paquette, B & Sanche, L. (2009). Polymer gel in rat skull to assess the accuracy of a new rat stereotactic device for use with the Gamma Knife. *Acta Neurochir (Wien),* Apr 18, ISSN/ISBN: 0942-0940.

Charest, G., Sanche, L., Fortin, D., Mathieu, D & Paquette, B. (2011). Glioblastoma treatment: Bypassing the toxicity of platinum compounds by using liposomal formulation and increasing treatment efficiency with concomitant radiotherapy. *Int J Radiat Oncol Biol Phys,* Accepted.

Chen, ZF., Kamiryo, T., Henson, SL., Yamamoto, H., Bertram, EH., Schottler, F., Patel, F., Steiner, L., Prasad, D., Kassell, NF., Shareghis, S & Lee, KS. (2001). Anticonvulsant effects of gamma surgery in a model of chronic spontaneous limbic epilepsy in rats. *J Neurosurg,* Vol. 94, No. 2, Feb, pp. 270-280, ISSN/ISBN: 0022-3085; 0022-3085.

Chung, HT., Chung, YS., Kim, DG., Paek, SH & Cho, KT. (2008). Development of a stereotactic device for gamma knife irradiation of small animals. *J Korean Neurosurg Soc,* Vol. 43, No. 1, Jan, pp. 26-30, ISSN/ISBN: 2005-3711; 1225-8245.

Desmarrais, G., Bujold, R., Fortin, D., Mathieu, D & Paquette, B. (Submitted).

DesRosiers, C., Mendonca, MS., Tyree, C., Moskvin, V., Bank, M., Massaro, L., Bigsby, RM., Caperall-Grant, A., Valluri, S., Dynlacht, JR & Timmerman, R. (2003). Use of the Leksell Gamma Knife for localized small field lens irradiation in rodents. *Technol Cancer Res Treat,* Vol. 2, No. 5, Oct, pp. 449-454, ISSN/ISBN: 1533-0346.

Duan, XQ., Wu, HX., Liu, HL., Rao, ZR & Ju, G. (1999a). Expression and changes of Fos protein in the rat forebrain after gamma knife irradiation targeted to the caudate putamen. *Neurosurgery,* Vol. 45, No. 1, Jul, pp. 139-45; discussion 145-6, ISSN/ISBN: 0148-396X; 0148-396X.

Duan, XQ., Wu, SL., Li, T., Liang, JC., Qiou, JY., Rao, ZR & Ju, G. (1999b). Expression and significance of three types of Fos-immunoreactive cells after gamma knife irradiation of the forebrain in the rat. *Neurosci Res,* Vol. 33, No. 2, Feb, pp. 99-104, ISSN/ISBN: 0168-0102; 0168-0102.

Dynlacht, JR., Tyree, C., Valluri, S., DesRosiers, C., Caperell-Grant, A., Mendonca, MS., Timmerman, R & Bigsby, RM. (2006). Effect of estrogen on radiation-induced cataractogenesis. *Radiat Res,* Vol. 165, No. 1, Jan, pp. 9-15, ISSN/ISBN: 0033-7587; 0033-7587.

Dynlacht, JR., Valluri, S., Lopez, J., Greer, F., Desrosiers, C., Caperell-Grant, A., Mendonca, MS & Bigsby, RM. (2008). Estrogen protects against radiation-induced cataractogenesis. *Radiat Res,* Vol. 170, No. 6, Dec, pp. 758-764, ISSN/ISBN: 0033-7587; 0033-7587.

ELEKTA. *In: Gamma knife treatment stats,* Date of access: 2011, Available from: http://www.elekta.com/assets/Elekta-Neuroscience/Gamma-Knife-Surgery/pdfs/Gamma-Knife-Treatment-Stastics-2009.pdf.

Herynek, V., Burian, M., Jirak, D., Liscak, R., Namestkova, K., Hajek, M & Sykova, E. (2004). Metabolite and diffusion changes in the rat brain after Leksell Gamma Knife irradiation. *Magn Reson Med,* Vol. 52, No. 2, Aug, pp. 397-402, ISSN/ISBN: 0740-3194.

Hirano, M., Shibato, J., Rakwal, R., Kouyama, N., Katayama, Y., Hayashi, M & Masuo, Y. (2009). Transcriptomic analysis of rat brain tissue following gamma knife surgery: early and distinct bilateral effects in the un-irradiated striatum. *Mol Cells,* Vol. 27, No. 2, Feb 28, pp. 263-268, ISSN/ISBN: 1016-8478; 1016-8478.

Im, YS., Nam, DH., Kim, JS., Ju, SG., Lim, DH & Lee, JI. (2006). Stereotactic device for Gamma Knife radiosurgery in experimental animals: technical note. *Stereotact Funct Neurosurg,* Vol. 84, No. 2-3, pp. 97-102, ISSN/ISBN: 1011-6125.

Jia, Q., Li, Y., Xu, D., Li, Z., Zhang, Z., Zhang, Y., Liu, D., Liu, X., Pu, P & Kang, C. (2010). Radiosensitivity of glioma to Gamma Knife treatment enhanced in vitro and in vivo by RNA interfering Ku70 that is mediated by a recombinant adenovirus. *J Neurosurg,* Vol. 113 Suppl, Dec, pp. 228-235, ISSN/ISBN: 1933-0693; 0022-3085.

Jirak, D., Namestkova, K., Herynek, V., Liscak, R., Vymazal, J., Mares, V., Sykova, E & Hajek, M. (2007a). Lesion evolution after gamma knife irradiation observed by magnetic resonance imaging. *Int J Radiat Biol,* Vol. 83, No. 4, Apr, pp. 237-244, ISSN/ISBN: 0955-3002.

Jirak, D., Namestkova, K., Herynek, V., Liscak, R., Vymazal, J., Mares, V., Sykova, E & Hajek, M. (2007b). Lesion evolution after gamma knife irradiation observed by magnetic resonance imaging. *Int J Radiat Biol,* Vol. 83, No. 4, Apr, pp. 237-244, ISSN/ISBN: 0955-3002; 0955-3002.

Kamiryo, T., Berk, HW., Lee, KS., Kassell, NF & Steiner, L. (1993). A stereotactic device for experimental gamma knife radiosurgery in rats. A technical note. *Acta Neurochir (Wien),* Vol. 125, No. 1-4, pp. 156-160, ISSN/ISBN: 0001-6268.

Kamiryo, T., Berr, SS., Berk, HW., Lee, KS., Kassell, NF & Steiner, L. (1996). Accuracy of an experimental stereotactic system for MRI-based gamma knife irradiation in the rat. *Acta Neurochir (Wien),* Vol. 138, No. 9, pp. 1103-7; discussion 1107-8, ISSN/ISBN: 0001-6268.

Kamiryo, T., Berr, SS., Lee, KS., Kassell, NF & Steiner, L. (1995). Enhanced magnetic resonance imaging of the rat brain using a stereotactic device with a small head coil: technical note. *Acta Neurochir (Wien),* Vol. 133, No. 1-2, pp. 87-92, ISSN/ISBN: 0001-6268; 0001-6268.

Kamiryo, T., Lopes, MB., Berr, SS., Lee, KS., Kassell, NF & Steiner, L. (1996). Occlusion of the anterior cerebral artery after Gamma Knife irradiation in a rat. *Acta Neurochir (Wien),* Vol. 138, No. 8, pp. 983-90; discussion 990-1, ISSN/ISBN: 0001-6268.

Kondziolka, D., Couce, M., Niranjan, A., Maesawa, S & Fellows, W. (2002). Histology of the 100-Gy Thalamotomy in the Baboon. *Radiosurgery.Basel, Karger,* Vol. 4, pp. 279-284, .

Kondziolka, D., Lacomis, D., Niranjan, A., Mori, Y., Maesawa, S., Fellows, W & Lunsford, LD. (2000). Histological effects of trigeminal nerve radiosurgery in a primate model: implications for trigeminal neuralgia radiosurgery. *Neurosurgery,* Vol. 46, No. 4, Apr, pp. 971-6; discussion 976-7, ISSN/ISBN: 0148-396X; 0148-396X.

Kondziolka, D., Lunsford, LD., Claassen, D., Maitz, AH & Flickinger, JC. (1992a). Radiobiology of radiosurgery: Part I. The normal rat brain model. *Neurosurgery,* Vol. 31, No. 2, Aug, pp. 271-279, ISSN/ISBN: 0148-396X; 0148-396X.

Kondziolka, D., Lunsford, LD., Claassen, D., Pandalai, S., Maitz, AH & Flickinger, JC. (1992b). Radiobiology of radiosurgery: Part II. The rat C6 glioma model. *Neurosurgery,* Vol. 31, No. 2, Aug, pp. 280-7; discussion 287-8, ISSN/ISBN: 0148-396X; 0148-396X.

Kondziolka, D., Somaza, S., Comey, C., Lunsford, LD., Claassen, D., Pandalai, S., Maitz, A & Flickinger, JC. (1996). Radiosurgery and fractionated radiation therapy: comparison of different techniques in an in vivo rat glioma model. *J Neurosurg,* Vol. 84, No. 6, Jun, pp. 1033-1038, ISSN/ISBN: 0022-3085; 0022-3085.

Kondziolka, D., Somaza, S., Martinez, AJ., Jacobsohn, J., Maitz, A., Lunsford, LD & Flickinger, JC. (1997). Radioprotective effects of the 21-aminosteroid U-74389G for stereotactic radiosurgery. *Neurosurgery,* Vol. 41, No. 1, Jul, pp. 203-208, ISSN/ISBN: 0148-396X; 0148-396X.

Kouyama, N., Katayama, Y., Hayashi, M., Tomida, M., Tokumaru, O & Kawakami, Y. (2003). On the survey of fonctional alterations in the rat striatum after gamma-knife irradiation. *Neuroscience Research,* Vol. 46 (Suppl 1), pp. S111, .

Lee, JI., Itasaka, S., Kim, JT & Nam, DH. (2006). Antiangiogenic agent, thalidomide increases the antitumor effect of single high dose irradiation (gamma knife radiosurgery) in the rat orthotopic glioma model. *Oncol Rep,* Vol. 15, No. 5, May, pp. 1163-1168, ISSN/ISBN: 1021-335X.

Lemay, R., Archambault, M., Tremblay, L., Bujold, R., Lepage, M & Paquette, B. (2011). Irradiation of normal mouse tissue increases the invasiveness of mammary cancer cells. *Int J Radiat Biol,* Jan 13, ISSN/ISBN: 1362-3095; 0955-3002.

Li, Y., Jia, Q., Zhang, J., Han, L., Xu, D., Zhang, A., Zhang, Y., Zhang, Z., Pu, P & Kang, C. (2010). Combination therapy with Gamma Knife radiosurgery and antisense EGFR for malignant glioma in vitro and orthotopic xenografts. *Oncol Rep,* Vol. 23, No. 6, Jun, pp. 1585-1591, ISSN/ISBN: 1791-2431; 1021-335X.

Liang, CD., Li, WL., Liu, N., Yin, Y., Hao, J & Zhao, WQ. (2008). Effects of gamma knife irradiation on the expression of NMDA receptor subunits in rat forebrain. *Neurosci Lett,* Vol. 439, No. 3, Jul 18, pp. 250-255, ISSN/ISBN: 0304-3940; 0304-3940.

Liscak, R., Vladyka, V., Novotny, J,Jr., Brozek, G., Namestkova, K., Mares, V., Herynek, V., Jirak, D., Hajek, M & Sykova, E. (2002). Leksell gamma knife lesioning of the rat hippocampus: the relationship between radiation dose and functional and structural damage. *J Neurosurg,* Vol. 97, No. 5 Suppl, Dec, pp. 666-673, ISSN/ISBN: 0022-3085.

Lunsford, LD., Altschuler, EM., Flickinger, JC., Wu, A & Martinez, AJ. (1990). In vivo biological effects of stereotactic radiosurgery: a primate model. *Neurosurgery,* Vol. 27, No. 3, Sep, pp. 373-382, ISSN/ISBN: 0148-396X; 0148-396X.

Major, O., Walton, L., Goodden, J., Radatz, M., Szeifert, GT., Hanzely, Z., Kocsis, B., Nagy, Z & Kemeny, A. (2006). Radiosurgery of isolated cerebral vessels following administration of paclitaxel in the rat. *J Neurosurg,* Vol. 105 Suppl, Dec, pp. 214-221, ISSN/ISBN: 0022-3085; 0022-3085.

Mathieu, D., Lecomte, R., Tsanaclis, AM., Larouche, A & Fortin, D. (2007). Standardization and detailed characterization of the syngeneic Fischer/F98 glioma model. *Can J Neurol Sci,* Vol. 34, No. 3, Aug, pp. 296-306, ISSN/ISBN: 0317-1671.

Milas, L., Hirata, H., Hunter, N & Peters, LJ. (1988). Effect of radiation-induced injury of tumor bed stroma on metastatic spread of murine sarcomas and carcinomas. *Cancer Res,* Vol. 48, No. 8, Apr 15, pp. 2116-2120, ISSN/ISBN: 0008-5472; 0008-5472.

Mori, Y., Kondziolka, D., Balzer, J., Fellows, W., Flickinger, JC., Lunsford, LD & Thulborn, KR. (2000). Effects of stereotactic radiosurgery on an animal model of hippocampal epilepsy. *Neurosurgery,* Vol. 46, No. 1, Jan, pp. 157-65; discussion 165-8, ISSN/ISBN: 0148-396X; 0148-396X.

Nilsson, A., Wennerstrand, J., Leksell, D & Backlund, EO. (1978). Stereotactic gamma irradiation of basilar artery in cat. Preliminary experiences. *Acta Radiol Oncol Radiat Phys Biol,* Vol. 17, No. 2, pp. 150-160, ISSN/ISBN: 0348-5196; 0348-5196.

Niranjan, A., Moriuchi, S., Lunsford, LD., Kondziolka, D., Flickinger, JC., Fellows, W., Rajendiran, S., Tamura, M., Cohen, JB & Glorioso, JC. (2000). Effective treatment of experimental glioblastoma by HSV vector-mediated TNF alpha and HSV-tk gene transfer in combination with radiosurgery and ganciclovir administration. *Mol Ther,* Vol. 2, No. 2, Aug, pp. 114-120, ISSN/ISBN: 1525-0016; 1525-0016.

Niranjan, A., Wolfe, D., Tamura, M., Soares, MK., Krisky, DM., Lunsford, LD., Li, S., Fellows-Mayle, W., DeLuca, NA., Cohen, JB & Glorioso, JC. (2003). Treatment of rat gliosarcoma brain tumors by HSV-based multigene therapy combined with radiosurgery. *Mol Ther,* Vol. 8, No. 4, Oct, pp. 530-542, ISSN/ISBN: 1525-0016; 1525-0016.

Novotny, J,Jr., Novotny, J., Spevacek, V., Dvorak, P., Cechak, T., Liscak, R., Brozek, G., Tintera, J & Vymazal, J. (2002a). Application of polymer gel dosimetry in gamma knife radiosurgery. *J Neurosurg,* Vol. 97, No. 5 Suppl, Dec, pp. 556-562, ISSN/ISBN: 0022-3085.

Novotny, J,Jr., Novotny, J., Spevacek, V., Dvorak, P., Cechak, T., Liscak, R., Brozek, G., Tintera, J & Vymazal, J. (2002b). Evaluation of geometric and dosimetric inaccuracies of stereotactic irradiation in the rat brain. *Stereotact Funct Neurosurg,* Vol. 79, No. 2, pp. 57-74, ISSN/ISBN: 1011-6125.

Ohuchida, K., Mizumoto, K., Murakami, M., Qian, LW., Sato, N., Nagai, E., Matsumoto, K., Nakamura, T & Tanaka, M. (2004). Radiation to stromal fibroblasts increases invasiveness of pancreatic cancer cells through tumor-stromal interactions. *Cancer Res,* Vol. 64, No. 9, May 1, pp. 3215-3222, ISSN/ISBN: 0008-5472; 0008-5472.

Omary, RA., Berr, SS., Kamiryo, T., Lanzino, G., Kassell, NF., Lee, KS., Lopes, MB & Hillman, BJ. (1995). 1995 AUR Memorial Award. Gamma knife irradiation-induced changes in the normal rat brain studied with 1H magnetic resonance spectroscopy and imaging. *Acad Radiol,* Vol. 2, No. 12, Dec, pp. 1043-1051, ISSN/ISBN: 1076-6332; 1076-6332.

Paxinos G, Watson C. 1986. The rat brain in stereotaxic coordinates.

Pellerin, M., Tremblay, L., Paquette, B & Lepage, M. (2006). Monitoring micro-vasculature damage induced by radiotherapy on mouse breast carcinomas using DCE-MRI. *Proc Intl Soc Mag Reson Med,* Vol. 14, pp. 2910, .

Precision X-Ray. Date of access: 2011, Available from: http://www.pxinc.com/.

Qian, LW., Mizumoto, K., Urashima, T., Nagai, E., Maehara, N., Sato, N., Nakajima, M & Tanaka, M. (2002). Radiation-induced increase in invasive potential of human pancreatic cancer cells and its blockade by a matrix metalloproteinase inhibitor, CGS27023. *Clin Cancer Res,* Vol. 8, No. 4, Apr, pp. 1223-1227, ISSN/ISBN: 1078-0432; 1078-0432.

Rad Source Technologies. Date of access: 2011, Available from: http://www.radsource.com/.

Rao, ZR., Ge, X., Qiou, JY., Yang, T., Duan, L & Ju, G. (2000). Expression and changes of HSP70 in the rat forebrain subjected to gamma knife (100Gy) irradiation targeted on the caudate putamen and survived for different times. *Neurosci Res,* Vol. 38, No. 2, Oct, pp. 139-146, ISSN/ISBN: 0168-0102; 0168-0102.

Rao, ZR., Li, T., Wu, HX., Qiou, JY., Wu, SL., Tang, T., Huang, SH & Ju, G. (1998). Expression and changes of glial fibrillary acidic protein (GFAP) in normal rat brain irradiated with gamma knife. *Chines J Minim Invasive Neurosurg,* Vol. 3, No. 2, 1998, pp. 106-111.

Regis, J., Kerkerian-Legoff, L., Rey, M., Vial, M., Porcheron, D., Nieoullon, A & Peragut, JC. (1996). First biochemical evidence of differential functional effects following Gamma Knife surgery. *Stereotact Funct Neurosurg,* Vol. 66 Suppl 1, pp. 29-38, ISSN/ISBN: 1011-6125; 1011-6125.

Rey, M., Valliccioni, PA., Vial, M., Porcheron, D., Regis, J., Kerlerian-LE, GL., Nieoullon, A., Millet, Y & Peragut, JC. (1996). Radiochirurgie expérimentale chez le rat par Gamma knife : Description d'un cadre stéréotaxique pour le petit animal de laboratoire. Commentaire = Description of a stereotactic device for experimental gamma knife radiosurgery in rats. Commentary. *Neuro-chirurgie,* Vol. 42, No. 6, pp. 289-293, .

Rofstad, EK., Mathiesen, B., Henriksen, K., Kindem, K & Galappathi, K. (2005). The tumor bed effect: increased metastatic dissemination from hypoxia-induced up-regulation of metastasis-promoting gene products. *Cancer Res,* Vol. 65, No. 6, Mar 15, pp. 2387-2396, ISSN/ISBN: 0008-5472; 0008-5472.

Speake, WJ., Dean, RA., Kumar, A., Morris, TM., Scholefield, JH & Watson, SA. (2005). Radiation induced MMP expression from rectal cancer is short lived but contributes to in vitro invasion. *Eur J Surg Oncol,* Vol. 31, No. 8, Oct, pp. 869-874, ISSN/ISBN: 0748-7983; 0748-7983.

Takahashi, S., Toshima, M., Fukuoka, S., Seo, Y., Suematsu, K., Nakamura, J & Nagashima, K. (1996). Effect of gamma knife irradiation on relaxation and contraction responses of the common carotid artery in the rat. *Acta Neurochir (Wien),* Vol. 138, No. 8, pp. 992-1001, ISSN/ISBN: 0001-6268; 0001-6268.

Theratronics. Date of access: 2011, Available from: http://www.theratronics.ca/product_gamma.html.

Tinnel, B., Mendonca, MS., Henderson, M., Cummings, O., Chin-Sinex, H., Timmerman, R & McGarry, RC. (2007). Pulmonary hilar stereotactic body radiation therapy in the rat. *Technol Cancer Res Treat,* Vol. 6, No. 5, Oct, pp. 425-431, ISSN/ISBN: 1533-0346; 1533-0338.

Tippayamontri, T., Kotb, R., Paquette, B & Sanche, L. (Ongoing research).

Tokumaru, O., Hayashi, M., Katayama, Y., Tomida, M., Kawakami, Y & Kouyama, N. (2007a). Gamma knife radiosurgery targeting protocols for the experiments with small animals. *Stereotact Funct Neurosurg,* Vol. 85, No. 4, pp. 135-143, ISSN/ISBN: 1011-6125.

Tokumaru, O., Hayashi, M., Katayama, Y., Tomida, M., Kawakami, Y & Kouyama, N. (2007b). Gamma knife radiosurgery targeting protocols for the experiments with small animals. *Stereotact Funct Neurosurg,* Vol. 85, No. 4, pp. 135-143, ISSN/ISBN: 1011-6125.

Tokumaru, O., Tomida, M., Katayama, Y., Hayashi, M., Kawakami, Y & Kouyama, N. (2005a). The effect of gamma knife irradiation on functions of striatum in rats. *J Neurosurg,* Vol. 102 Suppl, Jan, pp. 42-48, ISSN/ISBN: 0022-3085.

Tokumaru, O., Tomida, M., Katayama, Y., Hayashi, M., Kawakami, Y & Kouyama, N. (2005b). The effect of gamma knife irradiation on functions of striatum in rats. *J Neurosurg,* Vol. 102 Suppl, Jan, pp. 42-48, ISSN/ISBN: 0022-3085.

Vincent, DA., Alden, TD., Kamiryo, T., Lopez, B., Ellegala, D., Laurent, JJ., Butler, M., Vance, ML & Laws Jr, ER. (2005). The baromodulatory effect of gamma knife irradiation of the hypothalamus in the obese Zucker rat. *Stereotact Funct Neurosurg,* Vol. 83, No. 1, pp. 6-11, ISSN/ISBN: 1011-6125; 1011-6125.

Wang, JL., Sun, Y & Wu, S. (2000). Gamma-irradiation induces matrix metalloproteinase II expression in a p53-dependent manner. *Mol Carcinog,* Vol. 27, No. 4, Apr, pp. 252-258, ISSN/ISBN: 0899-1987; 0899-1987.

Wiant, D., Atwood, TF., Olson, J., Papagikos, M., Forbes, ME., Riddle, DR & Bourland, JD. (2009). Gamma knife radiosurgery treatment planning for small animals using high-resolution 7T micro-magnetic resonance imaging. *Radiat Res,* Vol. 172, No. 5, Nov, pp. 625-631, ISSN/ISBN: 1938-5404; 0033-7587.

Wild-Bode, C., Weller, M., Rimner, A., Dichgans, J & Wick, W. (2001). Sublethal irradiation promotes migration and invasiveness of glioma cells: implications for radiotherapy of human glioblastoma. *Cancer Res,* Vol. 61, No. 6, Mar 15, pp. 2744-2750, ISSN/ISBN: 0008-5472; 0008-5472.

Xstrahl. Date of access: 2011, Available from: http://www.xstrahl.com/.

Xu, D., Jia, Q., Li, Y., Kang, C & Pu, P. (2006). Effects of Gamma Knife surgery on C6 glioma in combination with adenoviral p53 in vitro and in vivo. *J Neurosurg,* Vol. 105 Suppl, Dec, pp. 208-213, ISSN/ISBN: 0022-3085; 0022-3085.

Zerris, VA., Zheng, Z., Noren, G., Sungarian, A & Friehs, GM. (2002). Radiation and regeneration: behavioral improvement and GDNF expression after Gamma Knife